Foundations of
Physical Activity

Foundations of

Physical Activity

Applications as Disciplines and Professions

Leonard A. Larson

The University of Wisconsin, Madison

Macmillan Publishing Co., Inc.
New York
Collier Macmillan Publishers
London

Macmillan Publishing Co., Inc.
866 Third Avenue, New York, New York 10022

Collier Macmillan Canada, Ltd.

Library of Congress Cataloging in Publication Data

Larson, Leonard August, (date)
  Foundations of physical activity.

  Bibliography: p.
  Includes index.
  1. Vocational guidance. 2. Exercise. I. Title.
HF5381.L323   331.7′02   75–12607
ISBN 0–02–367730–9

Printing: 1 2 3 4 5 6 7 8   Year: 6 7 8 9 0 1 2

Preface

This text deals with the foundations of physical activity in its roles as disciplines and professions. It is primarily for college students who plan to enter into a physical activity career. The opportunities for those who are properly prepared appear to be limitless. The individual, societal, and cultural needs for sports and physical activity have grown rapidly in the past three decades and, barring social and economic upheavals, will continue to grow.

This text is designed for the study of physical activity based on its positive qualities. Although it stresses the current status of physical activity, it also considers how physical activity should be. The future is viewed positively. The ideals and goals have yet to be reached, but they can be by those who truly wish to succeed.

The text is determined to some extent by what the present sequences in the advancement and operations of physical activity are, but it also proposes what they eventually should become. It describes how physical activity should start from basic considerations and should be developed into the various disciplines and professions that represent its value.

Part I considers the setting for physical activity and its applications. This provides the base in the world as it is today, the scope of physical activity as it is viewed within this context, and the potentials of physical activity as developmental phenomena within these settings. It represents the starting reference for a text on foundations.

Part II views physical activity as disciplines. These applications are now within the six basic disciplines of physiology, psychology, sociology, physical science, history, and philosophy. To fit this text better the disciplines were structured into four groupings: biophysical disciplines, sociopsychological disciplines, history, and philosophy. These are all-inclusive and more closely related to the phases of the disciplines that are now applied for the study of physical activity.

Part III discusses the professions that have been developed utilizing the medium of physical activity. There are now ten such structured professions, and each is discussed in its own chapter in Part III. Sufficient content with an emphasis on the conceptual structure of each application is provided in each chapter.

Part IV of this text views the perspectives and projections for activity. Following a full review of physical activity as disciplines and professions based on the most pertinent literature, it was considered reasonable to judge the future role of physical activity. This is summarized in the chapters on perspectives (Chapter 18) and perspectives applied (Chapter 19). These developments are foundations for physical activity, because the potentials for future development are related to the success of current uses and applications.

It is gratifying to review physical activity in the culture and to gain an understanding of the important functions it has served. Of more importance, however, are the roles open to physical activity for the future. The net result must be one of confidence for physical activity in the future in providing a very important service to the individual, society, and culture.

L. A. L.

Acknowledgments

The preparation of a text on foundations involves many people. A single individual could not complete the investigations for writing such a book in time for the text to be current. Consequently, research assistants have participated in the preparation of this text. Editorial reviewers, secretaries, and University of Wisconsin personnel have also helped.

During the early stages of preparation of the text, James J. Francis, from Wales, and Colin Martindale, from Barbados, served as research assistants. Their work consisted of a systematic review of the literature. In the later part of the preparation, J. A. Scott Kelso, a research assistant from England, prepared summary statements for each discipline and profession that contained support from the literature. These reviews include experimental studies and also clinical papers and writings from investigators who have devoted years to the application of physical activity for specific purposes. Full overviews could not have been prepared without the assistance of these researchers.

The preparation of the text for publication required editorial services. Research assistants participating in editorial reviews were Tom Grogg, Damon Burton, and Scott Kelso.

Preparation of the manuscript is always a difficult and time-consuming process. Secretarial personnel at the University of Wisconsin who prepared various parts of the text are Judith Siesen, Martha Fisk, Wendy Weber, and Catherine Wonn. The preparation of the text for publication would not have been possible without the assistance of these individuals.

Mrs. Helen Ringgenberg, administrative assistant in physical education at the University of Wisconsin, was responsible for personnel who assisted in all phases of the text.

L. A. L.

Contents

PART I

The Setting

Chapter 1

The Modern World

> One-third of mankind today live in an environment of relative abundance. But two-thirds of mankind—more than 2 billion—are entrapped in a cruel web of circumstances that severely limits their right to the necessities of life. They have not yet been able to achieve the transition to self-sustaining growth. They are caught in the grip of hunger and malnutrition, high illiteracy, inadequate education, shrinking opportunity and corrosive poverty.[1]

Significant changes have occurred throughout the world during the past quarter century. Human beings have always lived in a changing world, but never before have the changes been of the magnitude experienced in recent years. Life in the years before World War II was largely in a culturally homogeneous setting and followed traditional patterns. Certainly this is not true today.

Technical advances probably represent the primary cause for major changes in contemporary conditions in such areas as transportation, communications, and rapid population growth. The result is the interdependence of nations. Today the local community is not in an isolated setting, nor entirely enclosed within a state or nation. Social construction or reconstruction must therefore be considered within a world setting.

Mankind is now divided into two competing concepts of world order —one based on coercion, the other on consent. History has demonstrated that an order that stems from the people is more desirable than an order imposed by the coercion of a powerful individual or a small controlling

---

[1] Robert S. McNamara, "The Population Threat," *Today's Education,* Vol. 58, No. 9, 1969, pp. 20–23.

group. The former will govern the people to serve their needs, the latter is likely to govern to serve the needs of the government. In spite of its many weaknesses the fundamental validity of democratic order can hardly be questioned. It is through free associations among nations in bilateral, regional, and global diplomacy that world order can be achieved.

In a world community governed by democratic methods there will be conflicts of interests and opinions caused by cultural and other differences. But to avoid war, people and nations must rely upon the use of intelligence, upon free debate and discussion in order to find creative solutions to their problems, or at the very least to discover some shared interests that will make it possible for people in all nations to live together. Unless fundamental human rights and the values at their root are upheld and there is common conviction about the validity of the methods of intelligence in defending, extending, and reconciling them, war is unavoidable.[2]

The Role of the Individual. The individual is caught in a web of world conditions and more specifically the conditions that exist in his country. Both have significant effects. In government by consent, the individual has routes to initiate changes and improvements. In government by coercion, the individual can initiate change if the privilege is extended; if not, the method is civil war.

Questions of human and individual rights are now at the forefront of international and, in many instances, national attention. The conditions that violate human rights are many—the wall in Berlin, anti-Semitism in the Soviet Union, deprivation of human rights in communist countries, the setbacks of freedom in the less-developed countries, the struggle for racial equality in the United States, and so on. These conditions have stirred public opinion and certainly individual anxieties that have had profound effects on international relations. Certainly all individuals are directly influenced by such conditions—socially, economically, and politically.

Modern Society

World societies range in material wealth from abundance to levels of filth and starvation. It is imperative that all conditions be made known to all people in order to create a desire for change. The founders of the United Nations stated in the charter that to save nations from war and unacceptable social conditions, it is necessary to promote and develop better standards of living, including social conditions and personal rights

---

[2] Sidney Hook, "The Crisis of Our Democratic Institutions," *The Humanist*, July–August, 1969.

and freedom. It is reported that the promotion of the general welfare through economic and social cooperation now occupies more than four fifths of the men and money in the United Nations. Numerous other public and private agencies also devote funds and manpower to the improvement of conditions in the countries of the world. What are these conditions today?

Population Growth. According to McNamara [3] "the greatest single obstacle to the economic and social advancement of the majority of the peoples in the underdeveloped world is rampant population growth." McNamara states that although solution of the population problem will in no way substitute for the more-traditional forms of developmental assistance (economic, agricultural, educational, technological), nothing would be more unwise than to allow these projects to fail because they are finally overwhelmed by a tidal wave of population.

It is reported that it required 1,600 years to double the world population of 250 million, as it stood in the first century A.D. The 3 billion people on earth today will double in thirty-five years, at which time the world's population will be increasing at the rate of 1 billion every eight years.

In order to avoid mass starvation or political chaos, population planning for the reduction of the birth rate becomes a necessity. It is essential because the consequences of continuing the present population growth rates are unacceptable. Family planning is not designed to destroy families. On the contrary, it is designed to save them.

Technological Advances. It has become a commonplace that the world is experiencing a scientific and technological revolution, as expressed by such current terms as *knowledge explosion, second industrial revolution,* and *automation revolution.* Some believe that further growth in productivity will have serious effects on employment, because with increased speed of productivity, less manpower will be required. Whatever the causes, technological changes will have an impact on future social and economic problems.

Adjustments to technological advances by the individual and society are many, and they occur in nearly all communities. The changes must be anticipated and new skills and opportunities provided through future-oriented technical, vocational, and professional educational programs. Society and the individual should be ready for change when it comes.

Social Mobility. The belief in social mobility is an integral part of American thought. The class structure is open; the positions at the top are there for those with the talent it takes to reach them.

---

[3] McNamara, op. cit.

Loy [4] has reviewed social mobility as it applies to sports. He reports that it is difficult to determine the degree to which sport participation leads to social success because social mobility is a complex, multidimensional phenomenon. On a conceptual basis, Loy accounts for the sources of variations in social mobility in seven basic dimensions. The first is direction—horizontal or vertical. Horizontal mobility involves the transition from one social position to another; vertical mobility involves a rise or fall within the same social class. The second dimension is distance—or the distance one ascends within a social class. The third dimension is time—the amount it takes to move from one social position to another. The fourth is status change, e.g., occupational mobility. The fifth dimension is unit of analysis. This dimension of mobility applies to individuals, families, peer groups, or larger social groupings. The sixth dimension concerns the distinction between objective and subobjective changes in status—the change in salary is an example of the former, whereas gratification as the result of an increase in salary is an example of the latter. The seventh dimension deals with the social mechanisms underlying social mobility. Success in sports is an example of a mechanism involved in social change.

Understanding the nature of social changes and requirements for desirable change represents important preparation for all. Society should provide the opportunities and encouragement so that individuals can achieve the status needed for personal happiness and well-being.

Advances in Knowledge. Advancements in the sciences during the past few decades have established a body of knowledge that seems impossible to comprehend, much less master. The "explosion of knowledge" is a description that certainly fits recent advancements. One must search out advances in knowledge in various disciplines in order to understand the world and its people. Psychology aids in understanding the actions of individuals and groups; sociology in understanding the interactions of people and the development of groups; the humanities, literature, the arts, and philosophy in revealing the intellectual and creative contributions and abilities of man; and other sciences and medicine in providing understanding of the human organism and how current knowledge can improve health and provide a longer and more complete life.

Influences of the Physical Environment. During the past few years a thorough review of the experimental literature was made in connection with the development of the *Encyclopedia of Sport Sciences and Medicine* (New York: Macmillan, 1971). Twenty-three components of the physical environment were identified as having some effect on man's ability to do physical work and on his well-being. For more complete

[4] John W. Loy, "The Study of Sport and Social Mobility." Monograph paper, University of Wisconsin, 1968.

information, see the preceding work, but some generalizations will be given here. Factors that influence the human being are air conditioning (generally beneficial for sustained work), climate, seasons (favorable and unfavorable), clothing (thermal buffer—clothing should be regulated according to environment), diurnal reactions (bodily variations during the day—important in work adjustments), glare, lighting, shadows (related to work performance), housing (setting and changing of routines affect work performance and well-being), humidity (affects heat loss of body and related to work performance), magnetic fields (little research on humans; experiments on mice show effects on body physiology), noise disturbances (favorable or unfavorable to work performance—emotional level of individual an important factor), population (density related to work performance and general well-being), radiation (can be beneficial; degree of harm will depend on dose, dose rate, and volume of tissue exposed), temperature (temperate climate seems favorable to work performance; other atmospheric factors are important), tobacco smoke (toxic elements have unfavorable effects on work and body physiology), transportation (conditions will determine favorable or unfavorable effects on work and body physiology), underwater pressure (will influence work and health status), ventilation (favorable effects if desirable components are held in the atmosphere), weightlessness (removing gravity influences work performance and body physiology), wind (determines rate of heat exchange–will affect work performance).

Sociocultural Differences. The cultural nature of a nation is probably best described through its social institutions—the church, government, economic resources, education, politics, military, and communications and the artistic, ethical, and moral nature of the people. Of course, social characteristics are formed in a cultural setting. These elements include the description of man in his daily practices and associations with others —his attitudes, interests, emotions, intelligence, health fitness, leisure practices, occupation, security, human values, personal health practices, and so on.

The culture and social practices of a nation determine the environmental bases for health and work performance. The range of practices is so wide that understanding between some nations is not possible, without long, concerted effort, in practically every aspect of daily life. Efficiency and health levels also differ greatly, from nations with high production rates to those with hardly any high-production industries, and nations with excellent morbidity and mortality rates to those with considerably shorter life-spans and high disease rates.

Wealth and Poverty. Wide differences exist in the present distribution of world income. In a recent report the average annual per capita income in the United States was given as about $3,000, while in the other developed countries of the free world it is about $1,200. In the less-developed countries as a whole, it is about $150. In the vast majority of the less-developed countries—a majority that includes two thirds of humanity—it is less than $100.

The economic status of a nation and an individual (or family) is directly related to nearly all facets of human development—the mind, the body, the emotions, and the individual as a social being. Unfavorable influences lessen health levels and lower resources for sustained work and physical performance.

Work and Leisure. The balance between work and leisure has dramatically changed within a relatively few years. The advancements in technology have freed man for more leisure and have decreased the amount of hard physical work.

Current sociological literature seems to regard leisure as merely an adjunct to work. The pleasurable satisfactions provided by leisure activities tend to be treated as a means to an end—the end of gaining relief from the strain of work and of improving man's capacity for it.

It is reported that a distinct difference exists between "spare-time activities" and "leisure activities." In the former, the activities meet the requirements of household and family routines and the biological needs of the organism. In the latter, the activities are selected for pleasure and social interests and desires, for a change from the daily schedule. In leisure activities the regard for emotional satisfactions takes priority over all other considerations.

Unless we have the values, interests, skills, and opportunities to use increasing free time constructively, there will be more boredom, despair, and submission to the stimuli of drugs and unsocial activities. Entertainment enterprises are flourishing; sports and games for the spectator and many other sedentary leisure activities are high in popularity.

Government and Politics. Forms of government and political processes differ greatly in the various countries of the world, from democratic government with widespread participation in political activities to autocratic government with political activities restricted to a single individual or a few persons. The effects on the individual in these two social orders are most significant and easily observable.

In a democratic government the people can decide on leaders, and highly undesirable candidates will have little chance in an open election. In addition, the democratic tenets of government are also highly desirable principles for family life and human relations. Such tenets as respect for the human personality, equality of opportunity, reason and intelligence as a basis for problem solving, and self-government are sound grounds for personal living. They also represent the context for sports participation. Sports and physical activity constitute an integral part of the culture in democratic nations and assume important political roles. The place of sports and athletics in the life of the people is strong indeed.

Social Responsibility

In the preceding section brief descriptions were presented on the nature of the modern societies of the world. Probably most significant is the wide range of differences—from wealthy to poor, from democratic governments to autocratic controls, from resources of plenty to nations without the minimum requirements to sustain life.

Economic Factors. The poverty of less-developed nations is well known by affluent countries with resources in abundance. What is new is the determination of the poor to do something about it, in what has been called a revolution of "rising expectations." The uprisings have brought to a large part of the world a turbulence unique in history. Urgent demands for economic and social improvement are the dominant concerns in the poor nations of Asia, the Middle East, Africa, and Latin America. There is no longer any question of whether these countries will develop themselves; the only question is how.

According to United Nations reports, since the end of World War II, the United States has supplied over $40 billion in foreign aid to less-developed countries, and the amount is increasing each year. The United States is providing billions each year for low-interest loans for countries in Latin America, Africa, and Asia that have demonstrated the capacity to help themselves. Many other illustrations of economic help could be cited—food, clothing, industrial development, agriculture, education and school development, along with other aids, among which military security is the largest.

It is apparent that the economy of any nation, wealthy or poor, is viewed in an international setting. Sharing and developing national resources become the objective of each person and each community, regardless of size and national or governmental setting.

Educational Factors. Possibly the most basic need or right of an individual is preparation for a life of self-sufficiency or minimum dependency. Educational institutions are the teachers of the world and these institutions are more than the schools and universities; they include all institutions that attempt to improve the individual and society—the churches, social agencies, clubs, fraternities, and so on. According to Harold Taylor,[5] the institutions in a society hold the possibility of bringing a

[5] Harold Taylor, "The Crisis of Our Democratic Institutions," *The Humanist,* July–August, 1969.

sense of humane purpose and international unity from a fragmented collection of separate units of power. On the quality of the experiences of
individuals in educational institutions rest the quality or character of
our society and the quality of its purposes. Institutional graduates and
participants represent the resources for the solution of world problems—
far beyond the immediate physical resources of a nation. It is how the
resources are used and replaced that will determine the long-range security of a people and a nation.

With the exception of meeting the immediate needs of the starving
and those living under unacceptable conditions, preparing each person
for a life of gainful work and economic security is the major task for all
societies. Education or vocational preparation should be made available
to *all* persons, regardless of personal economic ability. The costs cannot
be paid in countries with little resources; aid must come from the countries with the economic resources. It is not a question of a will to help; it
is an obligation of each nation with the resources to improve the state
of the world. All are intimately involved and interdependent.

Political Factors. In the democratically controlled nations and governments, the individual has a minimum number of political restrictions on
personal achievements and goals. Within the wide scope of law (which
is determined by the people) the individual can plan for a professional
and personal life that is rewarding both economically and personally.

It is the responsibility of all nations to provide a setting for individuals to gain, through their efforts, the life requirements essential for
health and well-being. This extends to providing educational programs,
an opportunity for free enterprise, a setting for free communications and
social intercourse, a voice in the government, and leadership compatible
with the will of the people.

Social Factors. The ultimate aim of people from all nations, as a
basis for the solution of world problems, is world citizenship. The people
of the world must understand social and cultural differences and effect
agreements within these contexts. In the modern world of immediate
communication through transportation, radio, and television, understanding among people in varied social settings is not impossible nor is a
"United Nations" for the resolution of social and political problems. The
objectives are most valid. Constant effort on the part of people and
governments is necessary. Efforts to eliminate war are an excellent place
to start. Steps in this direction are constantly being taken by many
countries and certainly by the United Nations.

The socially integrated person or nation can be described by a few
important qualities—respect for law and order; respect for the human
personality regardless of national origin, color, or creed; self-sufficiency
in the resolution of personal and national problems to the limits of one's

resources; positive attitudes and actions toward self and others on all issues, whether social or political; and individual efforts toward self-government and economic and personal security for all the people, the nation, and the world. These are probably the most basic qualities underlying human understanding in building world unity and a desirable world order.

Cultural Factors. The traditions and mores, the ways of life, differ considerably within the various nations over the world. Cultural settings result from centuries of life in a nation, mostly in cultural isolation. In the modern world the setting is not isolation, but a cultural merging so rapid that individual and national adjustments have been unable to keep pace. The result is misunderstanding and national unrest.

In the democratic nations in particular, cultural differences and the conditions influencing differences are significantly similar. Travel among people of all nations, particularly democratic nations, is at an all-time high. Industries are rapidly being developed on an international basis. International athletic competition is becoming more common each year. All such activities have tremendous cultural and social impacts, resulting in a blending of cultures.

Cultural merging is the strength of a world society. It is not the destruction of a society that is the result of centuries of development; rather it is changing in each culture toward modern ways of life resulting from advances in technology and the sciences and medicine. Such worldwide applications may form the basis for a world society.

Health and Welfare. Probably the most costly program of a society or nation is the health and economic welfare of the people. For individuals who do not have the resources to provide for their well-being, this becomes a responsibility of society—local, state, national, and worldwide. Welfare budgets alone have reached a level in some communities in the United States that could bankrupt the community. The costs are staggering! The resources must come from the people through taxes and voluntary contributions. There are no other resources.

Socialized medicine is now available in many nations (not all, however), providing services to people in need at minimal cost. Individual economic resources under these conditions do not determine whether you receive needed health and medical services. Protecting the individual's health is indeed a major concern of a society, particularly when inflation, with spiraling costs, makes it difficult for an individual to be self-sufficient.

Communication and Human Relations. Communication among people is necessary for understanding. In the past, language and transportation acted as effective barriers. These barriers have essentially been

eliminated. It now becomes important to bring people of all nations together by making it economically possible to use available transportation.
The countries of the world are now apart by only a few hours.

Radio and television have been effective instruments in increasing
understanding between people and nations. Both media are strong social
forces. The programs reflect the desires and the values held by a majority
in a society or by those in control of the media. The effects have been
demonstrated in politics, economics, education, and culture and in social
conditions in particular. The results of political campaigns and discus-
sions will influence the people and political issues. This has been demonstrated. The importance of the media for advertising, distribution, and
sales is reflected by the large sums spent. Without results, the use of
these media would be dropped. The media are used as major sources of
information and news. An event in the most distant part of the world
becomes known in minutes and is reported at the first daily newscast.
Formal and informal education programs are presented by the networks.
The way people choose to entertain themselves, levels of taste, the place
they assign to creative works of art and literature, are all matters of
cultural significance. The social effects influence daily life and habits.
These potential effects on the family are generally positive, although
effects can be unfavorable.

The need for international understanding has never been greater than
it is now. All forms of media should be used to enhance understanding so
that nations may not only improve living conditions within their own
culture, but of equal importance, gain understanding within the context
of world cooperation on all problems.

Educational Responsibility

Educational responsibility has changed from a local to a worldwide
concern within less than fifty years. It is important in studying the foundations of physical activity and its professional applications (and education is one) that the various aspects of educational responsibility be
understood. World needs for educational services include the enhancement of human qualities that can be gained by the proper use of physical
activity.

The responsibility for education must go beyond the problems of
society, local or worldwide. Education must be directed and planned for
the individual with all the differences that will be found in a group. He
should be prepared to meet problems with courage and competence. Education should transform one from a life of self-centered desire to one of
devoted service planned within a democratic framework

Thus the setting for the understanding and professional applications
of physical activity has been illustrated. The activity itself will become

valuable to each individual and group, but from an educational reference, the activity becomes a means to an end. How it is used and under what leadership will determine its contribution to the preparation of the individual to live with his family, to his attitudes and efforts toward the solution of community problems—from local concerns to those of countries in Asia.

Chapter 2

Physical Activity: The Scope in World Culture

Physical activity is essential for life. If the organism is not physically active, the functions of the body will gradually but surely diminish from desirable levels until there is difficulty in moving even under minimal conditions. Without physical activity, the regression in bodily functions will continue until death results.

Life is sustained through physical activity. Circulation, respiration, heart action, muscular contractions, the neuromuscular system—indeed all systems, organs, and functions of the body—are highly related to the total organism's level of efficiency and quality of performance. These, in turn, are heavily dependent on the scope and quantity of physical activity engaged in. Of course, the human organism has other demands (e.g., food and rest) but these too are highly related to physical activity. The nature, scope, and worth of physical activity require study from the various scientific disciplines in order to ensure proper use of activity for favorable human development. This is, in fact, the basis for this book.

Classification of Physical Activity

In order to study and analyze a field of knowledge, it must be defined, conceptualized, and organized into meaningful structures. Systematic study or application of a single concept requires viewing the concept in all possible contexts. The only exception is when one is interested in the single concept itself, rather than any application it might have. Conceptualizing a body of knowledge, however, is in any case an excellent starting point. It provides greater understanding even when minute details are being dealt with.

Human movement is a most complex phenomenon. It involves the joints, the limbs, sections of the body, basic movement patterns of an infinite number, and strategies of combinations of movement patterns into games, sports, athletics, recreation, and other forms that have meaning, value, and direction. To facilitate understanding of the scope of physical activity, an attempt is made to structure the classification of human movement. An organizational structure makes the study and applications of physical activity more meaningful.

The most basic movements of the organism are the limb articulations. These movements represent the muscular contractions around the joints of the body. Regardless of the size, scope, or intensity of human movements, some limb articulations are involved. The work load of limb movements is minimal. Using the fingers, the hands can, without involving the total body, produce high-precision movements, with little physical exertion.

Movements of the limbs can be advanced to more complex fundamental movements of the total organism. These include the limb articulations in the larger movements of the body. These movements place larger demands on circulation, respiration, muscular systems, and other systems and organs of the body. The movements of running, jumping, and throwing are parts of the physical activities that are organized by strategies into games, sports, and athletics toward goals that give additional meaning to the activity.

The activities organized by strategies represent the most complex structures of physical activity. They are the most useful to the individual and within a society and culture. These are the activities that are designed for some social, cultural, or scientific purpose.

The classification of physical activities that are organized by strategies is difficult. It seems that the most reasonable criterion is "according to purposes in use, consideration, analysis or application to be made of the physical activity." The conceptual structure is then selected according to how activity is to be applied (List 1). Activities are then classified according to applied purposes.

List 1. Strategies of movement systems

1. Organizational type. (Classification is according to the degree and type of organization required to conduct the activity; degree of organization ranges from almost none, as in games where there are few rules and a variable number of players, to highly structured team athletics.)
   a. Low organization activities (playing catch, shooting baskets).
   b. Individual activities (swimming, gymnastics).
   c. Dual activities (fencing, tennis).

    d. Team activities (baseball, basketball).

    e. Group activities (calisthenics, relays).

    f. Aquatics (diving, synchronized swimming).

    g. Conditioning exercises and activities (weight training, calisthenics).

    h. Remedial activities (weight lifting, swimming).

2. Developmental potentials. (Appropriate physical activity, conducted correctly, can contribute to the development of the human organism in a variety of ways. Developmental potentials, then, are those dimensions of human physical performance that can be enhanced by activity.)

    a. Muscular power (long jump, kicking).

    b. Muscular strength (weight training, isometrics).

    c. Muscular endurance (push-ups, handstands).

    d. Flexibility (bending exercises, twisting exercises).

    e. Accuracy (batting, bowling).

    f. Balance (handstands, skating).

    g. General endurance (bicycling, skating).

    h. Speed (sprinting, throwing).

    i. Agility (obstacle course, dodge ball).

    j. Coordination (skipping, kicking).

    k. Alertness (tennis, baseball).

    l. Steadiness (foul shooting, putting).

    m. Timing (passing basketball, high jumping).

    n. Rhythm (modern dance, ballet).

    o. Reaction times (boxing, wrestling).

3. Professional applications. (This classification refers to the facets of physical activity where professional personnel, who devote their occupational careers to the pursuit of excellence in the various activities, are to be found.)

    a. Sports and athletics (hockey, baseball).

    b. Leisure and culture (hiking, camping).

    c. Education (dance, life-saving).

    d. Health (jogging, walking).

    e. Institutions (swimming, fitness activities).

    f. Dance (folk, social).

    g. Preventive medicine (jogging, calisthenics).

    h. Recreation (outdoor living, skiing).

    i. Rehabilitation (running, calisthenics).

    j. Sports medicine (treadmill running, jogging).

4. Objectives. (Although there may be a varied range of objectives for physical activity, this list refers to physical education in the broad sense of the term.)

    a. Individual health (calisthenics, swimming).

    b. Effective utilization of human organism in work, play, and rest (walking, relaxation techniques).

    c. Knowledge, understanding, and appreciation of the human organism and the process essential for development and maintenance (distance running, weight training).

    d. Social efficiency (team games, camping).

    e. Democratic qualities of leadership and fellowship (team games, outdoor living).

      f. The individual as a self-adjusting organism (self-testing, team games).

5. Applications as an academic discipline. (With the human organism in movement as the focus of attention, these broadly conceived disciplines seek to understand man in motion from their special vantage points.)
   a. Physiology (endurance activities, adapted activities).
   b. Sociology (team games, outdoor living).
   c. Psychology (competitive sports, individual sports).
   d. Physical science (kicking, jumping).
   e. Philosophy (sports, games).
   f. History (sports, physical education).

6. Administrative requirements. (This classification refers to the requirements for administering facilities needed to conduct various physical activities for a community.)
   a. Outdoor facilities (hiking, skating).
   b. Resident camps (canoeing, riding horseback).
   c. Indoor facilities (basketball, gymnastics).
   d. Recreation buildings (dance, badminton).
   e. Stadiums and fieldhouses (basketball, football).

7. Media. (Man in motion can be characterized by the media in which he moves: land, water, and air. Outer space could be a fourth, and will receive greater attention in the future.)
   a. Land (running, skiing).
   b. Water (water skiing, water polo).
   c. Air (sky diving, aerial trapeze).

8. Age requirements. (Educational and recreational institutions attempt to build their activity programs on types of movement most appropriate physically, psychologically, and socially to the age of the participants. Although chronological age does not always accurately reflect physical, psychological, or social level, it appears to be the most efficient indicator currently available, although this is changing.)
   a. Birth to three years (play).
   b. Three to five years (jungle gym, swings).
   c. Six to seven years ("it" games, throwing and catching balls).
   d. Eight to nine years (tag games, cowboys and indians).
   e. Ten to eleven years (soccer dodge ball, baseball).
   f. Twelve to thirteen years (softball, volleyball).
   g. Fourteen to fifteen years (swimming, tennis).
   h. Sixteen to seventeen years (distance running, dance).
   i. Eighteen to twenty-two years (ice skating, golf).
   j. Twenty-two to forty-five years (tennis, bowling).
   k. Forty-six years to sixty-five years (jogging, golf).
   l. Sixty-five years and over (walking, swimming).

9. Maturation requirements. (A minimal amount of muscular activity is necessary for normal growth and for maintaining the integrity of tissues during the years of physical maturation. Thus human beings must literally move to stay alive.)
   a. Infant [first year (gross motor movement, play)].
   b. Early childhood [first to sixth years (jungle gyms, climbing)].
   c. Late childhood [sixth to tenth years, boys only (team games, rough and tumble)].

      d. Adolescence [twelfth to twentieth years, boys only (fitness activities, swimming)].
      e. Postadolescence [twentieth to twenty-fifth years (golf, tennis)].
  10. Environmental settings. (A complete list of environmental settings would be endless; the present one refers only to the physical and sociocultural environment. Environmental variables, obviously, can affect physiological performance.)
      a. Geographic location (arctic: snowskiing; temperate: tennis).
      b. Climate (hot and wet: walking; hot and dry: baseball).
      c. Altitude (0 to 6,000 feet: sprinting; over 6,000 feet: golf).
      d. Urbanization (rural: horseback riding; urban: handball).
      e. Sociocultural setting (primitive: hunting; transitional: baseball).
  11. Energy expenditure. (Energy expenditure can be measured in terms of oxygen consumption or caloric cost.)
      a. Light [(2.5 to 5 kcal/min.) bicycling 5 mph, ping pong].
      b. Moderate [(5.1 to 7.5 kcal/min.) push ball, bicycling 10 mph].
      c. Heavy [(7.6 to 10 kcal/min.) touch football, karate].
      d. Very heavy [(10.1 to 12.5 kcal/min.) basketball, bicycling 15 mph].
      e. Exhausting [(12.6 kcal/min. and over) ice hockey, cross-country skiing at 6 mph on hard snow].

Organizational Type. Structured physical activity (according to strategies) can be considered or applied in several conceptual frameworks. The most common classification in the professional literature is by organizational type. This is possibly due to teaching uses to be made of physical activity. When considering an activity in an instructional program, the nature of the activity itself is probably the most immediate consideration, that is, whether it is organized as a team sport, dual activity, individual activity, and so on. The organizational type is highly related to instruction, facilities, pupil interests, and other administrative considerations. This classification, however, has value only for organizational considerations.

Developmental Potentials. Strategically structured physical activities can be classified by their potential for the development of the human organism. Classification of physical activity according to the development criterion gives information about the activity that is not provided when it is classified by organizational type. Information about developmental potentials has many uses—among the most important being instruction and achievement of selected developmental goals.

Professional Applications. Physical activities can be classified by professional applications. Part III deals with each of the ten professions organized around physical activity. Each professional group has more or less differing objectives, resulting in a differing choice of activities and consequently variances in classification. List 1 lists activities classified under the various professions. In sports and athletics, for example, activities are classified according to their competitive value along with the organizational type that constitutes their appeal. The essential criterion is competition—with sports (more informally applied) or with athletics (highly structured).

It is interesting to note the professional worth of physical activity. The scope is very large indeed. It is in many instances how the activity is professionally applied, more than the nature of the activity itself, that gives it value. There are, of course, some wide differences, as, for example, in the activities used in the dance and those applied in athletics. Similarities are noted in the activities classified under athletics and those under education. The difference is in their applications. In athletics the emphasis is on participation under competitive conditions. In education, of course, both concepts apply, but the emphasis is on educational goals and achievements rather than results of competition. However, a conflict of values between athletics and education should not exist; they simply use activity for different purposes and the results are valuable in both cases.

Objectives. Physical activities can be classified by the objectives that direct their uses. Because the developmental potentials vary with each activity, it is natural that activities will be classified differently in this context from the way they are classified in others. Activities are classified by six objectives [1]—individual health, the effective utilization of the human organism, understandings, the individual as a social being, the individual as a democratic leader–follower, and the self–group adjusting organism. Probably this classification is the most valuable, particularly when education is the professional goal.

Disciplines. Considered as a discipline, a physical activity is analyzed to determine its worth in human development. The activity is also studied to determine its inherent characteristics in order to understand the nature of the activity itself. The purpose is to gain knowledge about physical activity.

Study and analysis, of course, must have a starting point. In the case of physical activity, references are made to the established disciplines in the sciences and philosophies. These are presented in List 1, namely, physiology, sociology, psychology, physical science, philosophy, and history. Physical activity has been studied by applying all six disciplines, but the most intensive analysis is in physiology. Physical activity is reasonably well understood as a physiological phenomenon, and its study is considered to be an applied discipline or subdiscipline of physiology.

Recent developments include research on physical activity in psychology and sociology. Future developments will include the other disciplines

[1] L. A. Larson, *Curriculum Foundations and Standards for Physical Education* (Englewood Cliffs, N.J.: Prentice-Hall, 1970).

with increased emphasis, resulting in scientific and philosophic under-standings that will make the professional application of physical activity more meaningful for the teacher and the participant.

It will be noted in List 1 that although in some of the disciplines, a common factor is found in the classification of activities (sociology, and psychology), each discipline sets the requirements in content for the classification of activities into homogeneous groups for study, knowl-edge, and understandings in application.

Administrative Needs. Physical activity can also be classified by ad-ministrative requirements (List 1). It is most useful to know the facility needs of an activity prior to its selection. This is certainly necessary when it is used for instructional purposes, but can be equally important for individual selections. The administrative classification of activities in no way reflects their developmental or intrinsic worth. This classification simply places into homogeneous groups the required physical facilities.

Media. Participation in physical activity requires facilities. Physical development results when the individual attempts to overcome the forces provided by the environment. When physical activity is applied under educational auspices or for instructional purposes, the facilities are pro-vided that are necessary for participation in the activity (e.g., a swim-ming pool). In instructional programs, for the sake of time and efficiency, the media are simulated (the pool instead of a lake). But the ultimate purpose of instruction is the proper use of the environment for pro-tection, survival, and, of course, human development in a natural and desirable setting.

Age. Physical activity participation has an age requirement. The classification of physical activities by age therefore provides information on the appropriateness of the activity. Classification by chronological age is a common practice for professional workers in education, recreation, and other fields. If the individual does not have the skill or physical re-sources required by the activity, of course, successful or satisfying par-ticipation cannot result.

Age classification of physical activity or physical activity require-ments has a sequential structure (List 1). Participation results in the improvement of abilities, making it possible to advance to higher forms of physical activity. These sequences continue until finally one finds only a few (possibly one) persons who can reach the ultimate level for a given age (e.g., world champion in a 100-meter event). Age classification for physical activity is usually the starting reference for both the profes-sional worker and the participant. Regardless of the goals, the individual cannot achieve without the ability to participate.

Maturation. For the proper fit of an activity to the individual, maturation level is probably the most valid basis. This is classification by physiological age. During the years up to maturity, a difference is found between chronological age and physiological age. The differences continue, but for different causes (genetic and environmental influences and personal practices), after maturity has been reached.

Maturation levels during the growing years are generally described as prepubescent, pubescent, and postpubescent. Later, classification can follow several patterns, the most common of which is young adult, mature adult, and aging organism. Each of these periods represent a physiological status that is reasonably descriptive of the group and provides a useful basis for the classification of physical activities (List 1).

Environments. Classification of physical activities by social and physical environments, although possibly a little less objective, has many useful purposes. Participation in physical activity is related to the physical environment. This can be hot-wet, hot-dry, cold-wet, and so on. The physiological processes are affected by physical environmental conditions. In selecting appropriate physical activities, therefore, these conditions must be considered.

The social environment becomes involved when physical activity involves more than one individual. Activities are also more or less appropriate for the particular social environment.

The classification of physical activities by social or physical environments has many useful purposes. People generally form in some social group (family, friends) and seek activities in this setting. It provides additional strength for the setting if the activities are appropriate, that is, fit the group. People also live in a particular physical environment, and activities should be chosen that make the best possible use of that environment.

Energy Expenditure. Physical activities differ in the potential energy required for participation. It is possible and desirable therefore to classify activities on this basis. Classification also provides a guide in planning physical activity programs to balance caloric utilizations, as when attempting to maintain acceptable body weight. The classification of physical activities is in terms of caloric expenditures while participating at a defined unit of time and intensity.

The human body sustains life through energy provisions from food and it sustains life through physical activity that comes only from action resulting from the release of energy from foods. Each person will differ in requirements; age, maturation, body structures are some factors causing differences.

Physical Activity and Environmental Effects

Physical activity is influenced by and influences the environment, both physical and social. Some effects are desirable and therefore aid in the goals of physical activity. Others are undesirable and will have negative effects. The environmental relationships involved in human performance of physical activities are (1) the elements of the physical environment, (2) the elements of the culture and society, (3) social practices and characteristics of the people, and (4) individual and group limitations and handicaps.

Physical Environment. A number of elements in the physical environment influence the physical organism in physical activity. *Air conditioning* can be beneficial. The controlled temperature can help maintain the thermal balance and normal body temperature, favoring activity. *Altitude* can be beneficial or restrictive. The organism has adaptive powers in higher altitudes that aid in human performances. These adaptations benefit the mountaineer, the athlete competing at high altitudes, and others. Endurance activities, however, that require a continuously high rate of oxygen supply are handicapped by high altitudes. Adaptation can reduce the handicap, particularly under strenuous training.

Climate, seasons, and weather exert both positive and negative influences on the individual in physical activity. Efficiency and capacity of physical performance and susceptibility to fatigue vary with extreme changes in these environmental conditions, both favorable and unfavorable. *Clothing* acts as a thermal buffer between the environment and man's body surface. Clothing facilitates warm-up, protects the body from cold and heat, protects the body from abrasion and injury, and in these ways is an aid in physical performance. If improperly used, clothing can be a deterrent. *Diurnal variations* are the daily physiological changes in the human organism. These changes have both negative and positive effects. Performance is improved at the most favorable time of the day in each person. *Housing* is related to physical activity performances both favorably and unfavorably. Changes in the normal routine of an individual have adverse effects on physical performances. *Humidity* is closely related to physical activity. The principal effect of environmental humidity is on the rate of evaporation of water from the skin and respiratory tract. The effects of humidity, however, will vary with each activity.

Noise disturbances are related to physical performances in varying ways. Some are disturbing to the performer (sensitive individual in precision activity) and some are motivating (cheering at a game). *Radiation* is beneficial to human performances. The influence, however, of excessive amounts can be harmful; the degree of radiation exposure is determined by the dose, dose rate, and volume of tissue exposed. *Temperature* has both positive and negative effects on human performance. The effect is coupled with other factors—the degree of activity, relative humidity, wind velocity, and clothing. *Wind* can influence performance by affecting the rate of heat exchange between man and the environment. Influences will vary with the physical activity.

Cultural and Societal Environments. Cultural and societal settings affect the quality and quantity of human physical performances. *Attitudes and interests* of the group and the individual significantly influence human physical performances. The highly motivated person will perform at his optimal or near optimal level, the uninterested person will not. *Competition* is a common application of physical activity. In some instances it serves as a motivator and the individual will rise to higher levels of participation because of it. In other instances the individual may not be able to meet the personal pressures applied. *Economic and social* conditions of a society and an individual are also related to health status and the ability to perform at a high level. There are exceptions. Health practices and social living conditions during the growing years will influence the physical abilities and powers of the grown man. *Education* for understanding physical performance and its personal requirements will aid performance. Where strategy is complex, the understanding level is more significant. *Emotions* of the individual can hardly be unrelated to physical performances. Anxiety, stress, and tension are parts of the person involved in performance and will be related to performance levels.

The cultural and societal environments will also include the *fitness* of the individual, and society as a whole is related to the individual. Fitness, of course, is fundamental to performance. It is also highly specific to the activity. The individual can be prepared to meet activity requirements to the limit of his capacities. *Health* is related to the cultural and societal environments, and health levels are correlated with participation and will establish the level of participation itself. *Leisure* is another cultural factor affecting individual involvement in physical activity. The reduction of the workday has provided more time for physical activity. Those who use this time will be favorably influenced by the sociocultural-physical values and qualities that can be achieved by proper participation. *Occupations,* whether inactive or active physically, are factors that appear to be related to preparation for physical activity. Individuals who are not prepared are probably less likely to become involved, although there seems to be growing interest among sedentary groups to become involved physically. The beneficial results have been reported. *Security* is a basic quality in human performance. The insecure individual will not be able to reach levels of performance possible for him. Personal psychological understanding is needed to remove factors leading to insecurity, such as fear, feelings of guilt, and resentment. The established *values* of a society will improve or reduce the performance of the individual by affecting his attitudes.

Social Practices in the Environments. Social practices of the people in the various physical environments will affect the individual and thereby influence performances. The personal condition of *anxiety* plays a large role in physical performances (in athletics) and in some instances is a sole reason for participation. In athletic performances the attitude of the spectators will play an important role in the anxiety level of the individual. *Competition* can be viewed and practiced in a society as opposition to the social process or as a form of cooperation or advancement. How it is applied will determine the social outcomes, good or bad. *Drug usage* while participating in physical activity has negative effects or reduces the level of activity. Drugs designed to aid performance have been found to have little physiological value and are considered unethical. The social practices of the *family* change with the environment. Physical activity was once a part of survival, but today physical activity is a part of the family as a social institution. *Frustrations* resulting from social practices create many possible behavioral sequences. Physical activity, and the resulting performances, can remain the same, be impaired, or be enhanced, depending upon many complex personal reactions. It is a matter of personal adaptability to stress conditions.

The *health practices* within a social environment will influence the individual and his physical performances. The effects, however, will vary with each person. The differences are accounted for by personal physiology, tastes, psychological reactions, and individual cultural experiences and background. The increase in personal *leisure* is, of course, correlated with freedom to make personal choices in daily living. The individual tends to take on the social practices of a group or community, and if it values sports and physical activity, he is more likely to participate during leisure. *Smoking* is a social practice with a demonstrated negative effect on health, and eventually an unfavorable effect on physical performance. The respiratory and circulatory systems will function less effectively, particularly during strenuous performances. *Tension* within a society affects each person in various ways. Tension that results in frustration will adversely affect physical performance, but tension that makes a person sensitive, aware, and ready can sharpen a person and his physical resources for improved performances.

Individual and Group Limitations and Handicaps. Limitations and handicaps of an individual or a group are closely related to physical performances. The factors are many—anxiety, deformity, disease, injury, malfunction, drugs, body size and proportions, fatigue, frustrations, nationality, body weight, health habits, stress, and fitness are some important elements. There are personal conditions that are factors in the process of individual adjustment to the environment. Some stem from the environment directly and are enhanced or reduced in influence by individual reactions.

The studies dealing with *anxiety* show a relationship to the adjustment of the individual in physical activity, with too much anxiety resulting in interference with performances and too little also having negative effects. Anxiety in the form of concern can be a helpful condition. The *physical handicaps* of the body will influence personal adjustment and therefore personal performance. The reactions differ with each person and the adjustment to be made. *Drugs* manifest themselves in various behaviors and affect personal adjustment to the environment and certainly to physical activity. Excessive use of drugs is harmful. *Body size, structure, and weight* are highly related to performance and adjustment in physical activity. Deviations from normal growth and development patterns limit the adjustment possibilities of the person in physical activity.

The individual is limited in his adjustment to the environment and physical activity by *fatigue* levels. Fatigue can be caused by an extensive variety of physical, environmental, and psychological factors. Fatigue will negatively influence performance. It represents a distinct handicap both in personal adjustments and in performance in physical activity and other relationships. *Frustrations, tensions, stress* are correlated with personal adjustment. The three concepts are also interrelated. Tensions and stresses that lead to frustrations cause the individual to respond with a less than spirited reaction. *Nationality and social characteristics and qualities* have been a matter of review in sports for some years. The difference in sports performance of various social groups may be attributed to sociological causes. Socioeconomic conditions and social class are influential factors. Genetic factors influence the size of the individual.

Sociocultural Applications of Physical Activity

Physical activity is a part of a society and an integral facet of the culture. It varies in each nation, community, and group. It has been a part of the life of all people from early times to the present. The influence of international sports has made physical activity a part of life in all cultures and nations. It is now an integrating force among nations.

Physical activities and their organized forms in sports, as they are practiced and applied, influence society and the culture. Social and cultural interests also influence the kind of physical activity practiced and enjoyed by the people. Some of the most powerful factors that influence physical activity are found in social and cultured institutions.

The individual citizen is responsible for the conditions that exist in a society. The cultural mores are determined by man. If man wishes a setting that is conducive to growth, development, and adjustment, then the individual begins with the physical environment and with the practices and the life of the people in this setting. What is desirable must be determined and social procedures must be set in motion to accomplish the desired ends.

The only purpose of sports and physical activity as a part of social institutions is to achieve goals important to the individual and desirable for the society. Optimal health and well-being cannot result from a sick society, and a sick society must be corrected so that it enhances human development and adjustment.

The growth of sports, athletics, and physical activity has been more rapid during the twentieth century than at any other period in history. The increase in professional sports alone, in the United States, has reached a level unpredicted only twenty-five years ago. The application of physical activity in the personal life of the people, in industry, in religious institutions, in colleges and universities are only some examples. The potential of physical activity and sports as a social force, in these applications, goes beyond the imagination of the people, in general, and the scientists, in particular, who have only recently begun systematic studies.

Government. It is desirable for society to have the participation of all people in the affairs of the community, not only in social life but also in government. Full citizenship is the objective. The people must become concerned with community affairs—from physical conditions to life in a community as it is and as it should be. Participation is a responsibility for each person.

The processes of industrialization and urbanization have rapidly increased over the past years. As a result the government becomes more centralized and more powerful. It therefore assumes increasing responsibility for the welfare of the people. This responsibility has significantly increased in the years since World War II for the leisure life of the citizens. Recreation, sports, physical activities, and quality of life are all concerns of government, as shown in some instances by direct operations (federal parks) and in most instances by strong supporting sponsorships. Recognizing the effects of urbanization, leisure, and automation, with its resulting loss in physical activity, governments (on all political levels) are giving strong support to preserving land for outdoor life.

According to Alex Natan,[2] "Never has a state risen so swiftly to world power as has sport." In a period of about sixty years the rise of the influence of sport to world power has been accomplished. Natan compares this rise to empires that have required centuries for equivalent

2 John W. Loy and G. S. Kenyon, eds., *Sport, Culture and Society* (New York: Macmillan, 1969), p. 203.

power. Natan goes on to report that "at the same time no other world power has ever shown such considerable symptoms of decay in so short a span as has the sporting movement." The reason advanced is that sport has become, particularly on the international level, a means of propaganda and has therefore assumed an increasing political significance. His claim is that sport has become a tool of politics. In the United States the applications of physical activity, in many roles, have not been linked with political propaganda, but do receive political support.

Government involvement in sports and physical activity serves the basic function of sustaining the government as a strong democracy by leading people toward the highest levels of life through acceptable citizenship practices. What is considered good must be preserved. This is the premise of democratic governments. Sports and physical activities properly conducted add significantly to the understanding and practices of democratic action and behavior. Democratic principles of government are the same as those applied in sports and physical activity. A full discussion of the nature and scope of the applications has been presented earlier by the author.[3] These are briefly summarized here.

In order that democratic government remain strong, the principles of democracy must be applied in the home, school, and community and by all political levels of government.

1. *Respect for the human personality.* No social, economic, or political restrictions are placed on the individual or group because of race, religion, nationality, or economic status. All individuals are different and unique.

2. *Equality of opportunity.* Democracy allows individual freedoms limited only by the rights and freedoms of others, and the principle of equality means that freedom is limited only by one's ability to use it.

3. *Cooperation for the resolution of conflict.* Cooperation means the planning for individual needs and interests, but always as these needs and interests relate to the welfare of others and to society as a whole. Working together toward goal achievement is a valid procedure in a democracy. The talents and abilities of the individual will determine the quality and quantity of achievements.

4. *Reason and intelligence as a basis for the solution of problems.* Actions, judgments, and decisions are based on fact. Reason and intelligence in the use of facts form the basis for opinion.

5. *Self-discipline as a basis for responsibility.* Democracy provides maximum opportunities and choices for the individual. Democracy does not fit everyone into a single pattern, judged by a superior being. This means that the individual must have self-discipline before he can accept full responsibility for his freedom.

6. *Self-government through group planning.* Self-government follows the principle that those affected by an action or decision should have an opportunity to participate in its formulation. It is the use of the group process to establish its standards for community life.

[3] Leonard A. Larson, *Curriculum Foundations and Standards for Physical Education* (Englewood Cliffs, N.J.: Prentice-Hall, 1970), pp. 139–158.

The involvement of government in the power and potential of physical activity for citizenship development is evident. It not only leads to the desirable personal development of the individual (which is the prime purpose of government), but also strengthens the government in performing this function.

Professions. Physical activity is applied in professional roles. It is amazing, when reviewing the professional organizations now well established, that physical activity has such potential and flexibility.

Disciplines. The objective of the scientific disciplines as applied to physical activity is to understand the effects and relationships of physical activity on the individual and the group. A full discussion of the knowledge that has been acquired will be given in Part II.

Labor and Industry. The second industrial revolution that followed World War II brought about tremendous changes in industry and labor. It has become a commonplace that the world is experiencing a scientific and technological revolution. These great advances have caused serious social and economic problems, but have also given man more leisure and extended his control over the environment. Properly used, these advances could favor man both socially and economically.

One of the most persistent occupational trends in the United States is the growing demand for workers with increased general education and technical and professional education. A college degree is viewed by many as a minimum requirement for employment in more attractive positions. In the skilled and semiskilled categories the training requirement is not as high as in the technical and professional categories, and the growth rate is downward rather than upward. For unskilled workers the decline is very rapid.

Industrial and labor changes will influence the individual and society. These are probably the most important sociocultural changes in a society. What does this mean to life in a society and, of greater importance, the life of each person?

Leisure is directly related to advances in science and technology—in both increasing free time and in lessening physical work. Both are fundamental sociocultural problems if they are neglected. The constructive use of leisure and the development of physical abilities are essential for health and well-being. Physical activity therefore becomes a large consideration for the individual and for society. Man must have physical work or activity and society must plan for leisure with activities that are wholesome, interesting, and demanding.

The rapid increase in physical exercise programs, sports, athletics, commercial recreation, and health clubs is a direct result of industrial and labor changes during the past fifty years. These activities have become one of the largest cultural components of our society, as evidenced by the sports pages of the newspapers, the Saturday and Sunday TV sports programs, increasing numbers of community swimming pools, golf courses, and so on. From the standpoint of personal involvement, probably as much as 15 per cent of the population has daily routines, for two to three hours of a sixteen-hour working day. The requirements and demands for physical activity are indeed great.

Education. The role of education in a society and as a part of the culture is very considerable. In the United States, education takes the largest portion of the state's budgets. This expenditure is being increasingly supported by the federal government.

There are many reasons why physical activity and sports became important parts of educational programs, including contributions to health and fitness, preparation for an active role during leisure, the potential of sports in social integration, and wholesome entertainment. It is important that physical activity become a part of education not only for its inherent educational potentials but because it prepares one for physical activity in later life. It is first necessary to develop skills and interests in physical activity. Personal development is not simple; it takes time and precise instruction. Secondly, instruction in the schools represents all the children in the United States. It is the place to establish desirable cultural patterns. Sports and physical activity should be a part. Thirdly, sports and physical activity in educational institutions represent a part of the life of the community in addition to institutional life. Cultural interests can be directly developed. Fourthly, sports and physical activity in the schools represent a physical location for participation by the entire community. This is a very important requirement to advance physical activity into its proper cultural place. It has great potential in the preparation for a life of good health, well-being, and citizenship.

Communications. The role of newspapers, magazines, popular books, films, radio, and television in modern societies and cultures goes beyond the imagination. The media have the power to design the social patterns and the culture of the people. The space devoted to sports in the newspapers, the time on radio and television schedules, the books on sports and exercise programs, the films on sports indicate the role played by these communications media in modern societies.

Sports and physical activities represent a large part of programming time and space in the communications media. From a strictly commercial viewpoint, sports have increased the interest of the people in the various media. They are popular! The use of famous athletes for commercial ads will attest to the popularity of sports. Participation in sports and physical activity by all people is significantly supported by the communications media. Personal participation, in addition to viewing, is thereby increased.

Leisure. Technological developments have liberated man from routine and drudgery. They have given man mastery of time and space. They have given him leisure he had long desired. One of the most important considerations for leisure is what man should do with his time. It could be inactivity—rest, watch, do nothing. Such practices lead to regression of the physical organism and the human personality. Man must be involved in social and cultural affairs—which include, in part, the necessity for physical activity. Basically, man longs for struggle. He enjoys a struggle to master and conquer. He loves competition. Work alone does not provide this outlet. Certainly unused leisure does not.

Because of their potential for enjoyment and personal satisfaction, sports and physical activity now take up a large part of the time spent during leisure. The professional ideal is that the time spent in physical activity should contribute to the adjustment of the individual and society and add personal development that will increase the satisfactions of life.

Health. The health of the people and all individuals is a social and cultural desire for everyone. The strength of a society is nearly directly determined by the health and the physical resources of its members. Its health potentials are probably the most important reason for encouraging physical activity. One's daily practices in all aspects of life have an effect on the physical body, establishing health and fitness levels. The destiny of man is largely determined by what he does daily.

The role of physical activity is paramount in setting the health level of the individual. It is not only a question of a disease-free organism, but also of the level of energy available for enthusiastic and vigorous living. There are 60 to 70 per cent of the American people who are unfit for energetic living. Certainly this is a condition of poor health. Others who are physically active have developed resources of physical energy that sustain them on the job and with reserves to enjoy leisure. Whether the leisure interests are social or physical, one is unable to participate if exhausted.

During the past few years research has demonstrated the value of physical activity to health. The evidence is convincing. It ranges from ability to perform feats of skill and strength to sustaining the cardiovascular system in a normal functional state and preventing cardiac failure.

Religion. The moral and spiritual life in a society and a culture is highly correlated with the strength and the quality of living in the society. Religion contributes directly toward this end. The church is a social institution functioning in a culture in a manner similar to the school, the home, and other social institutions. The goals are much the same—an acceptable society with desirable social and cultural practices. It is possible, and most desirable, for the church and religious institutions to become concerned with human behaviors, social practices, and attitudes of people without interference with fundamental concepts of the various religions. The moral and spiritual values stemming from religious teachings tend to have common meanings to a society and a culture.

The role of physical activity and sports has increased significantly as a part of church programs during the past several years. The gymnasium, the swimming pool, playgrounds, recreation rooms in church buildings are designed for physical activity under the auspices of the church. The gains in human development of youth have been most noteworthy. The role is an important one for the church. Qualities of integrity, dignity, honesty, loyalty, and fair play are some moral values that can be gained by physical activity under church leadership and auspices.

Ethnic, National, and Racial Groups. The social and cultural integration of people toward common human understandings is a community and world problem of the first order. Differences that appear unsolvable because of color, race, and nationality have no base in fact. The place of sport and physical activity in contributing to the solution of these social problems has received wide special reviews and test applications over the past twenty-five years. The results appear favorable to the social institutions and governments using this medium for human understanding and communication.

Sports and athletics have been highly successful in racial integration since World War II. The motivation for success of the team is stronger than attitudes about race. The acceptance of human skill and achievement, as a basis for understanding, is also stronger than biased attitudes. It is safe to say that integration (including ethnic and nationality) had its first significant contribution from sports. It is only within the past few years that integration has been emphasized in other social, vocational, and cultural activities. Sports represented an ideal beginning because of the common goal held by all players—the strong desire to win.

The increase in international sports has been rapid only within the past few, short years. Transportation is one factor, but the emphasis on international understanding is another. It is a pleasure to observe the Olympic Games. Youth from all over the world compete in a setting of friendship and hard competition. There are only a few instances of unfavorable attitudes and behaviors. Success in the Olympic Games has stimulated competition among countries that now include the entire world.

The strength of sports as an integrating force has been satisfactorily observed in the past years. Its place in the social and cultural practices of each nation has been well established. It will increase in future years when economic conditions permit transportation of teams on a world-wide basis.

Physical Activity in a World Setting

Physical activity in its basic form (as simple exercise) and in its applied combinations (as sports, athletics, recreation, and so on) has a large place in the cultures of the modern world. Hardly a person or a social institution is not influenced by physical activity either directly or indirectly. Many kinds of work activities are involved, ranging from employees dealing with personal health and fitness to professional and scientific workers. Research programs in the science and medicine of sport and physical activity have increased rapidly within the past fifty years, and numerous social institutions and people are involved. Sports, athletics, physical activity in many forms are integrally woven into the cultures of all nations. The nature of physical activity and its many possible combinations vary with the traditions, ways of life, and mores of each country. The effects on the people are far-reaching socially, politically, and economically.

Social Factors. The social interests and practices of people within a culture have an infinite number of variations. The combinations differ to some degree in each culture, and there are differences between the various social groups within a nation and among nations. In some instances the social and political differences are highly significant.

All human behavior represents interactions between and among the forces of the environment, both social and physical, the conditions that the individual lives with each day. The most powerful force is the family; it is a social institution and the fundamental unit of a society. During the twentieth century the American family has undergone many changes in mores, location, stability, work schedules, economics, and additional leisure and free time from work. The freedom from work is highly related to sports, athletics, and physical activity.

The part that sports and physical activity play in the modern life of man as both participant and spectator is large indeed. The rapid growth of professional sports in the United States gives evidence of spectator interest. Sports and physical activity have become an integral part of modern life, and are now an influential social force.

Economic Factors. Not only have sports, athletics, and physical activity become important factors in a culture for reasons of fitness and health, but they have become important economically. Commercial sports is now big business. In the United States professional football, basketball, and baseball are all well established economically. They are professions for the player and certainly for the management. Athletics, sports, and physical education (required in the United States) represent one of the largest and most expensive parts of the school budget. Some of these funds are returned to the schools through commercialization of athletics. In universities and colleges an attempt is made to cover all costs of inter-collegiate athletics from gate receipts. The programs in colleges and universities—encompassing various sports, physical facilities, and paid coaches—represent staggering amounts of money when viewed nation-ally.

Without question, sports, athletics, and physical activity have en-tered into the economic world in the United States. This trend is now rapidly increasing internationally. Providing services to meet the grow-ing interests in physical activity will require professional workers and economic support.

Political Factors. Sports and athletics affect the politics of a culture and a nation, being involved in governmental operations, in the manage-ment of people, in providing desirable activities for the citizens, in ad-vancing the fitness and health status of the citizens, and many other political requirements.

Probably the most powerful political value of sports and athletics is their potential in the development of desirable citizenship. The team is a miniature society. It contains all the political elements needed for a good society—respect for the human personality, equality of opportunity, reason and intelligence for problem solving, self-government, and other political-democratic elements. These potentials represent part of the rationale for athletics in school programs. Athletics properly taught and organized in the schools prepare the individual for an understanding of democratic principles exactly as they can be practiced in the home and community.

Democracy as it relates to sports and athletics will be discussed further in this text. It is one of the major forces in a culture in preparing people for desirable citizenship on all political levels. It is now being em-phasized internationally, not only by an increased interest in the Olym-pic Games, but through a constant program of international sports. The People-to-People sports program is only one example. The political ob-jective is world citizenship through cultural understanding.

Educational Factors. In the United States in particular, sports, ath-letics, and physical activity are integral parts of school, university, and social agency programs. The potentials of physical activity have been found to be compatible with educational goals and the purpose of edu-cational institutions to prepare for citizenship.

In this book the relationships between the goals of education and the potentials of physical activity will be noted and supported. It will be observed that physical activity can contribute to all goals of education in varying degrees. In the preparation for good health, it makes a large and unique contribution. In helping to achieve democratic human under- standing and self-government, it makes a considerable contribution, along with other school subjects. In the development of the individual as a desirable social being, it adds significantly to the contributions made by other school programs.

Physical activity is a potent educational force in all cultures. The potentials, however, to be achieved require leadership—as with all school programs—that fully understands all educational goals and the processes required for their achievement.

Cultural Effects. The culture of a nation is determined by all its people and social institutions. The culture is the sum total of all com- ponents of a society, and sports, athletics, and physical activity as applied to the individual and as found as a part of the society are large parts of a culture. The role of sports and athletics in a culture is highly related to leisure. Leisure has increased and is increasing—so are sports and ath- letics. They are becoming a way of life—hunting, fishing, golf, tennis, and all forms of physical activity are part of our social institutions. They provide a change from professional and vocational routines, they provide a challenge, they provide refreshment, they provide ways of communica- tion that are relaxing and fun, and they provide for social status. Without question physical activity is a well-established, integral part of the culture. This is true not only in the United States, but in countries throughout the world.

Chapter 3

Physical Activity: The Scope in Human Development

When considering the developmental potential of physical activity, setting, culture, and social practices are fundamental starting references. Physical activity is one of the developmental media in a society. The full media are comprised of the culture and mores of the people. In a totalitarian government, for example, all developmental media are used to achieve obedience and acceptance of political objectives. On the other hand, in a democratic government, the role of the media is to develop understanding and responsibility among the people, so that they can participate in government. The roles are in complete opposition. It is of interest to note, however, that the physical activity medium can serve both roles with equal efficiency.

The individual, as a citizen, is responsible for the conditions that exist in a society. In a democratic society, the individual's responsibility begins with himself, then expands to the family, the immediate community, the state, the nation, and finally a concern for problems that exist in other countries of the world.

Cultural mores are determined by man. They are the results of daily practices. If man wishes a society that is conducive to growth, then his efforts must be directed to the solution of societal problems. A strong society is constituted by strong, dedicated, and disciplined individuals. A single person can have significant influences on the mores of a group

35

or community. He may start with his own family; disciplined children in a family represent good material for society.

Optimal individual growth cannot be achieved in a sick society. Positive development comes from the conditions that provide opportunities for individual participation in activities according to standards that represent the community as it should be. All societal forces will influence the participant, but the setting in physical activity is of particular importance. The total personality participates; therefore the total personality can be shaped within the context of physical activity.

Social Forces and the Cultural Setting

What is a good society? A more difficult question is, "How can a society be structured and its functions developed to make it good?" The factors of size, economic status and potential, and social differences, among many others, combine to make these questions most difficult to answer. Regardless of political structures, history is full of social failures. Poverty, disease, unfit living conditions, unemployment, ignorance, racial conflicts, and war are only some of the problems that the individual faces in work and adjustment.

Little doubt exists about the influence of social forces. Life in an unfit environment may not destroy the individual, but it will have a marked influence. There are, of course, individuals who have risen far above the setting in home and community. Unfortunately, these are exceptions.

The desirable human values inherent in an activity must have a favorable setting to yield favorable results. This is particularly true for physical activity and sports. In fact, the process of participation in physical activity follows the same cultural patterns that represent the experiences of the individual in the home or in the social group. The culture is advanced and perpetuated, therefore, by participation. The question that must be resolved is the following: "What are the basic social values in a culture that will draw the positive values from physical activity that will strengthen the individual, and thereby society?"

Health Resources. Most of the world's people live in poverty, ignorance, disease, and hunger. Such conditions do not contribute to the advancement of man's health.

Clinics, educational and social agencies, medical and dental services, playgrounds, swimming pools and gymnasiums are all important resources for the advancement of health and fitness. They should provide services that represent all facets of human development—physical, mental, social, and emotional—beyond family and personal responsibilities.

Educational Resources. Schools, colleges, and other educational institutions should provide opportunities for the development of skills and attitudes that will provide man with the essential resources for health and well-being. Knowledge of the human organism and of the influence of personal practices is essential. This should include the knowledge of the medical and scientific worth of physical activity for the development of efficient functioning and good health.

Ethical and Moral Resources. The community setting should provide a wholesome environment for each person. The informal setting and leisure life are important. Leadership is essential. Sports, games, and physical activity contain the potential for socialization. Provision for participation in such activities is a responsibility of society.

Citizenship Resources. Society must involve all people in the affairs of the community. This includes not only government but social life. In order to develop citizenship, community activities and participation by all must be achieved.

Economic Resources. A society must be secure. The degree of economic security is determined by the resources of the community and the people. Each person has a responsibility to provide for the needs of all the people. Educational, social, and cultural institutions and activities are essential for all the people. The ability of a community to support these activities will determine the potential for a good society.

Social and Communicative Resources. A good society is one in which all members can communicate with ease and skill. Inability to communicate leads to misunderstandings and eventually to harm. Without free, clear, and reasonable communication a true meeting of the cultural elements does not occur.

Communication involves more than words. It includes all relationships, including social activities, sports, and cultural programs.

Resources for Fullness of Life. Life is more than work. Today more time is available for leisure than is needed for work. Society has the responsibility to prepare its citizens for both work and leisure. Preparation for leisure activities is essential to adjustment in our present world.

Basic Needs

The basic needs are the same for all mankind, whether or not they are recognized as such by all individuals. Society must provide a setting in which the basic needs, listed in the following paragraphs, can be met.

Health and Fitness. No one is happy when he is ill, nor is an individual able to gain happiness when he is weak and lacking in energy. Good health is necessary to a full life and there are many factors that combine for it.

The individual is constantly exposed to elements that can be favorable or unfavorable to health. The results of negative environments are disease, undesirable health practices, tensions, stresses, insecurity, and a general setting that reduces health level and renders positive actions for health less effective.

The components for good health are not only physical but mental and emotional. The physical base, however, is most fundamental and supportive of health. Protecting the organism from disease is probably most basic. All resources of medicine and education are needed to prepare one to understand the protective needs of the body. The disease-free organism represents the desirable starting point for good health.

An individual, if he is to reach a level that will sustain him in all strenuous daily activities, must develop his body for physical strength and endurance and maintain normal body weight. He must observe sound health practices (for example, with regard to nutrition and rest) that will support the physiological process and not cause bodily losses.

Critical Thinking and Analysis. The ability to think, analyze, and solve problems is needed for all people in all life activities. Hope comes to people if social, political, and economic problems can be resolved reasonably and intelligently. Learning comes from striving. Solutions must be found that yield satisfactions. Judgments and patterns of behavior emerge through human endeavor. By adjusting, the whole individual participates in every perceptual act. In coping with his environment, he progressively alters his perceptions and develops complex ones that are more satisfying and effective.

From early childhood, progression stems from simple awareness of the environment to more complex discriminations. The complexity and the potential of the environment will influence both the quality and the quantity of discriminating powers. The human factors that determine individual powers are maturation levels, the quality of the human organism, the satisfactions gained, the purposes or motives, the quality of experiences, and the immediate meanings for the individual. One does not learn in a vacuum, but in environments that have potential challenges and satisfactions.

Moral, Spiritual, and Ethical Values. The moral, spiritual, and ethical values held by man are the most basic needs for the individual and for a society. An individual and certainly a society could hardly survive if those personal qualities were lacking. A system of moral and spiritual values is indispensable to group living. As social order or structures become more complex, as the welfare of all depends increasingly upon the cooperation of all, the need for common moral principles becomes greater. Especially in a society that cherishes the greatest possible degree of individual freedom, the allegiance of the individual to commonly approved moral standards is necessary. "No social invention however ingenious, no improvements in government structure however prudent, no enactment of status and ordinances however lofty their aims, can produce a good and secure society if personal integrity, honesty, and self-discipline are lacking." [1]

Responsibility. Responsibility and discipline are marks of maturity. They are also essential qualities for every person regardless of country or culture. One must develop the quality of responsibility and must develop discipline in all requirements for personal life and life within a society. The individual must be responsible for the consequences of his own conduct.

Man creates his society for his own good, but after the creation, he must assume responsibility for that which he has created. Society is dynamic, and it is man's responsibility to guide the dynamics of his institutions and social groups. Thus, as society evolves, it grows in complexity; it fosters integration patterns and social interrelationships, and it forces its members to specialize. Man is responsible for understanding and giving direction to these trends.[2]

For normal human development man cannot be separated from others. A human society, beginning with the immediate family in a home, is the most inclusive of all relationship structures. Groups (family or societies) are formed because individuals have needs that are best met by the organizations of groups of men. Group organization provides a sense of belonging and satisfies economic, political, and social needs that include the total individual and the total society, from the home to international relations.

Security. Security, both economic and social, is a basic need for man. During childhood the balance between protective authority and delegation of responsibility can provide the necessary sense of security while inducing growth toward maturity. As the individual develops and matures, he will acquire a large measure of self-reliance in his relationship with others. Security is derived from associations that develop self-confidence and personal responsibility. It begins with treating others with respect and consideration.

Social security represents something that society or the family does

[1] "Moral and Spiritual Values in the Public Schools." Educational Policies Commission. Washington, D.C., NEA, 1951.
[2] Celeste Ulrich, *The Social Matrix of Physical Education* (Englewood Cliffs, N.J.: Prentice-Hall, 1968).

for the individual. Personal security is something the individual does for himself. The former comes from outside the individual, the latter comes from within. Social security consists largely of acceptance and an individual life without damaging needs. Personal security is the result of the reactions of the individual to all outside conditions as they are meaningful to him. If one is able, under all conditions, to be reasonably independent, the basis for security has been achieved.

Fullness of Life. A full life not only is necessary for happiness and fulfillment, but is an important health factor. Boredom, unhappiness, and discontent in one's life role are not factors that add to health and full living.

Fullness in one's life comes from balance. Balance provides for differences, new experiences, enlargement of one's education, enlargement of human relations and of one's views. One should have a balance between work and leisure. Work must be pleasant and enjoyable. It is tragic to spend about one third of one's life in an occupation that is distasteful.

Leisure holds a major potential for fullness in life. It is the only time when personal choice is truly possible. Doing nothing certainly does not add to a full life, but activities that are challenging and enjoyable, and that contribute to personal advancement in interests and skills will add significantly to one's life.

Nash [3] has presented criteria that rate activities on their contribution to the effective and satisfying use of leisure. Of the criteria he has listed, when judged by long-range effect and personal satisfaction, several take on particular value. The activity itself makes little difference if it has a positive contribution and if it is the personal selection of the individual.

The third major component in the fullness in life is the physical recovery of the body from the drains and strains of life and work. Man needs rest and sleep. This phase generally represents about one third of the day for each person. Again there are differences. The degree of stress and tension of the day is a major factor. The recuperative power of the organism is another. But, in common to all, man does require rest and sleep to recover from the stress of the day. Whether recovery is complete depends on the individual's ability to cope successfully with the other two thirds of his life.

Citizenship. Citizenship is not only another basic need of man, but a social obligation. One should have standards of what the group should be. It is not enough to have ideas or ideals; one must assume responsibility for their implementation. One must practice what he believes, and this is applied in the home, in small groups, and in the community, which extends from the local community to the countries of the world.

[3] Jay B. Nash, *Philosophy of Recreation and Leisure* (St. Louis: Mosby, 1953).

Citizenship also includes the process of acceptable living in a social order. This requires the personal application of the fundamental principles of a democracy. The principles include (1) respect for the human personality, (2) equality of opportunity, (3) reason and intelligence in problem solving, (4) discipline to assume responsibility, (5) cooperation in the resolution of conflict, and (6) self-government through group planning.

In a democracy dedicated citizenship is an absolute requirement if the government is to be planned to serve and protect the citizens. Each person must be prepared in knowledge, skill, attitudes, and understandings about the government and all social institutions if life in a nation is to be pleasant and secure.

Human Understandings. The brotherhood of man, in its relationship to human understandings, takes precedence over self-interest. The respect for the human personality is a basic factor in human understandings. The democratic tenets cited in the preceding paragraph are also important personal guides. They provide an opportunity for individual freedom to pursue life activities.

Human understanding starts in the home, with the parents. Teachers also play a very large role as models for the children in their charge.

Interpersonal relations on all social and political levels require good faith and personal integrity. Suspicion and fear will cause individuals and nations to withdraw and become defensive. The individual and national objective should be full understanding of differences and respect for them. The achievement of happiness is not gained by a single procedure or pattern. Wide cultural differences exist in the world, and all have the right to exist. If this can be recognized by each person, in each nation, the ability of people to live together throughout the world will be significantly advanced.

The Potentials of Physical Activity

Physical activity can help improve patterns of growth during the growing years, health, motor efficiency, and longevity. The extent of such results is determined by the physical state of the person himself, daily hygienic practices, and frequency, intensity, and duration of physical activity. The nature of the activity itself also affects the nature of the development. Different activities will affect the organism differently.

The human organism, at rest or in physical activity, is influenced by its habitat, both social and physical. A social environment (home, school, work) that is pleasant and where the ways of life add to the health status of the individual will be far more likely to produce good results from physical activity than an environment with undesirable social conditions, such as stress and unacceptable health practices. The effects of the physical environment will also affect the growth and development of the individual.

This book is devoted to the study and analysis of physical activity. It does not include the nature of the physical activity itself and how it should be taught, how the movements may be learned, but deals entirely with the potential of physical activity.

As an overall review or introduction to this text, the author has classified the goals or objectives that can be achieved through physical activity. Physical activity as a discipline (Part II) and physical activity as a profession (Part III) are discussed with the premise that these are the basic goals that represent currently, according to experimental and clinical evidence, what physical activity can do for the person. The foundations for physical activity as a discipline and as a profession are thereby established.[4]

Individual Health. Health is influenced by knowledge and understanding of the organism as reflected in daily care. Health is also social and emotional. Personal interests and practices set the level of health. Reactions to stresses, environmental forces of all kinds, will affect the social and emotional behavior of man and will also affect the physical body itself. Constant internal emotional stress is not a favorable setting for desirable health levels.

Disease and its control are closely associated with physical activity. Physical activity can be a preventive measure, for the development of a strong, vigorous organism will result in less susceptibility to certain types of disease. Moreover, if disease should strike, a strong body will be more capable of withstanding the debilitating effects of illness than will a weaker one. Correction of disease or injury damage is a physical process. The objective is to regain as much functional power as possible and also to overbuild compensatory functions as an aid to normality.

Physical defects, as a health factor, are both structural and functional. The loss of a body part represents a structural defect; the deviation of a bodily function represents a functional defect. The former may be corrected in part by prosthetic devices; the latter in many instances may be corrected or improved by properly applied physical activity or exercises. Defects and rehabilitation of the individual can usually be improved or corrected by properly applied physical activity.

Organic vigor is probably the most valuable effect of physical activity. It is the ability to sustain and resist the forces that act and react on a person and also the power to continue the functions of the body at normal or above-normal levels. It is the basis for good health. An indi-

---

[4] See Leonard A. Larson, *Curriculum Foundations and Standards for Physical Education* (Englewood Cliffs, N.J.: Prentice-Hall, 1970), for a more complete presentation of the goals for physical activity.

vidual has good health when his total physical capacity can function smoothly in generous excess of his peak regular requirements. Physical, mental, emotional, and social frustrations should then never be more than temporary and are not likely to exert harmful influences.

Body weight and body symmetry are factors in the health of the individual. Both influence a person's efficiency and his resources in energy for action. Cumulation of the by-products of obesity or overweight will lower the vitality of the organism and will lead to ill health, inefficiency, and earlier death. Proper nutrition and diet cannot be separated from physical activity; both deal with caloric energy, stored or used.

Poor body symmetry and posture gradually lead to maladjustments in the body, with effects on mechanical efficiency and body physiology. Both are closely related to health.

Fatigue can be both temporary and chronic. Nearly all people are temporarily fatigued as the result of work or stress. With a person in good health, temporary fatigue is canceled by physical activity, rest, and relaxation. Chronic fatigue will eventually destroy the organism, particularly if it is physically weak. In a strong physical organism the possibility of chronic fatigue is greatly lessened.

The Effective Utilization of the Human Organism. Another major potential of physical activity is the preparation of the human organism for effective, efficient, and energy-conserving work. The human body is a machine. It operates on fuel consumed at a rate set by size, weight, skill, and all factors that deal with movement and its efficiency.

The human organism responds to the laws of mechanics, just as any system of weights and levers does. Physical activity can develop the body mass or weight so that it can be efficiently manipulated in all daily tasks so as to gain the desired result without fatigue or with minimal expenditure of energy.

Neuromuscular development unfolds on a clearly progressive schedule. The process begins at birth and continues throughout life at differing rates. The *first period* occurs from birth to entry in school and includes physical development and the beginnings of skill mechanics of movement.[5] These skills include sitting, crawling, walking, and so on.

The *second stage* of neuromuscular development involves development of the basic elements that underlie all fundamental skills, which include accuracy, strength, agility, and so on.

The *third stage* of neuromuscular development involves the fundamental skills that constitute the components of games, sports, and physical activities. These are the skills of running, jumping, throwing, catching, and so on. Success in developing these skills comes from the proper physical base, proper development of the basic elements and an under-

[5] Ibid., chap. 7.

standing of the mechanical patterns in order to practice and continue to use these fundamental patterns in physical activity.

The *fourth stage* is the application of the developed patterns of human movement in games, sports, and physical activities of all kinds. The individual has now reached mature neuromuscular development. He has the ability to participate in games, sports, and athletics that will continue to advance neuromuscular levels and to sustain and develop the physical body.

Understanding the Human Organism. Performing well in physical activity, preparing for it, and understanding the factors related to successful action are not possible without knowledge. It is an essential requirement and it is a result of physical activity and the individual's participation.

The understanding necessary for applications of physical activity begins with the objectives. The philosophic and scientific nature and worth of the objectives in physical activity are major components. The scientific nature of achievement (physical, mental, social, and emotional) represents another component in the use of physical activity. This includes all systems and functions of the body. Understanding of the organism includes the factors (environmental) that facilitate or restrict human development in physical activity. It also includes all the mental facilities of the person in learning and understanding.

The Individual as a Social Being. The individual is a social being. When participating in physical activity, he is closely associated with others in social relationships. Over a period of time, all the elements of the social discipline will be related to other individuals. The potential for change, adjustment, and development of the individual as a social being is very much a part of the strength of the physical activity medium.

No society can survive without social order. A system of social values is indispensable for both individual and group living. As society becomes more complex and as individuals become dependent upon cooperation for survival, the social and moral development of the individual become increasingly important.

The author has delineated the components of the social individual that directly apply to physical activity.[6] These elements are not unique to physical activity. They represent the social individual who is a desirable citizen. These components are respect for law, regulations, and social standards; individual self-sufficiency; individual positive actions; individual regard for self; individual regard for others; and individual vitality.[7] Under proper leadership and in good social and physical settings, the social individual and group can participate according to the

[6] Ibid., p. 126.
[7] The elements contained in each component are listed in Larson, op. cit., p. 126.

defined actions of social behavior. If continued, physical activity will add significantly to the development of the individual as a social being.

The Democratic Individual and Society. Physical activity (and all its combinations and applications) contains all the elements of democratic human relations, democratic governing structure, and democratic controls. Within this framework one has freedom to develop physically, mentally, emotionally, and socially.

Opportunities for democratic human behavior are associated with the administrators, teachers and leaders, coaches, captains of teams, players, students, managers, press, cheerleaders, officials, and spectators, along with the community as a whole. The basic democratic components that should be practiced in human associations are respect for the human personality, equality of opportunity for optimal development, cooperation for the resolution of problems, discipline as a basis for responsibility, and self-government through group planning and action. All the elements are essential to give strength to the individual and to the group.

Individual and Group Adjustment. Another major contribution possible through physical activity is individual adjustment to the group and group adjustment to the individual. Strength in one will give strength to the other. They are completely compatible.

The constant struggle of man is to survive. The many strong forces that work in opposition to this objective cannot be entirely eliminated. Man can modify environments to meet personal objectives, particularly if he is strong. Adjustments are then made to meet individual designs.

One cannot live apart from his environment. Even if it were possible, it would not be desirable, because one's environment can bring out the best in man.

The ultimate of all preparation is to be ready to meet all conditions in life with a highly satisfactory result. One then will enjoy meeting new situations each day. The confidence that comes from understanding and skill is the objective for each person. Preparation begins in the home, continues in the schools, and is the objective of social and religious agencies in the communities.

Developmental Factors Related to Physical Activity

When considering human development in a physical activity context, environmental considerations become necessary. Their effects are demonstrated in activity participation, in normal life, and in the outcomes from participation. Some environmental conditions will be presented and briefly reviewed.

Stresses, Strains, and Fatigue. Stresses, strains, and fatigue have unfavorable effects on the individual generally and while he is participating in physical activity. The stresses that drain one's energy or that interfere with conserving or developing needed energy resources, of course, reduce levels of participation. They will therefore interfere with human development levels possible under more favorable conditions.

Health Practices and Habits. The strains on the human organisms are many—disease; physical defects; constant tension; lack of proper rest or sleep; poor diet; overindulgence in food, alcohol, and smoking; accidents; constant use of self-medication and drugs; poor human relations; unwise exercise or no exercise; and chronic fatigue. Practices that lead to these unfavorable conditions will lower physical resources and will render the results of physical activity ineffective, even in maintaining the status quo.

A fundamental requirement for favorable results from physical activity is the proper preparation for physical activity. In sports it is called training. Only if those practices that conserve energy in physical activity are followed can the individual develop progressively as the result of consistent physical activity.

Physical Activity Practices. The individual who avoids physical effort at all times during each day cannot be prepared for vigorous physical activity when it is needed. Of greater consequence is the slow but constant retrogression of the physical organism that such inactivity entails. The organism needs activity to sustain life. In daily practice, one should walk rather than ride when this is possible, should take every opportunity for physical exercise while at work, when riding, or when in any sedentary position (for example, tensing the muscles while sitting).

Lack of exercise is an ingredient for physical inefficiency. Moreover, a sluggish organism does not have clear and efficient reasoning power and performance.

Human Relations. Unhappiness, tension, social unacceptance, and constant rejection are not the ingredients for positive human development. They reduce the beneficial results of physical activity. Under undesirable conditions the mind and emotions become harmful to the physical condition of the body. The result is physiological maladjustment and an increase in bodily deterioration.

Human relations and personal associations that are pleasant, satisfying, and challenging aid human development. Not only do they have favorable effects on the physiological processes, but they represent a part of social and emotional development.

Knowledge of the Body. Knowledge of the human body should be a part of the education of all people. Such knowledge should include awareness of the effects of various environmental forces, the effects of daily health practices, the requirements in the care of the body, and the requirements for human development that will advance or maintain the organism at normal or above-normal states of functioning. Judgments are made each day and they must be made with knowledge of the human body and its operations and functions. Lack of knowledge and understanding will result in practices, in many instances, that are health-destroying.

Social and Economic Conditions. Social and economic conditions that cause people to live on an economic level that is not physically sustaining; that result in ignorance, disease, and poor health; and that do not provide for necessary health and medical services are all health-destroying. Physical activity to improve one's physical condition can make little progress in such conditions.

Interests and Motivations. Every individual needs a goal, both immediate and long-term. There is a well-established principle that unless one wants something deeply achievement will be inadequate. This is true in all areas of human activity. With proper motivation one will always be reaching for new ideas, skills, and experiences that will help one to grow.

Prevention, Protection, and Security. Prevention of disease and poor health conditions is important. Security is an important element in prevention. In order to grow and develop one must feel secure.

Protection applies to physical activity. One must have the health and the physical requirements needed to participate so that accidents will not occur. Favorable results can come from physical activity only when the gains are not lost by unwise participation.

Opportunities for Human Development

The worth of physical activity to the individual and the group is far greater than most people realize. The developmental worth of physical activity is also underestimated by most teachers, leaders, and coaches. Physical activity is necessary for prevention of disease and poor health; it is also necessary to sustain the organic functions of the body needed to live day by day without loss of energy necessary to work successfully.

All people need physical activity, but the energy-producing characteristics of this activity must be sufficient for physical activity to be successful. One must know each individual's requirements; all are different to some degree. Age, sex, and traditions are some individual factors to consider.

Human development from physical activity is both qualitative and quantitative. It is not enough to realize the ingredients of needed development from physical activity; we must determine the levels of development necessary or desirable for each individual. These are quantitative judgments and are founded on the daily activities of man. What he does, the requirements for work and leisure, are factors that will set quantitative goals. The individual who wants to be a "weight lifter" must practice many hours per day to reach the level of a champion. For daily living needs, such effort and goals are unnecessary. Beyond the minimal needs for health and well-being, the quantitative levels are determined by personal desires. High levels of achievement, of course, are not harmful. They may also be very satisfying to the participant.

PART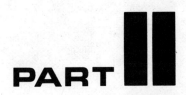

Disciplines

One must understand physical activity before it can be applied as a profession. Physical activity is designed to improve the human organism in every way possible. Goals set the directions for the outcomes from physical activity; they can only be set on the basis of fact and philosophy. The questions are, "What do we want for the individual?" and "How can physical activity contribute toward these ends?"

Part II is planned entirely as fact finding and interpreting, with physical activity as the reference. What is the worth of physical activity? The presentations will deal with physical activity without reference to any professional uses.

Research on physical activity has been largely within the professional contexts. It has dealt largely with the "how" and the "why" of physical activity in numerous professional relationships and applications. The "body of knowledge" about physical activity has been, therefore, limited to a framework that will not fully describe the scientific and philosophic nature of physical activity.

The sciences and philosophies of man have a broad history and encompass extensive research. Within these basic fields little research has been concentrated on physical activity. It has dealt largely with man as a person and with his relationship to his social and physical environments.

The plan for the chapters in Part II is to develop a "conceptual structure" with the concepts from the foundational sciences and philosophies that appear to be relevant in describing the scientific and philosophic nature of physical activity. This involves "borrowing" from the well-established sciences and philosophies until research in physical activity per se has a chance to deal with the concepts directly. The relationships are very close. In fact, the applications of the sciences and philosophies become more than hyoptheses; they can become very useful indeed in the professional planning for physical activity.

50

Research in professional physical activity is going on, and research in the conceptual study of physical activity has grown during the past few years. In physiology, studies have been numerous during the twentieth century throughout the world. Recent studies have been undertaken in other sciences and philosophies.

The selection of the sciences and philosophies and the organization of the content in the four chapters in Part II result from some of the studies directly made on physical activity and from a rationale that the selected sciences and philosophies are necessary to explain the behavior of man in physical activity. The sciences have been arbitrarily integrated or merged strictly on the basis of physical activity and what appears to be the value of the concepts in physical activity. With additional research, no doubt, the sciences and philosophies may appear in their original basic state, rather than integrated.

Experimental and clinical writings have involved the disciplines of physiology (a component of biology), sociology, psychology, history, physical sciences (largely physics, mechanics, and chemistry), and a number of the basic philosophies. The writings have been direct within a professional context and have been theoretical in a sense of dealing with the concept itself without any professional references. These six sciences and philosophies will be presented in four chapters, dealing with the biophysical sciences (physiology and the physical sciences), the sociopsychological sciences (sociology and psychology), history, and philosophy. In each instance the conceptual structure will set the framework for writing to provide an understanding of the scope of physical activity as a phenomenon and to provide a basis for professional physical activity in the ten professions organized at this time. These ten professional applications of physical activity will constitute the chapters in Part III.

Chapter 4

Biophysical Foundations

In the human body, as in a machine, movement cannot occur without energy. To understand fully the two concepts of movement and energy, reference is made to the sciences of human motion (physical sciences) and of human energy (physiology). Because in physical activity it is most difficult to deal separately with these two concepts, we will consider the "biophysical sciences of physical activity." It is recognized that other sciences besides the physical and the physiological sciences also involve movement or physical activity. They will be considered in subsequent chapters.

If the body moves in defiance of the laws of mechanical efficiency, the cost in energy is higher than if it moves in accord with them. If the body is unsynchronized, it is mechanically less efficient. Thus physical activity should be understood mechanically. Physical activity then becomes a biophysical phenomenon and a science of physical activity.

The body reacts, like any mass, to the laws of mechanics. It has mass (weight), levers (bones), and energy-producing and moving mechanisms (muscles, nerves, and the physical and chemical equipment for the development of energy). The objectives in using the body are efficiency, power, form, accuracy, control, and the least possible energy expenditure. Basically, two principles are involved: (1) the proper use of the body and its parts in the most mechanically efficient way and (2) the minimum expenditure of energy in movement to accomplish a given task.

The activity or movement patterns of the body are common to many forms of activity. The mechanical and energy principles are therefore common. This is true whether the movement is applied to work, sports, household duties, or recreation. Understanding the science of mechanics and energy building of physical activity has therefore numerous professional applications. It is a most basic science, stemming from the appli-

53

cation of the physical and the biological sciences. It is clearly a subdivision of these two disciplines.

The Biophysical Science

The biophysical science is an applied discipline of the parent disciplines of biology and the physical sciences. It is a scientific discipline aimed at understanding man in physical activity. The content of this science is essentially the mechanics of the human organism in physical movement or physical activity and the content related to the energy requirements and other physiological functions essential for action and for sustaining physical activity. It would be most difficult to plan, train, and prepare for physical activity without knowledge of the content of this science. Physical activity is basically a biophysical phenomenon.

The biophysical science is closely related to factors in physical activity, in addition to mechanics and the physiological resources of the organism. Physical activity is influenced by body build and body flexibility. The inflexible individual will have difficulty in physical activity and his activity will cost more in energy. Other closely related factors are muscular strength and power, and reaction time is important in many movements.

Spatial ability is another factor related to efficient movement. This is the ability to judge, in space, the pattern the movement should take. If judgment is inaccurate, the action will be reduced in effectiveness. One must also be able to make quick adaptive movements in sequence. In addition, the emotional factors of will power and desire are important. The negative emotional elements of disturbance, frustration, and uncertainty are closely related to movement inefficiency.

Broer [1] has placed into an organizational structure the various prerequisites and controls correlated with human movement and efficiency. The central control is the nervous system, which is the regulator of the body functions. The movement of the body occurs through the functioning of the nervous system to produce balance, timing, accuracy, and other neuromuscular controls. Also, the functional powers are regulated in an appropriate application to produce efficient action. Success is determined by the manner in which the forces are applied. Success in reaching one's full potential is due to the application and coordination of the mental, physical, and emotional resources of the organism. Broer has presented the basic mechanical principles underlying efficient movement. These principles, in application, will determine the physiological require-

---

[1] Marion R. Broer, *Efficiency of Human Movement* (Philadelphia: Saunders, 1960).

ments of the organism. Properly applied, the requirements will represent the minimum for physical activity or any specific movement.

For an understanding of movement, knowledge of the center of gravity of the body is needed; power and efficiency of movement are directly related to this. Balance, as it is determined by the center of gravity in relationship to the supporting base, will also influence movement. The nature of motion and the conditions related to it are also factors in human mechanics. Such conditions involve direction and speed. The lever in movement and the way the movement is applied to the lever constitute the difference between an efficient and an inefficient action. Mechanics of movement includes an understanding of objects in action, such as a ball in flight. The pattern of flight is determined by the force developed by the human organism. Other factors that are correlated with work and efficiency are load, rate, speed, training, skill, age, nutritional status, and attitudes.

The Biophysical Conceptual Structure

The Setting

The objective in conceptualizing the biophysical science of physical activity is the identification and organization of its content. With an acceptable conceptual structure, the biophysical content that should be known to use physical activity properly is then established. The objective is full knowledge and understanding, but not how the content can or should be applied professionally.

In conceptualizing the content of the biophysical science one could have several starting points. One could start with the conceptual structure of the already established physical sciences and then relate, appropriately, the conceptual structure from physiology or the biological sciences. The reverse process could be followed by relating the physical sciences to a basic structure from physiology. Both procedures seem to be inadequate for the identification of content in biophysical science. As a background, however, a brief review of these approaches will be presented.

In the science of biomechanics a conceptual structure has been reported by Alley, Cooper, and Counsilman.[2] The concepts and principles were drawn from physics (general physics), mechanical engineering (mechanics of solids, mechanics of machines), hydraulics (mechanics of fluids), aeronautics (aerodynamics), electrical engineering (electronics), photographic and cinematic techniques, and anatomy. Biomechanics is, according to these authors, a study of the organism in action from both

[2] L. Alley et al., "Biomechanics." A mimeographed report, University of Iowa.

an internal analysis of actions and the external forces that act on the body for favorable performance. This is through the discipline of biomechanics.

Margaret Fox [3] has also conceptualized the content of the *mechanical* facet of the biophysical science of physical activity. The conceptual structure is constructed on the basic mechanical principles that applied to the organism in action. The structure is composed of five categories. These are

1. Newton's laws of motion (inertia, acceleration, counterforce).
2. Force (concurrent forces—resultants absorbing force, centrifugal, equilibrium, balancing, center of gravity, buoyancy).
3. Motion (linear, rotatory, rotation, friction, air resistance, water resistance, momentum).
4. Machines (levers—balance, speed, force, pull, for example).
5. Miscellaneous (projectiles, angle of incidence, and reflection and elasticity).

This conceptualization, topical outlines and the classification of concepts by other authors, served as a starting reference for conceptualizing the body of knowledge in the biophysical science.

The question that needed resolution was, "What should constitute the structure for the body of knowledge that adequately represents the basic reference for understanding the biophysical nature of physical activity?" The question was resolved by the development of a context including all identifiable elements of human movements or those movements that are basic (starting reference) for all combinations of the physical activity possibilities for man.

The Structure

The basic categories of movements applied in all combinations of physical activity provide the framework for the conceptualization of the biophysical science (List 2). It is recognized that each of the thirteen categories can be further delineated into smaller units or concepts. However, no additional category would appear to result from such analysis, and further delineation would serve no additional purpose in understanding the conceptual structure of this science. For understanding in depth, it is, of course, necessary to deal with minute details of each category. This is not the purpose of this chapter or text; we want to understand the nature of physical activity from an overall viewpoint.

List 2. Conceptual structure: The biophysical science of physical activity

1. Muscular power. (*Definition:* ability to release maximum muscle force in the shortest period of time. *Example:* standing long jump.) Applica-

[3] Margaret G. Fox, "The Body of Knowledge in Physical Education—Mechanical." A mimeographed report, Academy of Physical Education.

tion of physical principles: The physical principles here revolve around the two mechanical principles of time and force.[4]

a. Influencing factors:
    (1) Direction of the force: The most efficient pull is one that is 90° to the force.
    (2) Point of application: In opening a door one pushes on the end for minimum energy expenditure and hence maximum force.
    (3) Distance over which the force is applied: The shorter the distance, the greater the power, given constant force.

b. Newton's laws of motion: [5]
    (1) First law: Taking another stroke in swimming before all momentum is lost.
    (2) Second law: Revolving in a hammer throw to increase momentum.
    (3) Third law: When a runner pushes against the ground, he achieves the same forward force as that which he applied backward.

2. Muscular strength. (*Definition:* maximum strength applied in a single muscular contraction. *Example:* grip strength applied to a manuometer.) Application of physical principles:

a. Magnitude of force:
    (1) The greater an object's mass, or any resistive forces, such as friction and the surrounding media of air and water, the greater the inertia and the more force necessary to move it. (It is harder to move in water than on land.)
    (2) The greater the mass of an object imparting the force and the faster it is moving, the greater the force imparted, all other things being equal. (A soccer ball has greater force than a tennis ball.)

3. Static strength. (*Definition:* ability to sustain maximum force over a fixed resistance. *Example:* holding a weight-lifting position for a required time.) Application of physical principles:

a. Principles of force: sustaining force in a tug of war.
b. Point of application: holding mass with balance maintains a more optimal force.
c. Friction: using cleated shoes in field sports.
d. Principles of equilibrium: [6] the tripod position in a headstand.

---

[4] *Principles of force:*

$$\text{Force} = \text{mass} \times \text{acceleration}$$

$$\text{Acceleration} = \frac{\text{Force}}{\text{mass}}$$

$$\text{Velocity} = \frac{\text{distance}}{\text{time}}$$

$$\text{Power} = \text{Force} \times \text{velocity}$$

[5] *Newton's laws of motion:* (a) Law of inertia: an object continues at rest or in motion at the same speed unless acted upon by a force. (b) Law of acceleration: when a body is acted upon by a force, its resulting acceleration (change in speed) is proportional to the force and inversely proportional to the mass. (c) Law of counterforce: to every action force there is an equal and opposite reaction force.

[6] *Principles of equilibrium:* (a) a body is balanced when its center of gravity is over its supporting base; (b) the nearer to the center of the base the line of gravity falls, the more stable the body; (c) the larger the base, the more stable the body;

4. Dynamic strength. (*Definition:* ability to exert an explosive force against a resistance. *Example:* handball.) Application of physical principles:
   a. Newton's first law of motion: It is more difficult to move a heavy object than a light one.
   b. Newton's second law of motion: A runner's speed is in part determined by the magnitude of the force he exerts against the ground.
5. Muscular endurance. (*Definition:* ability to continue muscular exertions of maximal or submaximal magnitude. *Example:* chinning.) Application of physical principles:
   a. Principles of leverage: [7] in chinning, swinging indicates fatigue.
   b. Principles of equilibrium:
      (1) Avoid swaying in running.
      (2) Tripod position maximizes endurance in headstand position.
      (3) Blocking in football.
   c. Laws of force: Keep the horizontal component as long as possible when pulling an object.
6. General endurance. (*Definition:* moderate contractions of muscle groups for relatively long periods of time, which require an adjustment of the circulatory-respiratory systems to the activity. *Example:* long-distance running or distance swimming.) Application of physical principles:
   a. Laws of gravity and buoyancy: [8] keeping the legs up to avoid "drag" in swimming.

(d) the base should be enlarged in the direction of the moving or opposing force; (e) the lower the center of gravity, the more stable the body; (f) forward (or backward) rotating motion increases stability.

[7] *Principles of leverage:* a lever is used to gain mechanical advantage so that a small force exerted over a great distance is converted into a larger force operating over a lesser distance or speed is gained. (R = resistance; F = force.)

First-class lever:

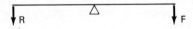

Force arm longer: favors force
Resistance arm longer: favors speed

Second-class lever:

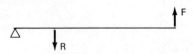

Third-class lever:

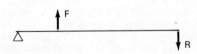

[8] *Gravity and Buoyancy:* (a) Law of falling bodies: in the absence of air friction, all bodies, regardless of size and weight, will fall with the same acceleration. (b) Archimedes' Principles: a body wholly or partially submerged in a fluid is buoyed up by a force equal to the weight of the displaced field.

b. Principles of equilibrium: riding a bicycle.

c. Laws of motion: taking another stroke in swimming before all momentum is lost.

7. Agility. (*Definition:* speed in changing body position or in changing direction. *Example:* dodging run.) Application of physical principles:

   a. Laws of gravity and buoyance: keeping the center of gravity low when turning.

   b. Principles of leverage: keeping the body "neat" when turning.

   c. Air resistance: "streamlining" when diving.

   d. Principles of equilibrium: wide stance when landing.

   e. Newton's third law: when diving, movement of one part of the body causes a similar compensatory movement in the opposite part.

   f. Principles of projectiles: [9]

      (1) After takeoff the path of the center of gravity cannot be changed.

      (2) In jumping, one lands at approximately the same angle as one takes off.

      (3) Long jump flight is determined by the angle of lift and the magnitude of force applied at takeoff.

8. Speed. (*Definition:* rapidity with which successive movements of the same kind can be performed. *Example:* 50-yard dash.) Application of physical principles:

   a. Principles of gravity and buoyance: avoid swaying in sprinting.

   b. Principles of equilibrium: use of arms in sprinting.

   c. Newton's first law to overcome inertia.

   d. Laws of force: "leaning over" to kick a soccer ball.

   e. Principles of leverage: streamlining to maximize speed.

9. Flexibility. (*Definition:* range of movement in a joint or sequence of joints. *Example:* touching floor with fingers without bending the knees.) Application of physical principles:

   a. Laws of equilibrium: wide base when performing many flexibility exercises.

   b. Principles of leverage: most human levers are third class.

10. Precision of movement. (*Definition:* the ability to control voluntary movements toward an object. *Example:* diving.) Application of physical principles:

    a. In precision movements the basic mechanical principles mentioned above are used extensively. In addition, the principles of angle of rebound and spin are utilized: facing a racquet in stroking a tennis ball.

11. Coordination. (*Definition:* ability to integrate movements of different kinds into a single pattern. *Example:* a tennis smash.) Application of physical principles:

    a. Principles of gravity and buoyancy: law of falling bodies.

    b. Principles of refraction: spear fishing or diving for a weight.

    c. Principles of angle of rebound and spin:

       (1) A soft basketball does not rebound in the same way as a fully inflated one.

---

[9] *Principles of Projectiles:* (a) The path of the center for gravity is determined at takeoff. (b) An object approaches the ground at approximately the same angle as that at which it was projected. (c) The path of the center of gravity of an object through the air is determined by the magnitude of the projecting force and the angle of its projection.

(2) Spin has more effect in curving a tennis ball than it does in curving a baseball.

    d. Principles of projectiles: the time it takes an object to fall is equal to the time it takes to reach its highest point.

12. Balance. (*Definition:* the ability to control the organic equipment neuromuscularly. *Example:* gymnastic beam exercises.)
    a. Principles of equilibrium.
    b. Principles of leverage (first class): effect of light and heavy persons on teeters.
    c. Laws of force: centrifugal and centripetal force, solid stance to maintain balance when throwing.
    d. Principles of light and sound: looking straight when balancing.

13. Rhythm. (*Definition:* ability to execute a movement with smooth and relaxed motion. *Example:* hurdling.) Application of physical principles:
    a. Principles of equilibrium: a good, balanced position is essential for rhythmic movements.
    b. Principles of leverage: joint movements.
    c. Principles of motion (Newton's third law): If one side of the body moves forward, the other side compensates by moving backward.

The Biophysical Science of Physical Activity

The biophysical science is an integration of two basic disciplines [physical science (mechanics) and biological science (physiology)] in order to gain an understanding of physical activity. It is most difficult and quite undesirable to deal separately with these two basic disciplines in physical activity, for they are so closely related that one can hardly deal with the physiology of human movement without relating the action to the mechanical principles applied in it.

The biophysical science conceptual structure (List 2) is organized on the basis of the fundamental movements of the human body that underlie all combinations of movements in physical activity. This structure is described as a biophysical science in relating the mechanic principles and laws applying to each facet of the movement structure and then relating the biological resources or requirements essential for the movement itself. The requirements of human movement are integrated on the assumption that the two are necessary for movement and each will determine the physiological resources needed to perform. Success in applying mechanical principles will be directly related to efficiency in using organic resources. One must be considered in relation to the other.

An attempt is made to relate body physiology directly to each of the thirteen fundamental factors underlying physical activity. Such an analysis is desirable to judge what the movement can accomplish in human development and what the requirements for the movement itself are. It also correlates the mechanical principles necessary for the movement and the physiological relationship with each mechanical principle or combination of principles. The analysis is difficult, for in no instance does physical activity utilize a single mechanical principle or a single organ, system, or function. All mechanical principles are related to nearly all activities to some degree. This is also true for physiological requirements. In the review and summary of what research has accomplished in the biophysical science, we will view the biophysical science as a whole.

Prerequisites. Human movement requires physical resources or energy. Human movement also requires mental insight and the ability of the movement pattern to direct the physical resources for appropriate action. In addition, movement is closely associated with emotional factors that will disturb or stabilize movement toward the most desirable pattern. These requirements taken as a whole represent the biophysical science of physical activity.

In considering the scientific bases for human movement and in reviewing the supporting literature, we begin by analyzing the prerequisites and then by considering mechanical laws and principles that give efficiency or grace to the movement. This is a more effective way to present the literature. The presentation should add to the understanding of the biophysical science.

The prerequisites are classified into three major categories, namely, the physical requirements for human movement, the mental requirements or insights into movement patterns, and the emotional factors that either aid or disturb the pattern in action. Each category will be briefly reviewed.

The *physical factors* are organized into five divisions for the purposes of analysis:

1. The muscular system (strength, endurance, power, static and dynamic).
2. The general endurance of the organism (essentially circulatory, respiratory, or cardiovascular).
3. The directional abilities of the organism (agility, speed, and flexibility).
4. The neuromuscular control of the organism (precision, coordination, and balance).
5. The response of the organism to exterior stimuli (rhythm).

The *muscular system* is required for all movements, large or small. It is the contraction of the muscle that causes the movement. The range is from power and endurance to movements of control (for example, precision). The muscle will increase in size as a result of exercise. The gain in muscle size is accomplished by a loss in adipose tissue. Because muscle tissue weighs more than adipose tissue, there will be an increase in body weight. When the muscle gains in size, there is also a gain in strength, and strength increments are usually proportionately greater than increases in muscle girth. Increase in muscle size is the result of the thickening of the sarcolemma, increase in the connective tissue, and increased density of the muscle. Strength gains resulting from physical activity are the result of a greater number of fibers in action and muscular endurance is the result of increased periods for muscle contractions resulting from more readily available fuel; fuel and oxygen are in more abundance because of improved circulation and respiration. Muscular strength, power, and endurance are also improved, because of more available hemoglobin, increased activity of the capillaries, and improvement of the transmission of nerve impulses. Placing a heavy load (overload) on the muscle will improve power and the volume of the muscle.

The second classification of the physical factors is *general endurance*, dealing essentially with the respiratory, circulatory, and cardiovascular systems. Physical activity will cause a slight increase in the heart size (thickening of the heart muscle) and will increase the minute and stroke volume of the heart and circulation, increasing fuel resources for longer physical activity. In a physically trained individual the heart rate is decreased as much as ten to twenty beats per minute, with an increase in fuel supply, and the heart rate will return to normal more rapidly. The decrease is the result of physical activity with a more powerful heart and a larger stroke volume. Blood pressure will also be lowered as the result of consistent physical activity. The result of these improvements is larger oxygen supply to the muscle and a more efficient return and release of waste products. Respiration is improved because of increased volume of the chest and lungs; the rate of breathing is slower and fuller and more economical. The oxygen supply to the muscle and the utilization of the oxygen by the muscle are improved with appropriate physical activity and one is able to withstand a larger oxygen debt. The slower heart rate provides a longer time for the heart to reach its maximum, with the return to the resting pulse more rapid providing for longer periods of physical activity due to circulatory improvements.

The third classification of physical factors as prerequisites to physical activity and human mechanics is the change of *direction abilities of the human organism* (agility, speed, and flexibility). These are the abilities in successive · ·vements of the body or the abilities to change the movements in various directions and in space. These abilities are in part the result of circulatory, respiratory, and muscular resources, but they are due essentially to the nervous system and one's neuromuscular abilities or resources. Speed activities require muscular power in addition to neuromuscular responses. Agility and flexibility activities will require muscular endurance if continued for long periods of time, but they are essentially neuromuscular and structural in nature. The neuromuscular response is the result of improvement in movement or ability of reaction time in response to stimuli. Physical activity of this type (agility, for example) will improve nerve connections for more effective coordination. Kinesthetic sense is related to directional abilities.

Continued practice in physical activity will result in a reduction in the concentration on a task from the higher centers of the nervous system. In addition, physical activity will reduce the adrenergic responses that result, in cumulative effects, in higher blood pressures, higher pulse rates, increased blood fats and blood sugar, and other conditions predisposing one to coronary heart disease. Normal sympathetic–parasympathetic balance is maintained through physical activity, thus releasing tension and emotional stress that are unfavorable to cardiac functions. Adrenergic response and activity are desired in most activities. Adrenergic action is a preparation to meet danger; it can also be precipitated by the need for higher levels of performance. In adrenergic action the mind becomes more acute, vision and hearing keener, reflexes sharper, muscles tensed and ready, blood pressure increased, heart rate faster, heart contractions more forceful, and flow of blood to the muscles of action greatly increased. These changes are the requirements for action. Following action, however, the body should return to normal.

The fourth classification of the prerequisite physical factors is the *neuromuscular control of the organism in action* (precision, coordination, and balance). The ability to control physical movements stems from the nervous system and the muscular system in coordination and in response to stimuli. The control of human movements is nearly entirely a matter of nerve and muscle and regulation in the intensity and direction of stimuli. The success of human control is a result of the contraction of the action muscles and relaxation of the antagonist muscles in coordination or in response to proper stimuli.

The fifth section of the physical factors or prerequisites for physical activity is the *response of the organism to exterior stimuli* (rhythm). This ability involves the sensorimotor system in coordination. It is the coordination of external stimuli to the internal mechanisms of the central nervous system and the muscular system in timing, response, and coordination. The higher brain centers of the organism are very much a part of ability in activities of rhythm, which involves the rate of identification and understanding of the external stimuli and the ability to transmit the nature of the stimuli to action patterns of physical activity through muscular contractions and relaxations.

The prerequisites for human physical activity involve more than physical factors. Mental and emotional factors are very much a part of any physical action. Any response of stimuli requires an interrelationship between the nervous system and the muscular system. Muscle contraction and work result from stimuli from the nervous system. In addition to mental involvement in activity patterns, emotional factors will influence mechanical patterns.

Insights and abilities in human movement—the *mental factors*—require an understanding of the movement pattern. One must visualize the pattern part by part before putting it into action. The movements of the individual reproduce the visualized pattern. The action of the organism includes also the ability to make adaptive decisions; to understand spatial relationships; to judge movement in distance, speed, height, and direc-

tion; to determine rhythmic sequences and movements, along with kinesthetic insights and abilities of all factors that support the successful
accomplishment of the physical movement.

Mental abilities and capacities develop, in general, along with and at
about the same rate as the skeletal and muscular systems. The harmonies
that promote the development of the bones and muscles also influence
the development of the psychomotor and psychosensory centers. Many
abilities are involved: one must be able to judge space, have good timing,
make decisions, visualize mechanical patterns, and transmit past experience into action that eliminates conditions that interfered with prior
action. Mental ability is the ability to transform sensory perceptive impulses into abstract movements. The mental concept or picture of what
is going to happen in a movement must accompany or direct muscle
reaction. Intellectual ability is a major factor or prerequisite to success
in physical activity. One must also have ability in the physical prerequisites and, of course, the mechanical skills needed to execute the movement patterns with effectiveness and efficiency. With keen insights,
however, optimal mechanical abilities will be achieved by the individual.

The *emotional factors* or conditions underlying human performance
are both positive and negative. One's emotional status can greatly influence learning and level of performance. Disturbing conditions may
result in failure to perform a skill that should be well within grasp. The
desire to succeed is a most positive factor in performance. Stress under
motivation can have very positive effects. One is the ability to introduce
all needed resources under such conditions. Stress, however, under conditions of emotional disturbance, may reduce performance and cause
failure. External factors play a role in human performance and differ in
their influence. Altitude, temperature, wind, terrain, spectators, and dress
are physical conditions that influence human performance. It is necessary
not only to understand the character of the pattern but also to understand what to emphasize in order to make the most appropriate decision
in preparation. Adaptations are often necessary.

The biophysical science of physical activity deals with human movement. The components of movement are the prerequisite factors and are
physical, mental, and emotional in nature. The requirement must be equal
to the needs of the mechanical patterns of the skill itself if successful
movement is to result. These considerations represent the content of the
biophysical science of physical activity.

Mechanical Principles or Laws. After achieving an understanding of
the prerequisites of human movement, it is necessary to have an understanding of how the physical, mental, and emotional resources can be
applied to movement for effectiveness (motor success) and for efficiency
(energy conservation). Both requirements are needed in physical activity.
They vary with each activity.

The most fundamental laws and principles of mechanics, as needed for an understanding of physical performance, are presented in List 2 and footnotes 4–9. These principles are also applied in List 2 for a mechanical understanding of the thirteen basic movements of physical activity that underlie all physical activity. These are the references for the discussion that follows.

Force. Force is energy harnessed to generate movement. The action of forces is both internal and external. Internal force is generated by the innervation of the muscle by nerve stimuli to contract the muscle into action. The strength of the impulse and the muscle groups will determine the force exerted on an object. External force requires also internal generation of energy; in addition, it involves the mechanics in the movement of the object. Properly applied, movement will have its optimal result.

Many conditions determine the nature of a force. These are illustrated, in relationship, in the formulas (footnote 4).

For efficient physical movement it is necessary to understand the nature of the developing force, the conditions under which it is applied, and the factors that cause favorable and unfavorable actions on movement after the force has been applied. These are both internal (within the organism) and external (environment).

Motion. Motion is the movement of the body. It involves both direction and speed. When force acts, the resulting speed will be proportional to its magnitude and inversely proportional to the mass involved. The heavier the load, the more force is needed to attain a given speed. Reference should be made to List 2 and footnote 5 for definitions and illustrations of the Newton's laws of motion.

The principle that for every action there is an equal and opposite reaction is applied in many activities. In sand, the force exerted by the runner is dissipated, moving the sand backward. The reaction force is unchanged, but it is now being divided into at least two components, one acting on the runner to propel him forward and one on the sand to shift it backward.

Several factors influence the magnitude and direction of movement, of which friction, air resistance, water resistance, and gravity are major forces. These conditions vary with each physical activity. For efficient physical activity, the forces that interfere with optimal movement must be minimized when they act in opposition to action. They can be exploited when in favor of the action.

Motion itself is a change in position of an object that can be horizontal, vertical, or circular and that requires a force to produce it. Linear motion is movement of an object with points in a straight line. Rotary movement is around the center of an object in an arc about the center.

The movement of force is the place at which the force is applied to the body to produce movement. The closer to the center of gravity the force is applied, the greater will be the motion or linear movement. The law governing freely falling bodies affects all in the same way regardless of size or weight or shape, providing air resistance is discounted.

Equilibrium. Equilibrium of the human organism is the basis for human balance. A body is balanced when the center of gravity is over the supporting base. The larger the base and the nearer the body to the center of the base, the more stable the body. Both these requirements depend upon the same principle that the further the center of gravity has to travel to pass outside its supporting base, the less likelihood there will be that it will get into a position of instability. In physical activity, therefore, the base must be large enough to allow movement without loss of balance.

Whenever the effective base is widened for stability purposes, consideration must be given to such factors as the direction of movement of the object or body, the direction of the propulsive braking or supportive forces exerted by the individual, the movements of the body relative to its center of gravity, the weight carried, and the height of the center of gravity. If external forces are not absorbed by the body within the confines of its base, the body will lose its balance. The body is realigned constantly in order to maintain the center of gravity close to the center of the base and thereby maintain stability. This realignment of the body is carried out at a level below consciousness, although higher control can be exercised. Thus balance is maintained only as the result of a complex interaction between the muscle and joint sense organs, specific organs of balance in the inner ear (the semicircular canals), visual cues, and a complex system of reflective proprioceptive and kinesthetic pathways.

Leverage. Leverage is a major factor in walking, running, lifting, pushing, and other activities that involve power and force. The crowbar, for example, is applied to lift a heavy object by using a long arm from the fulcrum.

The human body has levers (bones), fulcrums (joints), and forces (contracting muscles). Any action or movement, of course, is influenced by both internal resistance (body weight) and external resistance (air and other environmental conditions).

With few exceptions the levers of the body are of the third class. They have a shorter force than resistance arm because the muscles insert close to the joint and the weight is concentrated further from the joint. The human lever system is constructed to favor velocity over force; however, physical laws that control human movement favor force over velocity. Strength and reaction time, therefore, are the most important factors in physical activity.

Gravity and Buoyancy. Gravitational forces act on all bodies (except in space). This force must always be taken into account, because it can have a profound influence upon movement. It acts on every particle of the human body, but is considered for all practical purposes to act on the weight centers of each body segment or of the body as a whole. The body balances or rotates around this center of gravity.

The body in motion meets with air resistance. The resistance varies with body size and shape and with the speed of movement. The larger the cross section in the line of travel, the greater will be the influence of air resistance. In the absence of air friction, all bodies, regardless of size and weight, fall with the same acceleration.

An important consideration in aquatic activities is the buoyancy of the body. In water the body is buoyed by a force equal to the weight of the water displaced. If the water an individual displaces weighs more than he does, he will float; if not, he will sink. The density of the human body is thus the only consideration in whether the individual floats. All human tissue, except fat, sinks. Even lung tissue sinks if the air is removed. Consequently, buoyancy in man depends upon tissue factors, namely, fat and air. The density of the body is especially important in all swimming activities but also in other physical activities of power, strength, and endurance. In these events the individual with low density is favored but the density of muscular tissue is a needed factor for power and strength.

Projectiles. Projectiles are objects given an initial velocity great enough for them to escape from any restraining or supporting force. Once in flight the forces that act upon a projectile are the gravity, air resistance, force that caused its motion, and any other internal forces that it may generate itself. The distance that a projectile (a shot put, for example) travels is determined by the initial speed and the angle at which it is projected. Distance and speed are factors in projecting an object. The greater the speed of an object and the lower the angle at which it is thrown, the greater the distance it will travel. The weight and surface area of an object are factors in determining the amount of air resistance. In addition, an object will approach the ground at approximately the same angle as that at which it was projected. The path of the center of gravity is determined by the projecting force and the angle of projection. The greatest distance is obtained when an object is propelled at a 45° angle, because of the equalization of the horizontal and vertical forces. If speed is a major factor, the angle of projection should be small in order to gain optimal distance.

Spinning and *rebounding* follow mechanical laws. A ball will rebound at an angle equal to that at which it strikes a hard surface. Barring other factors, such as spin, a ball with a backspin stays in the air longer, has a shorter roll, and has a bounce that is higher and shorter than normal. The opposite is true in a forward spin of a ball.

An Overview

The human body works as a machine and is therefore subjected to all the laws and principles of physics and mechanics that must be applied to gain efficiency in work operations. The discipline necessary for understanding the physical nature of the body, as a machine, is the biophysical science of physical activity. It has a body of knowledge of its own that has resulted from direct research on work done by the human body and it has drawn principles and laws from the basic science of biology (particularly physiology) and from the physical sciences (physics, mechanics, and chemistry).

The skill and efficiency of the human organism at work is a combination of the movement pattern and the physical resources available for the pattern to be placed into action. There are, of course, other factors (knowledge and understanding, for example), but for a review of the biophysical sciences, these factors must be considered in another context. Here we are concerned with the requirements for movement, from the biological resources to how they are used.

The biophysical science is discussed in this text first on the basis of the fundamental movements that serve all combinations of movements or physical activity (List 2). This analysis follows with the application of the mechanical principles that apply to each of the *thirteen* basic movements or skills. Examples are presented in each instance. This is followed with a summary of the physiological descriptions or facts that explain the requirements for each of the *thirteen* movements. This is an attempt, of course, to relate the various components of the biophysical science.

This science is also presented by listing the prerequisites of human movement (largely physical and environmental but also emotional and intellectual) and then reviewing the movements in terms of the mechanical principles and laws that apply to physical activity. This makes the presentation more functional, as it is most difficult to review by components, because of the large amount of overlap that occurs in the requirements of the basic movements in both the mechanics and the physiology of work.

Finally, as a perspective for this discipline of human performance, it is reasonable to conclude that we cannot understand any physical action of man without these basic disciplines applied to physical activity in the formation of an applied discipline—the biophysical science of physical activity. It is applied not only to athletic and sports activity but to human movements that cause stresses on the organism that need to be understood.

Chapter 5

The Sociopsychological Foundations

Psychology is generally defined as a science of human behavior. It is concerned especially with the complex organization of behavior as expressed by the human personality and the human organism. It embraces such concepts as learning, motivation, perception, personality, development, maturation, motives, group interaction, and ability levels, along with subdivisions of these basic concepts. Sociology, a closely related science, also deals with human behavior, but with the system of social values and concepts indispensable for individual and group associations and with the social characterization of the individual and the group. Concepts descriptive of a social system are socialization, social stratification, social institutions, human ecology, social systems, human values, and social behavior. These basic concepts have subdivisions that further describe the discipline. In this chapter these two basic sciences are treated in integrated form as the sociopsychological science of physical activity.

Human physical performance is more than a biophysical phenomenon, important as that aspect is. Scientists and educators have long had an interest in the sociopsychological nature and potentials of physical activity. Research, over the years, has been largely clinical and experiential, with little solid experimental evidence. There are many reasons for this. It is difficult, and sometimes inadvisable, to set controls to study human reactions and behaviors in physical activity. Clinical observations have therefore been planned with observation schedules and protocols that provide systematic bases for observation and judgment. Thus the literature does provide a basis for the description of physical activity according to sociological and psychological concepts.

In general, physical activity and sports have reached an important place in the social and cultural mores of people throughout the world. Their value is widely recognized. It is also recognized that sports and physical activity contain potentials for human communications that go beyond language. It has been noted by international scientists and sportsmen that sports and physical activity can attract the enthusiasm, interest, and discipline of youth in world competition. These qualities are most valuable for improved human understanding among the nations of the world. And it has been noted that the sociopsychological concepts or characteristics of the individual are closely related to the biophysical concepts of human physical performance. This science has worthwhile contributions to make to understanding the human personality.

The Conceptual Structure of the Sociopsychological Science of Physical Activity

In order to reason about or apply the elements of any discipline, the concepts must be defined and organized into divisions and subdivisions that present their relationships. This is of particular importance here, because the sociopsychological science is a new application of two basic sciences to physical activity. In its most basic form sociology is the study of human social behavior and its related factors. Psychology is the study of human mental processes and behavior and their related factors. Social psychology combines sociology and psychology to study human behavior (social and mental) as it is influenced by and influences the behavior of others as individuals or in groups. The conceptual structure for the sociopsychological science of physical activity includes concepts from sociology and psychology that apply to physical activity and, in addition, applied concepts from social psychology (List 3).

List 3. Conceptual categories: The sociopsychological domain of physical activity

1. The individual as a social being.
   a. Personality, anxiety, needs, aspirations.
   b. Attitudes, values, beliefs.
   c. Roles.
   d. Self-image.
   e. Perception, cognition, skill abilities.
   f. Deviance.
2. Social institutions.
   a. Family, community.
   b. Religion, religious groups.
   c. Education, school groups.
   d. Business, industrial groups.

  e. Government, political groups, military.
  f. Recreation, health groups.
 3. Sociopsychological processes.
  a. Involvement.
  b. Competition.
  c. Cooperation.
  d. Small group dynamics.
  e. Complex organizational dynamics.
  f. Stratification and mobility.
  g. Cultures and subcultures.
 4. Sociopsychological environment.
  a. Competition, individual, team.
  b. Cooperation, individual, team.
   (1) Small informal group.
   (2) Formal organization.
   (3) Institution.
  c. Audience, small or large, passive or active.
 5. Learning and development.
  a. Attitude, values.
  b. Motivation (to start).
  c. Incentive (to start).
  d. Level of aspiration.
  e. Skill level.
  f. Attention.
  g. Perception.
  h. Cognition.
  i. Retention.
  j. Fatigue.
  k. Boredom.
  l. Motivation, persistence.
  m. Transfer.
  n. Knowledge of results (feedback).
  o. Distribution of practice.
  p. Inhibition.

It is important to realize, that although a clear rationale exists for developing a conceptual structure, this development represents a single organization and others may choose to organize this material differently. However, the important consideration is the basic concepts, not the organizational structure. The conceptual structure, however, is completely developed and can be followed with confidence. It represents an organizational or conceptual structure that clearly fits physical activity as it should be studied and applied.

The Setting. Physical activity represents a medium for the individual and the group that has potentials for human development and adjustment. It offers a dynamic setting for the individual. The process itself has commanding effects on the human personality. The desire for success and respectable performance in activity is strong. It is highly motivating. This medium, therefore, has significant potential for social and psychological development and adjustment of the individual. The particular application of the social and psychological concepts to physical activity represents a special consideration. Sociopsychology must organize suitable concepts into a structure that fits physical activity and that has validity in application. It must describe human performance as a sociopsychological phenomenon in a manner that gives meaning and value to improved performance. This is the purpose for the structure and its application to physical activity.

The Structure. The concepts of the sociopsychological science of physical activity are classified into five major divisions. Thus it is possible to present this applied science as a science of (1) the individual as a social being, (2) social institutions, (3) the sociopsychological processes in physical activity, (4) the social and psychological environments in a setting of physical activity, and (5) the learning and the development that result from participation. These divisions will be briefly described in the following section of this chapter and the evidence that gives content to this applied science will be presented.

The Individual as a Social Being. The individual is very much a social being in physical activity. His status will influence participation and participation will influence his status—good or bad. Physical activity has social requirements for participation, and participation will systematically influence the social being.

The sociopsychological concepts that apply to physical activity and relate to the individual as a social being are given in List 3. The personality of the individual, his security, attitude, health are all part of physical participation, and add to both its quality and quantity. One's role, status, reaction to changes in activity are also social characteristics and qualities. Participation of the individual as a social being is also influenced by group mores, customs, behavior, and deviant emotions. The individual reaction will determine the effects these conditions will have on personal development and adjustment. Personal motivation is a large factor in physical participation and has social influences. One's perception of patterns and strategies of participation are factors in success, satisfaction, and resulting social development.

Social Institutions. Physical activity is a part of our social institutions in many varying forms. The social institution sets the stage for the physical activity, and the physical activity influences the nature and purposes of the social institution (List 3). The family, the community, and the nation are large factors as social institutions. Physical activity is a part of those social institutions, influenced by the institution itself. How physical activity is used by the participant will determine the influence on the social institution. Religious, educational, political, recreational, military organizations are strong and large parts of all societies. They influence all activities of the individual, including sports and physical activity. The setting is very much a part of these institutions, and their particular use of physical activity will, in part, characterize the institutions. Class structure and the internal culture of the group or community are most important social institutional elements. Physical activity becomes a part of these settings.

Sociopsychological Processes. The social and psychological processes of the individual, the group, the community, the nation, and the world have a major influence on each person and group. The processes result from years of traditions, customs, and life of the people. Only recently, as the result of transportation, have these processes tended to be influenced by strong nations, cultures, and groups. Change, however, is slow in coming, and, of course, the desirability of change is dependent on the needs of the individual and the group.

Group stratification and individual mobility are important sociopsychological processes of major significance to the individual, having a large influence on his interests and ways of life, including physical activity (List 3).

To sociopsychological processes of competition, individual involvements, group structures, and organizations set the possibilities for the individual and his choices. Leadership of group activities has a strong sociopsychological influence on the individual and the group.

All the elements of the sociopsychological process are not only part of the life of the people in their daily activities, but part of the influence on physical activity. The activities chosen and the nature of participation in turn determine the social and psychological effects on each person.

Sociopsychological Environments. Sociopsychological environments have particular and significant applications to sports, athletics, and physical activity in all forms, directly and indirectly influencing the quality and quantity of physical activity performances. Association in physical activity with other individuals and within a group (as a team) has strong effects on the individual. His personal associations will affect the performance of the individual. Other elements of the social environment (social institutions, mores, traditions, customs, subcultures) have marked influence on the individual in all his activities, including physical activity. The nature of the activity itself (soccer in Europe, football in the United States) results from the mores, cultures, and certainly the interests and attitudes of the individual.

In addition to the social environment, the physical setting is closely associated with physical activity and interests. Winter sports in the cold climates, boating in lake and ocean regions, mountain climbing and hiking in hilly terrains are some examples. It should be the objective of each person to apply the physical setting to personal physical activity for personal well-being. Understanding the physical world is a most desirable objective, and using natural facilities for human development will add significantly to this objective.

The sociopsychological environments are a major facet of the sociopsychological science of physical activity. Physical activity has both a social and a physical environmental setting, and an understanding of the environments is essential for optimal participation.

Learning and Development. One of the major components of the sociopsychological science of physical activity is learning and development. Requirements and participation patterns should be understood before participation is begun. Knowledge of the developmental worth of each activity is also useful.

Learning and human development in and through physical activity have many elements (List 3). These elements include aspects of the physical organism (health, fatigue, maturation, skills, aptitudes) that set the limits and determine the rate of learning and development from participation. They include also the emotions and the intellect (security, confidence, inhibitions, motivation, boredom, and so on). The sociopsychological abilities and traits will set the stage for the quality and quantity of learning and development. Individuals will differ in aptitudes.

Physical activity requires many social and psychological abilities in participation, regardless of the level of play. Depth of involvement in the activity is an important personal quality, having significant influences on participation. The desire for competition is another relevant quality. Perceptual ability in the strategies of play and in play itself will determine, to a large degree, the quality of participation. Mental traits and abilities, such as retention, mental practice, and imagery are closely related to play and participation. Motivation, of course, is fundamental if the resources of the organism are to be put into participation.

Thus this is the conceptual structure of the sociopsychological science of physical activity. The basic elements of this science that apply to physical activity are classified into five divisions with elements delineating each division (List 3). This science adds to the biophysical science of physical activity in preparing for physical participation and in understanding the factors related to participation.

Foundations for the Sociopsychological Science of Physical Activity

As discussed earlier, the elements of the sociopsychological science are classified into five major divisions derived from sociology and psychology. Although there is inadequate scientific evidence from strictly controlled experiments, clinical and experiential references and data lend support to the elements presented in the conceptual structure of this new applied science. Furthermore its rationale involves the transfer of findings made in different settings to a sports or physical activity setting. The medium is different and therefore so will be the associations of individuals. These effects will be extensions or depressions of results, certainly not a new sociology or a new psychology. The medium differs because physical activity has a different set of requirements than the daily activities of the individual. The nature of these differences will be presented as each appears in physical activity, and we shall discuss their influence.

The Individual as a Social Being. Physical activity has the potential for causing individual social changes and adjustments in the social character and behavior of the individual. The organization, structure, and activity classification (team, dual, and so on) will determine, to a large degree, the changes that occur. A summary of possible effects will be presented.

1. *Physical activity has socializing effects.* These effects do not occur automatically: participation, regulation, and direct leadership are required. Physical activity can have negative results. It has been demonstrated that consistent participation in sports and physical activity leads to better-adjusted individuals, with more outgoing personalities, who are more socially skilled and better liked than their nonparticipating peers. Probably this is due in athletics to the greater social visibility of athletes; however, sports require positive social relationships for success.

2. *Physical activity favors social mobility.* Individuals with superior skills and physical abilities in sports and physical activity exceed their peers in social mobility. Physical activity brings individuals from various socioeconomic levels together into a new social class established as the result of sports participation. There are many examples of poor youth who have advanced to the highest levels of leadership in social and political groups.

Physical activity often involves an integrated social group in which there is a great deal of interaction. People are bound together by a common goal (to win) and a deep feeling about the sport. The result is a close association and integration of individuals that may result in lasting social changes.

3. *Physical activity has a positive influence on social behavior, adjustment, and development.* Physical activity and sports and athletics in particular have demanding requirements for participation. The individual must meet these requirements if he wishes to be successful or, in fact, able to continue with play. The result is a modification of behavior toward the team requirements, with a resulting improved adjustment to the group or team.

Behavior is a dynamic process by which the organism meets its needs. Physical activity provides the setting for release of tensions, but also requires a favorable attitude toward the team, individual players, and others associated with the success of the team. This may result in a lasting change in behavior, for this new adjustment to the group and group requirements will apply to similar situations. Some evidence indicates that sports participation does lead to a closer and more favorable attitude about others in group settings. For example, the mixture of racial groups in sports reduces prejudices, certainly within the team. Racial integration in a society is more likely to occur if racial integration is successfully accomplished in all school and community sports and physical activity play.

4. *Social roles, traditions, and mores are closely associated with sports and physical activity. Social change is a two-way channel.* The individual is influenced by his home, family, and friends during the early years of growth and development. If the home and the community are socially homogeneous, little change will result in the individual's social qualities. If great variance exists, then barriers must be broken for social integration. The school makes a large contribution—but schools too are constituted by social classes. It is only when activities have deep interest and high social status that integration of social groups can occur. Athletics is one of these activities. The dynamics of participation make this medium a most desirable one for social change.

Roles, traditions, and customs are subject to change. A strong coach can bring into the sport what is most desirable in the team members. The individual on a team can serve many roles—first player in a position, captain, aide to the coaches. Social changes do occur in this setting. A well-organized athletic team has significant potential for bringing about desired social changes within the individual and the group.

5. *Physical activity has a positive effect on deviance, antisocial behavior, and maladjustment.* Personal frustrations and insecurities are recognized in play. Aggressive, destructive, and unsocial attitudes and behaviors are demonstrated in play. Physical activities provide an opportunity to release strong impulses and feelings in substitute responses that can result in the modification of behavior through reduction of personal frustrations. Success in physical activity and physical satisfactions also aids in making a normal social adjustment. Involvement in sports and physical activity alleviates conflict-induced drives and provides experiences that enable participants to meet the demands of a complex social system.

Antisocial and delinquent behavior is a result, in many instances, of a lack of interest, bad home life and experiences, inability to meet school requirements, poor socioeconomic conditions, and few positive experiences in life to give hope. Sports, athletics, and physical activity have high social status in most communities. Certainly, school, college, and professional sports command the interest of many people. The individual does have a chance in this setting. It is possible to gain satisfactions, personal respect, and dignity by successful participation. This is enough to channel interests and personal desires into acceptable social channels, causing changes in many young boys and girls who otherwise might have taken to antisocial and delinquent behavior.

6. *Physical activity contributes to security.* Physical activity represents a unique and commanding social structure. It contains all the elements to gain confidence and become a satisfying member of the group. It provides the potentials for social security. Success in play, leadership roles, acceptance by others, personal satisfaction in accomplishment are social and psychological experiences essential for social learning. If sports is under democratic leadership, then sportsmanship becomes the setting for participation, producing favorable attitudes and personal satisfaction. It appears that the security one gains in social groups in the school (including sports) does provide a base for one's associations in the home, community, and, as one matures, in larger social and economic situations.

7. *Social mores and customs are closely associated with sports and physical activity and influence participation.* Physical activity cannot be divorced from the society it serves. The contribution made by physical activity is bisocial; the resulting experiences and development affect the participant as a member of social groups and society as a whole. The valuable socialization that occurs can be generalized to other activities, and the teacher and coach can be strong socialization agents.

It has been stated by school administrators, particularly in the high schools, that the physical activities programs reduce the number of dropouts considerably. The attraction of these programs is strong. The coach and physical education teacher have the opportunity to help avoid delinquent behavior, and it is important that they be properly prepared for this valuable role.

Attempting to change traditions, customs, and mores becomes an object only if they are unsocial and unacceptable for normal life and development. Difference is an acceptable part of all cultures; it should be nurtured and advanced in quality. Sports and physical activity can contribute to this objective.

8. *Physical activity can contribute to social maturity and to the individual personality.* Social standards in physical activity, and in other social groups, can contribute to the social adjustment of the individual through accomplishments in sports and athletics. Human personality is a group concept as it is a part of the culture or mores of the group, is molded by the social order, and is continuously influenced by social relationships. The setting and leadership of the team are therefore major concerns for individual social development and maturation.

Because social development and maturation occur through social relationships, one cannot learn the ways of the groups or society away from people or the group. Social development and the shaping of the personality occur through social interaction, along with the process of physical maturation. Maturation and social development go hand in hand. Physical activity and sports can contribute to both in an integrated way and will add quality to the human personality. This can be accomplished by design. The process, however, must be carefully planned and executed. In fact, a badly planned program can produce negative results.

Social Institutions. The second major division of the sociopsychological concepts of physical activity is social institutions. These are the organized forms within a society that provide for the needs (usually the most basic ones) of all individuals and groups. It is the social order within a society essential for management and social control and responsible for advancement of the individual.

1. *The family is a basic unit of society and must contain all needed elements for proper social development and adjustment.* The family is the most powerful unit in the development and adjustment of all members of the family. It is therefore essential that life in the family become a miniature society—with all the ingredients of government and life activities. This most certainly includes physical recreation, play, and sports. It is in the home that the child learns to play, learns the patterns followed in play, learns the ideals of sportsmanship and the first skills that must be learned in play. The attitudes and standards of the mother and father are so strongly impressed on the child, that they are most difficult for the school to change. The home unit cannot be underemphasized in social development, and it must have strong support from society.

In addition to activities in the home, the family should participate as a unit in out-of-home activities. Recreation and family fun and enjoyment are essential ingredients for the development of all members of the family. Physical activity in the form of recreation and sports provides an informal setting that contains all the elements for the social and psychological development of the child. High standards should be practiced in all activities in the home; democratic participation is one important social practice.

2. *The school, the church, the social agencies are social institutions closely related to the individual and society.* In addition to the family, the school, the church, social agencies, and peer groups have a strong influence on the individual and on the group. The school and the church are particularly influential, with the school having longer and more intense contacts. Each of the social institutions influences social and psychological qualities in the direction of its own patterns and sets of values.

In school the child has many experiences and roles. The student becomes a member of class groups, sports teams, social clubs, and other groups, all having their influence. The athletic teams, in particular, have requirements that include not only intense physical participation and discipline, but also rules and regulations on behavior and attitudes as they influence the morale of the team.

The social agencies supplement the family during the early years and become a large part of social life in later years. Programs, leadership, attitudes, and climate determine results, ranging from unacceptable human behavior to outcomes that give strength and security to the individual and, in turn, to the community as a whole. Great care is needed in support and direction of social agencies by community leaders and local governments.

Sociopsychological Processes. The community mores, culture, customs, and traditions are determining conditions for the social and psychological climate of social activities, including sports and physical activity. The mores of a society are strong forces in human development and adjustment. The culture of a society represents the basic beliefs and values of the people that come from deep roots in the community, group, or home. The individual lives in this setting from birth on until he moves into another cultural group, and forces in the new setting influence him. It appears that moving into a desirable cultural setting is about the only way that the individual can make cultural changes.

His mores and cultural background go with the individual into all his life activities, including sports and physical activity. For example, a democratic climate produces democratic values, and a sportsmanlike climate produces attitudes of sportsmanship. The social and psychological values or qualities desired for the individual and for society must be kept in mind. It is not success at any cost, but success in the acceptable social and psychological settings that should be taught. Certainly this applies most intensely to sports and athletics.

The social and psychological processes contain a number of major developmental concepts. Involvement in a group, as in sports, is valuable for individual development. Under acceptable leadership, the involvement has greater significance. How one competes is most important in sports. Sports is competition, and competition, properly learned, is a quality that applies in all life activities. One must understand the nature of competition, because life and survival are processes of competition. This concept must be properly taught, and sports is probably the best setting.

The direct learning of social skills in the process of play, sports, or competition is a parental and later school leadership responsibility. The social and psychological skills, relationships, and understandings are as tangible as the physical skills of play. And they are as important in play as in citizenship.

As part of social and psychological development the individual also learns such qualities as cooperation. This is a specific process and is essential in any human relationship if it is to endure and, of more importance, if the individual is to survive on a level of satisfaction and well-being. One can learn the process of cultural thinking and analysis. Another such quality is responsibility. It is of major significance in the development of all persons. One must be disciplined to accept and to understand responsibility, not only for oneself but for others. A good citizen goes beyond self. The culture should provide the setting for living as it should be.

Sociopsychological Environment. The sociopsychological environment consists of strong forces in development and adjustment. The human being is not separate from his environments—social or physical. He is not only an element in these environments, but he also is influenced by and influences them.

1. *The individual will react to and be influenced by his social environment.* Group attitudes, behaviors, and aspirations all function in a social setting. These social elements are found in the athletic team; they exert strong influences—in most instances, more powerful than those of any one individual.

In sports, the audience or the spectators are a large part of or, in fact, represent the immediate social environment of the individual. An audience favorable to a team or a particular individual will have significant effects on play. In sports, playing in the home surroundings involves not only the physical setting, but also the people who give strong support. Their support reduces the inhibitions of the player, supports his desires and advances his initiative in play, and has significant effects on emotional arousal and drive for success.

2. *The social institutions in a culture have direct influences on social and psychological development.* The agencies in a community are planned for the people of the community. Their objectives are service and their services are for the improvement of life in a community, beginning with the individual in most instances. References have been made to the home and the school. These are the two most powerful social institutions that will influence the individual during the early years of his life. What occurs in these two social institutions will determine to a major degree the social and psychological qualities and values held by the child.

There are other social institutions in the community that have strong influences—the church, the social groups, the clubs that are of importance during the adolescent and adult years. These institutions do have effects on change, but the group generally brings the cultural mores to the social institutions rather than the reverse.

3. *The social structure of the social institutions has significant influences on the social and psychological being.* Social systems and structure have sociological and psychological significance for the life of the individual, in the system and in all personal activities, including sports and physical activity. The structure itself and the management are strong forces. This ranges from how the family lives together in its daily management of responsibilities to the political management and structure of the school, community, state, nation, and world. Certainly, basic values are clearly reflected.

The social order will define human freedoms and restrictions by law, regulations made by the people to give individual freedom without interference. The scope will be determined entirely by the preparation and the maturity of the individual and the people to live without law and regulations on personal and social behavior.

4. *The physical environment has direct influence on the social and psychological individual and the group.* The physical setting in the home, the school, and all social institutions and organizations is closely related to the social and psychological attitude and behavior of the individual. Concern should be directed toward the effects of the settings on social, physical, and psychological well-being.

The physical setting is a major concern in sports and in physical activity. The objective is to use the physical environment as a participation facility and to enjoy the setting for participation. Mountain climbing is an example. The finest forms of physical activity have a setting in the physical environment—not always the gymnasium. The gymnasium has its role as an efficient mode of preparation—not as a lifetime setting for one's physical activity.

Learning and Development. The fifth component of the sociopsychological science of physical activity is learning and development. This component contains the elements essential for understanding the activities that make up one's life. Without insight and understanding, participation would be inadequate and lacking in personal satisfactions.

1. *Personal attitudes, confidence, aspiration, initiative are concepts that underlie learning and development.* Personal desires and ambitions are psychological concepts important in learning and development. One must want to achieve. These qualities are not directly a part of learning, but they underlie and give support to the rate and level of learning and development. In fact, they determine whether or not learning will begin.

The personal elements are of particular value in sports and physical activity. Physical activity is fun when one enjoys playing the game. But the personal enjoyment is the underlying motivation. The exercise alone that is contained in the sport would be most difficult to perform without the pleasure of participation. This is a major reason why physical activity should be planned as games and sports with motivational potentials.

2. *The social and psychological concepts are closely related to the learning and development of skills for participation.* Motor learning and development are significantly influenced by social and psychological concepts. These include perceptual ability to gain insights into the movement sequences of motor patterns and the inhibitions that may delay, interfere with, or otherwise affect motor learning. Attention, security, and arousal are factors related to learning and development. The confident and secure person is able to introduce into learning a skill the abilities directly related to achieving.

Skill learning and development are motor or neuromuscular achievements involving the nervous system, the muscular system, and the perceptual abilities and insights of the individual. These concepts must be applied in learning by an individual who possesses the social and psychological abilities to give support and direction to the acquisition of skill patterns. The motor learning resources must be in a setting of complementary social and psychological qualities.

3. *The ability to associate, relate, apply psychological factors in learning and development.* Learning and development are more than a single concept. They are related to many concepts closely associated with each skill or learning pattern. These concepts are of particular worth in applying learnings to skill patterns and requirements in various physical activities. A person who has been successful in one activity does have a resource to apply to another.

Motor or skill patterns in physical activity have high specificity. There are, however, common experiences and learnings that do apply to other physical activities. Activities will vary in the degree of association, but all are associated in some degree. Learning and development in a cross section of the various physical activity types will provide the individual with resources that will aid learning and development in an unfamiliar physical activity.

4. *Individual motivation, physical resources, and potentials are basic factors in motor learning and motor development.* The level of physical and psychological motivation will set the stage for the rate and level of motor learning. Upon maturity, the physical and psychological level of achievement will determine the resources for higher levels of achievement. Fatigue, tolerance, health levels, body type, and physique are all factors.

The neuromuscular patterns in physical activity occur within a human organism that will give support or will tend to reject the motor pattern, aiding or hindering achievement. Body type alone is a large factor; for example, an endomorph is handicapped in high jumping—the motor pattern cannot reach the highest levels of performance.

An Overview

Physical activity requires more for effective participation than the physical requirements and neuromuscular skill needed for the performance itself. There are numerous other forces, human qualities, that are part of performance. The biophysical factors needed for each physical activity are reasonably well known, and the professional worker can use this information to prepare one for effective performance in any activity. Biophysical requirements differ with each activity. The current knowledge of the biophysics of physical activity comes from applications of the physical sciences, physics, mechanics, and chemistry, in particular, and the biological sciences, particularly physiology. When applied to physical activity, however, it is nearly impossible to separate material into two independent areas—a physical science of physical activity and a physiology of physical activity—although independent studies are made. Physical activity combines the physical resources and the mechanical processes in such a closely integrated manner that it is most difficult to analyze movement "as a whole" without the resources of the combined basic sciences.

A nearly identical setting exists in the application, on an independent basis, of the sciences of sociology and psychology. Thus in this chapter a conceptual structure is offered that utilizes the resources from these two social sciences as they apply to physical activity. In performances of physical activity, it is difficult and, indeed, undesirable to separate these two sciences in application to human movement: thus the development of the sociopsychological science of physical activity, conceptualizing sociological and psychological concepts into an integrated applied science that fits the individual "as a whole" by considering the factors that complement the biophysical requirements to aid or advance participation to higher levels and add to satisfaction in physical activity.

The sociopsychological science of physical activity currently has the status of a discipline, largely in the professional field of physical education. Studies are being made that deal with concepts from the two basic disciplines, to give further understanding to the sociology and psychology of physical activity. It is desirable to plan studies that apply concepts in sociopsychological form, particularly when the results are directed to the professional worker to help in improving performance. For the average person improvement comes through increased satisfaction from activity; for the highly skilled individual, from the heights attained. Little doubt exists that the sociopsychological science will serve as an important resource.

Further advancement of the sociopsychology of physical activity can come from various applications and studies in physical activities. Because no two activities are physically alike in their requirements, it is likely that no two abilities are sociopsychologically alike in their requirements. At least, this is a reasonable working hypothesis. Some examples are presented of further studies that are needed in this area.

1. *The individual as a social being in physical activity.* The sociopsychological concepts as they apply to the individual as a social being are classified in the conceptual structure for physical activity (List 3). A review is presented in this chapter of the concepts as they apply in physical activity. These applications, for the most part, are inferential reviews within the context of physical activity. Some research evidence gives support, but much comes from clinical and experiential observations of the individual, as a social being, in physical activity. In final judgment, the concepts of the individual as a social being must come from carefully planned and controlled studies. In the meantime, the individual as a social individual can be judged and actions taken with reasonable confidence.

2. *Social institutions and physical activity.* Physical activity as a part of social institutions has a higher level of supporting evidence than other applications of sociopsychological concepts. Physical activity has been a part of family life throughout the ages. It has served to unify the family, giving pleasure that has favorable effects on the security of each individual. Similar experiences have resulted in the use of physical activity to meet institutional objectives, as in the YMCA, YWCA, and the Boys Clubs.

As the concepts of sociopsychology as related to social institutions are applied and studied, this will provide additional information on how this discipline can be used in professional and social applications.

3. *The sociopsychological processes and physical activity.* The social and psychological concepts as structured in this applied science have had many applications and observations in physical activity. Social behavior as seen in competition has had many tests. The observing and sensitive coach can pattern the social behavior of his players if he is accepted and has a strong influence on the players, as demonstrated in many instances of successful coaching.

The effects of mores and cultural practices have also been observed. Movement within cultural strata can be very dramatic in sports and physical activity. It is recognized, of course, that concepts such as involvement and leadership methods, among others, need to be studied within various classifications of physical activity to secure data that give additional evidence of the nature of the influence of those sociopsychological concepts on the individual in physical activity.

4. *The sociopsychological environments and physical activity.* Current writings on physical activity and the sociopsychological environments stem from many observations, as they are a fundamental part of physical activity participation. The sociopsychological effect of the audi-

ence is an example. The influences are strong in sports participation. The social group and the team are miniature societies, with their regulations on play and behavior.

The sociopsychology of physical activity within the social and physical environments is fundamental to participation in physical activity. Social settings affect the quality of performance and there is much evidence demonstrating the effect of the physical environment. Of course, further evidence and supporting data are needed to determine the effects of the sociopsychological environment in many settings with reference to physical activity of all types. Investigating the differences between individual and group activity is one example.

5. *Learning, development, and physical activity.* Studies and observations are available applying the various elements of learning and development to physical activity. Psychological elements such as perception, attitude, and inhibitions are clearly observable in their effect on physical activity. Training procedures are instituted as a result of observations. There are other psychological elements that are important in physical activity, particularly in athletic competition—for example, mental fatigue, boredom, aspirations, and retention. Physical activity is a psychological phenomenon of major importance.

Physical participation not only is a biophysical science of preparing for physical movements with skill and efficiency, but is a sociopsychological science of preparing the individual mentally and emotionally for participation. Without the latter, participation cannot be satisfying and certainly cannot reach the heights of success, if this is an individual or team objective. In athletics, success is the goal, but individual satisfaction is also a worthy goal.

Chapter 6

The Historical Foundations

The chapters in Part II consider physical activity within the context of the academic disciplines that can be applied in its study. In this chapter we will focus not on historical facts about physical activity, but rather on the potentials of physical activity in a historical setting as a discipline. This goal will be considered by examining whether physical activity is influenced by environmental and cultural forces and whether it plays a significant role in shaping and influencing people in their ways of life and practices. If physical activity does indeed play an important role historically, then it is worthy of study as a discipline. The time, effort, and emphasis placed on physical activity throughout the history of civilization have been immense. Because of its significant place in the various cultures and throughout the evolution of man, there is considerable reason to believe that it has played a vital role in people's lives. Certainly, the cultural influences on both man and physical activity represent a part of civilization that should be studied to determine their place in various cultural and historical settings and relationships.

Physical Activity Viewed Historically

Human beings are greatly influenced by the traditions and mores of a culture. Culture is deeply rooted in the history of a people. It passes from one generation to another with some variation within each generation, but remaining essentially unchanged. The differences among the various cultures are to be found in the fundamental characteristics of the people. The knowledge gained by analyzing the various elements of a culture and the role they play will provide a basis for understanding and explaining the traditions, the personal beliefs, and the forces affecting the daily lives of the people.

The foundations of physical activity in history are deep, for physical activity has been a part of all civilizations. The manifested range of activity has been from its nearly full involvement in the survival of the people to its application in sports and games as a part of leisure and enjoyment. This range represents the evolutionary change in the role of physical activity in the cultural life of man.

Nearly all applications of physical activity as a profession have their beginnings in early civilizations. The Greek and Roman periods are particularly noteworthy. During the pre-Christian period, many of the great philosophers emphasized that the development of the physical body was a social responsibility. For the past 2,000 years, the history of civilization shows, man has been engaged in various forms of physical activity. In many instances, success in physical competition (i.e., success in war) reflected the political strength of a nation. Success in war has been largely due to the physical ability of the people, which is indigenous to the culture.

In modern civilizations physical activity has become not so much an essential part of survival as a part of people's leisure time in such applied forms as sports and games. This change in emphasis came about largely during the nineteenth century in Europe and was carried to the United States. During the twentieth century, particularly in the United States, physical activity has been applied primarily as a medium for human development. It already has evolved through three definable periods and is now rapidly entering a fourth period.

In the United States the original professional application of physical activity in the schools and in communities was referred to as *physical culture*. This period had its beginning during the latter part of the nineteenth century and continued on into the 1920's. It is interesting to note that the term *physical culture* continues to be used by some newspaper writers and news commentators. For professional teachers and workers applying physical activity to achieve professional goals, this conceptualization was discontinued soon after World War I.

Physical culture applied physical activity in a formal context. It was designed to develop the human organism in symmetry and in physical balance. Perfecting the exterior lines of the human body was the objective. Anthropometry (the measurement of man) was an important facet of physical culture. During this period gymnastics was particularly important because it could be applied to develop independently different segments of the body. The physical activities used were essentially muscular.

The second historical period in the application of physical activity for professional purposes emphasized the concept of *physical training*. The term first emerged during World War I and continued in use through the 1930's. It was also the professional classification of physical activity applied in the various armed services during World War II. This term also continues to be used by some newspaper writers and commentators. The conceptualization of physical activity as physical training was proper in the armed services. In these programs physical activities were designed to train and condition service personnel for military duty.

Physical training had a broader interpretation and application than did physical culture. The program of activities was less formal. Sports, games, and athletics were large parts of the program. Formal activities such as calisthenics were continued, particularly for special training or for conditioning purposes. Formal gymnastics were part of school programs as a basic preparation for physical conditioning and as preparation for sports, athletics, and games. The main concentration was on improving abilities and aiding physical performances.

The third period began in the middle 1930's and has continued to the present time. Its main concept has been that of *physical education*. The scope of physical activity was enlarged, with sports, athletics, and games constituting the central core of all programs. The guides for the application of physical activities were educational objectives. It was a very important development for physical activity and for programs designed for the development of the human organism and the human being as a total personality.

Physical activity as a part of educational programs has the same goals as those for total education. The primary difference is in the unique contributions made by physical activity in the development of the individual. The process of participation and leadership in the applications of physical activity is important.

The fourth period in the application of physical activity is now beginning to emerge. Its primary concern is understanding and applying physical activity from a scientific perspective. It deals with human development according to scientific evidence in an effort to meet defined or determined human developmental goals. Philosophy becomes a directing force in setting goals and standards for human development.

Using scientific disciplines to develop greater understanding of the role of physical activity in human development is rapidly advancing both in the United States and in other parts of the world. The biological sciences have over the years played a large role, and that is now rapidly increasing. Physical activity is now also studied within the context of the social and psychological sciences. Likewise, the physical sciences are rapidly becoming more important in directing the application of physical activity.

The history of physical activity and its various applications is long and deeply rooted, and is a significant part of the culture, traditions, and mores. Governments have placed much emphasis on physical activities for survival. In recent years, educational applications have been more prominent. Education in and through physical activity has been found to contribute to modern goals. The ancient ideal of wholeness is considered important, but within the context of the age of technology and science. Goals have varied within each historical period. Because of our technology, a modern need is simply for physical activity per se—a goal that was not important during earlier years.

The preceding discussion is a brief setting for the review of the history of physical activity that will be presented in this chapter. In all periods physical activity was applied to achieve some personal or cultural goal. It was essentially professionally applied. The emphasis in this chapter will be on the strength of physical activity as a medium or facet of the culture. We will dwell on the nature of physical activity from a scientific and philosophical perspective, rather than on professional applications, goals, and accomplishments.

The Historical Structure for Physical Activity

In order to give direction and completeness to this review, a conceptual structure is presented that defines the scope of the analysis and provides a description of the nature of the analysis itself (Table 1). The conceptual structure has two major divisions—the sociocultural correlates of physical activity and the historical classification of the social, political, and cultural correlates of physical activity as represented in ten major historical periods.

The Sociocultural Correlates

The study of physical activity involves the sociocultural setting of the people. Physical activity is individually correlated and applied (man as an individual); man and physical activity applied to the group (man and society); and man and physical activity in a setting of the physical environment (man and the physical environment). The conceptual identification of the elements within these three settings will give meaning to the nature of physical activity (Table 1).

Man as an Individual. Physical activity is a human phenomenon. It involves all experiences in the life of the individual. He must move to live; the physiological functions sustaining life depend on it. His nature as an individual will determine the kind and scope of physical activity. Occupation, health, and security are factors in determining the kind and amount of physical activity (Table 1). Participation in physical activities will also affect personal qualities and characteristics. It is man as a person, as he differs from other individuals in his interests, choices, and life

TABLE 1

PHYSICAL ACTIVITY, CULTURE, AND MAN: RELATIONSHIPS

The sociocultural correlates of physical activity	The cultural setting for physical activity: cultural contexts for physical activity	
	Historical period	Cultural determinants

1. Man as an Individual
  a. Human Values
  b. Occupation
  c. Security
  d. Health
  e. Education
  f. Leisure
2. Man and Society
  a. Government
  b. Occupations
  c. Labor and Industry
  d. Education
  e. Communications
  f. Leisure
  g. Health
  h. Religion
  i. Ethnic, National, or
    Racial Composition
  j. Racial Composition
  k. Population
  l. Family
  m. Technology
  n. Military
  o. Cultural
  p. Stresses
  q. Security
3. Man and the
  Physical Environment
  a. Housing
  b. Climate, Seasons
  c. Clothing
  d. Humidity
  e. Transportation
  f. Population
  g. Sanitation
  h. Protection
  i. Pollution
  j. Altitude
  k. Land, Water, Terrain
	1. Primitive Period
	
	2. Biblical Period
	  (2000 B.C.–
	  600 B.C.)
	3. Grecian Period
	  (600 B.C.–
	  90 A.D.)
	
	4. Roman Period
	  (90 A.D.–1300)
	
	5. Middle Ages
	  (600–1600)
	
	6. Renaissance
	  and Reformation
	
	7. Colonization
	  (1620–1790)
	
	8. National Period
	  (1790–1860)
	
	9. Immigration
	  (1860–1900)
	
	10. Twentieth
	  Century, USA
		Survival: Food and shelter within a religious context.
		Learning: Knowledge for improved life and livelihood.
		Cultural Development: Improvement of the culture, including human development as a total personality.
		Conquest: The building of the Roman Empire through land conquests.
		Religion: Emphasis on the Christian Church with stress placed on the mind and the human spirit.
		Inquiry: Emphasis on knowledge and understanding man and the philosophic basis for his life.
		Freedom: Desire for improved life and living with a large degree of self-determination.
		Government: Emphasis on organization of the people and their life activities.
		Growth: Early growth in the USA with immigrants largely from European countries.
		Development: The development of all facets of society in the USA involving all aspects of life, living and society.

activities, that is the starting point or reference in our historical study of physical activity.

Man and Society. Man influences society and society in turn influences man. These forces include physical activity. Physical activity and man are both parts of a society. In this instance physical activity is as much a part of man as man, collectively, is a part of society.

Society is a collection of its parts. Its structure encompasses the functions required to survive and to give order to life. This includes all organizations and agencies essential to providing each person and the group with the needs necessary for survival (occupation, government, and education are some of the components). Requirements are set by the needs of the people. Physical activity is a part of the needs and is found in society in many forms (sports, games, and so on).

The individual as a part of society influences the groups in which he works. It is a mistake to think in terms of just a one-way interaction (i.e., that groups affect individuals and not vice versa). In fact, the changes effected by the individual will often determine the nature of the group or society. Individual efforts will determine the nature and scope of physical activity and the opportunities provided by the society.

Man and the Physical Environment. The individual is influenced by the physical environment but the physical environment in turn is influenced by man. These two-way interactions are of particular importance when looked at from the point of view of physical activity. Physical activity can significantly reduce the unfavorable effects of environmental forces on the organism. In fact, the physical environment can be used to provide favorable conditions for positive human development.

Participation in physical activity requires certain conditions from the environment and its physical resources. The nature of the environment will determine to some degree the nature of the activity itself and certainly the effects of participation on the organism. Some important physical environmental factors are climate, humidity, terrain, and protection (Table 1). The two-way relationships involving environmental factors can also favor human development. Physical activity is not just sports and games but also physical work needed to provide a favorable environment. There are many examples—walking or bicycling rather than riding in an automobile; physical work in providing safe playgrounds and play equipment; physically preparing for the effects of humidity and other climatic conditions; and so on.

The physical environment is the long-range setting as a facility for physical activity. The individual prepares in gymnasiums, in swimming pools, and on athletic fields for a physical life in the lakes, streams, mountains. It involves learning to utilize the natural physical environment as a facility so as to obtain enjoyment of life through the nature and beauty of the physical world. Hiking in a beautiful mountain setting is an example. Physical activity in these instances is the means to an end rather than an end in itself.

Applications of the Historical Structure

Physical activity and its history are presented as they apply to man within his culture. The rationale for the individual and physical activity within the various periods in history is found in the preceding section. The objective is to present evidence that will yield an understanding of the worth of physical activity as a part of man's life and culture.

The Primitive Societies. The life of primitive man was essentially one of struggle for survival. It was concerned with finding protection from the physical elements and securing and preserving food. The cultivation of the soil and the development of products essential for life were the major activities. Social life took place within the family, and physical activity was largely associated with work. Games and sports did not make up a significant part of the life of man during this period.

The Biblical Period (2000 B.C.–600 B.C.). The life of the people continued to be centered around physical survival—work and food—during the Biblical period. Religion had a strong impact on the life of the individual. Government and education were matters of concern. Physical activity was not a large part of this cultural period. Any physical activities were closely associated with the daily life of survival. Religious dogma was not favorable to physical activity.

The Grecian Period (600 B.C.–90 A.D.). The Grecian period is considered to have given birth to the Western culture and saw physical activity assuming increasing importance. It can also be considered to have given birth to organized physical activity as a part of culture for leisure, enjoyment, and physical well-being. The culture itself became more formal and had many cultural activities—art, music, science, and philosophy. Physical activity was an organized part of the culture. It was applied for the strength of the body and for enjoyment, and physical activity as sports, games, and athletics became a firm part of life.

The Roman Period (90 A.D.–1300). The place of physical activity in the culture of the people made significant advances during the Roman period. It was manifested in military conquests by the Romans and the building of the Roman Empire. Rules and rulers were established in various segments of the empire, representing an organized form of government over a large number of people and territories. Physical activity was favorably considered by the people and the government. It played a significant role in military life and in preparation for war and conquest. It was also a part of religious festivals and the free life of the people. The goals for physical activity were preparation of the body for war and for a physically active life of sports and games. Organized games and sports had a large place in the culture.

The Middle Ages (600–1600). Religion was again a major cultural influence during the Middle Ages. The Christian Church dominated the cultural life of the people. Physical activity developed during the Roman period was significantly reduced. Forms of physical activity came largely as a part of daily life under religious influences. Scholasticism considered physical activity unimportant, with the mind and the spirit assuming major roles. The concept of the total development of man was reduced significantly.

Renaissance and Reformation. The decline of religious powers and advances in science, education, and inquiry occurred during the period of the Renaissance and Reformation. The university had its beginnings, with emphasis being placed on inquiry and knowledge. War was still a part of the culture; it was not used for territorial gain, but resulted mostly from religious and philosophic differences. Physical activity gained a larger place in the culture as religious influences waned, especially as a part of war activities. Sports, games, and gymnastics were parts of physical activity. Their place in the culture, however, was not large.

Colonization (1620–1790). The period of colonization was a time for the pioneer and the individual with a desire for freedom and an improved standard of living. It was also a period of hardship for those seeking a better life. Life for the pioneers in America was hard. The people lived in small groups, with education centered in the home. The English influence was strong in the culture of the people as well as in physical activity. English games and sports were part of life, but physical activity was mostly related to survival in the hard life that was experienced. It took hard work to eke out a decent living for a majority of the people. Interest in sports and games was not large, except for people in the wealthy class, who had more leisure time.

The National Period (1790–1860). The national period was a time for rapid growth and development of cultural activities. The industrial life of the people advanced beyond the less-organized forms. Life changed for many from rural to urban. Government was more formally organized into democratic practices. Life needs became more demanding. Physical activity also grew significantly. Sports and games became important parts in man's life. Influences from European countries significantly affected the forms of physical activity. Gymnastics and free exercise became parts of school programs. Physical activity started to become part of educational programs. The British influence on physical activity continued also.

The Immigration Period (1860–1900). The immigration period was a time of rapid industrial growth and development. The Civil War had a major impact on the future of the United States. Following the war, growth was rapid in industry, agriculture, education, and transportation. Science was beginning its rapid development and it had increasing impact on daily life. Physical activity began on a large scale in agencies, schools, and colleges. Numerous national associations were organized to promote sports and athletics as well as recreation. Legislation for physical education in the schools was initiated. Formal preparation for leadership in physical education and sports also began in the United States during this period. It is a period that saw the formal beginnings of modern physical education, sports, and athletics.

The Twentieth Century—United States (1900 to present). All changes in the United States during the twentieth century were greatly influenced by the two world wars and two Asian wars involving the aid of the United States. These wars greatly affected the economy of the nation. The modern era can be divided into five periods representing significant emphases, influences, and changes. The first is the pre–World War I period, which saw significant advances in industry. Recreation as a part of community life had its major beginnings. School programs in physical education and athletics started in the United States, particularly in the eastern part of the country. Sports became a major part of college educational programs.

The second period included the postwar developments from 1918 to 1930. There was renewed economic development in the country. Work, life, and education were all improved. Work was plentiful and higher wages made life more pleasant for most people. Sports, games, athletics, and recreation greatly advanced in all agencies—schools, colleges, universities, and communities.

The third period, 1930 to 1940, represents one of serious economic difficulties and depression. Economic conditions influenced all aspects of life. Community activities, including all forms of physical activity, were affected. Government recreation programs were started to provide relief for the depressed. Governmental work projects were organized to offer work. Advances in nearly all areas of society were depressed.

During the period from 1940 to 1950 war was again a major force influencing the life of people throughout the world. People were mainly involved in preparation for war and, after it had ended, in making adjustments to peacetime living. Science played a prominent role in the war efforts. In the United States this period represented the onset of the scientific age, which has come to have a tremendous impact on all the activities of man, including sports and the preparation for leadership. Athletics experienced a major expansion during this time.

The period from 1950 to the present has witnessed many major developments resulting in high levels of prosperity for nearly all the people in the United States. The scientific age now is in full development, with the space achievements representing a good example of the advances made in science. The technological developments that science made possible have influenced all facets of life—industry, medicine, education, recreation, health, and others. During the current period recession has set in and adversely affected the standard of living, mainly because of the wars in Southeast Asia. The high cost of these wars has created inflation and much unemployment. Nonetheless, all forms of physical activity have advanced significantly during this time, particularly professional sports, which is now one of the major cultural components of life in the United States.

List 4. History classified as social, political, and cultural correlates of man

1. The primitive societies.
   a. Man and his culture: Communities established leading to a stratification of social classes. Implements were fashioned to facilitate cultivation of the soil and aid in the manufacture of crude domestic necessities. Animals became domesticated. Religion was based upon mythology and the image of man as a warrior.
   b. Physical activity within the culture: Physical prowess was essential for survival and the securing of food. However, with the establishment of communal living and innovative inventions, survival became a little less exhausting, so that leisure activities consumed an increasing proportion of time. Physical activity was also closely allied with religious rights.
2. The Biblical period (2000 B.C.–600 B.C.).
   a. Man and his culture: Knowledge increased dramatically in science, agriculture, and medicine. Man began to philosophize and to turn to monotheism rather than polytheism. Government was in the hands of a ruling class responsible in part for establishing a caste system. Education emphasized the necessity of achieving competence in reading, writing, and mathematics.
   b. Physical activity within the culture: Physical activity was of a utilitarian nature, although a wide variety of activities were indulged in.
3. The Grecian period (600 B.C.–90 A.D.).
   a. Man and his culture: Greece was the birthplace of Western culture. Society was based upon class stratification, although the nature of the government depended upon the city-states, i.e., Athens was democratic, Sparta, totalitarian. Greece was a patriotic civilization and bequeathed a rich, cultural inheritance of sculpture, pottery, architecture, music, history, philosophy, drama, and gymnastics. Education was conceived of as a program of progressive adjustment.

b. Physical activity within the culture: The emphasis was on the man of action, exhibiting the qualities of strength, endurance, and bravery. A strong patriotic spirit necessitated that every citizen be prepared to accept, in time of conflict, the role of soldier. There was a real awareness of beauty, harmony, and joy that could be achieved through physical activity and all-around physical development. Recreation was found in a spectrum of activities, namely, chariot racing, wrestling, boxing, foot racing, throwing events, and gymnastics. Professional athletics originated in this era.

4. The Roman period (90 A.D.–1300).
    a. Man and his culture: A nation of "empire builders" who absorbed the culture of the lands they conquered and transmitted it to the world. The Roman empire was characterized by its industrial, organizational, and administrative expertise. Laws were framed, a school curriculum formulated, and the foundation of Christianity laid.
    b. Physical activity within the culture: Physical fitness was a prerequisite for a nation so preoccupied with empire building. The military, through emphasis on the activities of running, jumping, swimming, javelin throwing, and fencing, established a precedent of efficiency that has rarely been surpassed. Physical activity, through its profound influence on society, eventually became the domain of the military and professional athlete. Religious and agricultural festivals were the main leisure pursuits of this period, featuring chariot races and gladiatorial contests.

5. The Middle Ages (600–1600).
    a. Man and his culture: The Christian Church exerted a profound and often overpowering influence on life. It was the age of the "isms": feudalism, monasticism, scholasticism, and asceticism.
    b. Physical activity within the culture: There was a general lack of interest in physical activity because of the preoccupation with asceticism. The recreational activities that were indulged in were generally crude or brutal. Hunting, falconry, ball games, games of chance, and forfeit games were the most popular. Tournaments, symbolic events in the education for knighthood, were popular until their eventual prohibition by the Church.

6. The Renaissance.
    a. Man and his culture: The spirit of inquiry dominated the period. The advent of the printing press awakened an interest in the works of Aristotle and led to an era of intellectual inquiry and scholasticism. Three great philosophic movements originated: humanism, which emphasized the harmonious development of the individual; moralism, which found its outlet in puritanism and protestantism; and realism, signified by a dependence upon scientific inquiry.
    b. Physical activity within the culture: The humanistic movement emphasized the harmonious development of the whole personality. Gymnastics, physical exercise, and a variety of games originated during this period. Moralism relegated physical activity to a relatively inferior position in the hierarchy of values. Physical activity, characterized as health and recreation, was looked upon as a means to moral and spiritual objectives. Realism saw physical aspects of man as an integral part of the personality.

7. The colonization period (1620–1790).
    a. Man and his culture: The pioneer spirit germinated from a deep desire for freedom. A rural population that experienced a life full of hardship depended on cooperation and tenacity for survival. Education, which eventually copied the English system, was the function of the home.
    b. Physical activity within the culture: Physical prowess was essential in overcoming innumerable environmental hardships and in securing food for survival. The populace combined recreation with useful labor. Many English games were adopted, which in time took on an almost uniquely American interpretation.
8. The national period (1790–1860).
    a. Man and his culture: Industrialism supplanted agrarianism as the main feature of life. Urban communities housed the new industrial classes that consumed the manufactured goods. The repercussions of industrialism were soon evident; new wealth brought about exploitation, the extension of voting powers, and preoccupation with generating an export trade. In Europe nationalism was rapidly emerging.
    b. Physical activity within the culture: The "factory system" was instrumental in reducing the necessity of physical prowess as a means of securing a livelihood. Man now sought his recreation through physical activity. In Europe physical activity took on a militaristic outlook, especially in France, Russia, and Prussia. Jahn, Spiess, Ling, and Nachtegan all contributed to the "intellectualizing" of physical education.
9. The immigration period (1860–1900).
    a. Man and his culture: This was the period of transition in which the inventiveness of the American nation was nurtured. The Civil War was directly responsible for enormous industrial growth. Railroads, electricity, and the mechanization of agriculture all contributed to unrivaled economic growth. Ethnic groups, by introducing the culture of their homeland, contributed to the development of a unique American culture.
    b. Physical activity within the culture: During this period there was an enormous growth in the interest shown by the public in sports. This movement was accentuated by the birth of the popular press and various other news media. Intercollegiate sports were established, as were many national sports associations. Teacher preparation in physical education followed the adoption of the German and Swedish systems of gymnastics.
10. The twentieth century.
    a. 1900–1918.
        (1) Man and his culture: Exaggeration in the shift from rural to urban living. A nationalism evolved that manifested itself in a vigorous international policy. The domestic market was so fully supplied with products that American industrialists sought new international markets. A policy of neutrality guided American policy at the outbreak of war in Europe, but as time wore on this attitude changed to one of active participation. The emancipation of women was a major political step forward during this era.
        (2) Physical activity within the culture: Recreational activities achieved prominence largely because of the need for relaxation

after the drudgeries of factory employment. At the outbreak of war there was a general awareness of the necessity of physical fitness.
  b. 1918–1930.
    (1) Man and his culture: This was a period of unparalleled benefits and a new standard of living. Unrestricted immigration was ended. Unprecedented school construction programs marked an emphasis on education.
    (2) Physical activity within the culture: Popular interest was generated in physical activity during this period because of an increase in leisure time, more spending money, the rise of the sporting page, radio, and the ease of transportation offered by the automobile.
  c. 1930–1940.
    (1) Man and his culture: This era was characterized by the Great Depression, which affected all facets of economic and social life. Unemployment had enormous effects on the morale of the populace.
    (2) Physical activity within the culture: The Depression accentuated the emphasis put on leisure activities as a release mechanism.
  d. 1940–1950.
    (1) Man and his culture: The overriding influence during this period was war. A resurgence was evident in the industrial domain and a feeling of internationalism fostered.
    (2) Physical activity within the culture: There was emphasis on programs of physical fitness to withstand the requirements of war.
  e. 1950–1970.
    (1) Man and his culture: This was an age of prosperity in which nuclear power and space exploration dominated. Migration was toward the large cities, creating numerous problems associated with urban living. Environmental concerns, soul-searching wars, and an ever-expanding educational system all contributed to cultural evolution of this era.
    (2) Physical activity within the culture: During this period there was growth in spectatorship, but actual participation declined. Radio, television, and ease of communication all contributed to this decline. Disillusionment with the star system, a high degree of specialization, and the overorganization of sports create a movement toward unstructured leisure-time activities.

Relationships Between Physical Activity, Culture, and Man

Physical activity, in various forms, has always been a part of culture. The nature of its manifestation has depended on the nature of the social setting in a given culture. The setting is determined by the needs of the people or the prevalent social issues, which in turn change the lives of nearly everyone. Some examples from history are war, which is the most common, depressions, and religious dogmas. All have served as major cultural contexts for physical activity. The immediate needs of life have always set the stage for physical activity. Physical activity therefore has not served as an end in itself but as a means to a larger end.

It is indeed important to note that the form of physical activity within a society is, to a major degree, set by the culture of the society. The reverse is not likely to be true. It is also of interest to note the wide variability in the forms in which physical activity has manifested itself— from manual labor to commercial sports and skills of the highest order.

In order to view physical activity in a total historical context, a summary of historical data is presented (List 4), noting the conditions that set the stage for physical activity and the cultural relationships that existed during each period. Only recently has physical activity in the form of sports and athletics become a rather independent cultural facet of society, that is, become more of an end in itself than a means to some end. However, cultural conditions will continue to have a strong influence on the development of sports and its importance to the people.

An Overview

Physical activity is viewed in this chapter as a fundamental element of culture, and the framework for review (Table 1) is developed on this premise. The historical periods were selected to represent distinct cultural periods involving significant changes associated with the physical activity of the people. The relationships considered were man as an individual in his culture, man as he is related to his society, and man as he lives in his physical environment. The review included facts and judgments on physical activity within these two contexts. We have tried to yield the relationships without making an attempt to give a complete review of historical facts. The various roles of physical activity in history were considered so that we might determine whether physical activity is an important element of the culture worthy of continuous study.

The study of man and physical activity in his culture included elements that were considered important in the study of physical activity. The search includes statements about the nature of each element in order to yield an understanding of the period. The attempt is to demonstrate how physical activity was applied by the people. In reviewing List 4 it is noted that physical activity varied significantly from period to period. In each case, it was closely associated with the life and traditions of the people.

An attempt to highlight the major factor or force affecting man, culture, and physical activity is presented in Table 1. The question to be answered is, "What is the major cultural determinant of the setting for physical activity?" During the early periods of history, man survived through physical work. In later historical periods physical activity would fit the prevailing cultural emphasis. In the period of emphasis on the spirit and the mind, physical activity played a very small part in the lives of the people. Learning, conquest, religion, inquiry, freedom, growth and development of the nation and the people were all cultural forces causing changes in physical activity and its uses by the people. These changes demonstrate that physical activity is a firm part of the life of man and that its form is directed by social forces. The primary question in this review is whether physical activity is worthy of study as an essential element in understanding culture. Little doubt remains as to its cultural importance. The potential of physical activity to influence the life of man makes it a suitable subject of study by historians.

Chapter 7

The Philosophic Foundations

Man requires guides for his thoughts, actions, and life conditions (home, family, associates) in daily living. Philosophy requires facts for analysis if it is to establish theories and principles concerning the nature of reality. Philosophy is basically concerned with developing an understanding of the essence of human existence. In this pursuit it develops theories. Philosophy cannot be contrary to fact or unsupported by fact. Philosophy is basic to understanding, and thus is related to science. The difference between philosophy and science is that science is concerned with analytical procedures, identifications, and descriptions, whereas philosophy is concerned with synthetic interpretation.

Philosophy, utilizing obtained facts, applies systematic thought and analysis to provide explanations that are satisfying to the individual and that point to patterns of life that are not in conflict with what the individual considers worthy and valuable. An established pattern of thought and reasoning is utilized in achieving these explanations. The fundamental aspects of reasoning are logic, ethics, aesthetics, politics, and metaphysics. Logic deals with methods of thought, ethics with conduct, aesthetics with beauty, politics with social organization, and metaphysics with the ultimate nature of reality. Utilizing these various systems of analysis, philosophy attempts to interpret and to seek out the true meaning of life from a number of different viewpoints concerning the nature of reality, each of which may yield a satisfactory, logical explanation of the universe, society, and the individual.

Philosophy speaks in terms of aims and thus is concerned with results. It organizes and attempts to give meaning to all elements of life. It addresses itself to attitudes about one's work and one's life in general.

Philosophy, as a result of systematic reflection and science, provides a way of actualizing one's beliefs. Science gives us facts, but only philosophy can give us wisdom. Knowledge involves the comprehension of facts, wisdom the evaluation and integration of facts. Philosophy implies the pursuit of wisdom and its formulation into logical patterns or systems of thought. Full meaning is achieved when philosophy is fully applied.

Philosophy puts forth a description of reality based upon logical systems of thought and reasoning. It emphasizes cultural thinking and reflection, in contrast to science, which is concerned with the acquisition of knowledge or facts. The philosopher is concerned primarily not with details but with relationships. The scientist must be concerned with details that fit together into larger bodies of knowledge. Philosophy is not a body of specialized knowledge but a body of thought systematically organized. It is a sustained process of thinking directed toward ultimate understanding. Philosophy is man's struggle to understand the universe in some coherent, systematic, and meaningful way.

Philosophy and science, however, are closely related, because one of the basic aspects of philosophy is reason, which is also integral to the conduct of science. Philosophy not only precedes science to set directions, worth, and values but comes after it in order to determine the meaning of its findings. Fact and worth can hardly be disassociated; human values come before fact or science.

The Nature of Philosophy

There have been many attempts to classify contemporary philosophies. Zeigler [1] has reviewed both Windelband's work on the history of philosophy and Butler's classification of philosophies into larger bodies of thought in an endeavor to present a more comprehensive view of philosophy. Viewed historically, philosophy in its early formulations had no significant divisions. Later, divisions of logic, physics, and ethics of philosophies were developed. These classification systems were followed by a threefold division: logic, ethics, and aesthetics. Zeigler outlines Butler's classification and his rationale for setting up four branches of philosophy. This review appears to give adequate integration to the various individual philosophies that fall into the four branches. Butler's four branches are subsumed under the categories of speculative philosophy (metaphysics and axiology) and critical philosophy (epistemology and logic). Metaphysics deals with questions about reality; epistemology with questions concerning the acquisition of knowledge; logic with the exact relationship between ideas; and axiology with the various systems

[1] E. F. Zeigler, *Philosophical Foundations for Physical, Health and Recreation Education* (Englewood Cliffs, N.J.: Prentice-Hall, 1964).

of values. The speculative branches deal with the postulation of first principles and the subsequent recognition of values, whereas the critical branches deal with explanations about how man acquires knowledge and how thought becomes verified. A most interesting formula is presented relative to the four branches of philosophy:

Present Values + Scientific Advances + Conditioning of the Emotions = What We Do

Metaphysics in dealing with the nature of reality is concerned with all thoughts and actions of man. This philosophy deals with man as a human being: his problems in relating to other individuals and to his own freedom; his beliefs and practices; matters dealing with the nature of reality itself and the possible changing of that reality; and more fundamentally, his purpose for living. It is a philosophy or system of thought that attempts to interpret the meaning of man's existence in the universe. Establishing a clear conception of reality is most satisfying to many individuals and becomes one of their main objectives in life. It provides a way for viewing their experiences and a basis for making their plans.

Epistemology as a philosophic branch is concerned with inquiry into the nature of knowledge and the means by which it is acquired. It is a system of thought concerned with types of knowledge stemming from deductive and inductive reasoning. It deals with how knowledge can be gained.

Logic is concerned with thought itself, i.e., with establishing the validity of ideas. The systems of induction and deduction are applied to establish this validity. Problem solving and experimentation are processes fundamental to the system of logic.

Axiology, one of the four major branches of philosophy, is directed toward the synthesis of knowledge and the results of philosophic thought. The emphasis is on values: Are they dependent or independent? Are they linked with the individual's existence? Are they based on ethics and ethical judgments? What are the various kinds of values? Are they consistent with prevailing beliefs? The end result of the application of axiology is to establish a rational basis for the individual to assess all his experiences and to plan his daily activities.

There are many subdivisions, classifications, and combinations of the four branches of philosophy reviewed in this section. Two further categorizations will be utilized to give additional structure to the analysis of philosophic thought. The first category deals with philosophies that are rationalistic, spiritualistic, and idealistic. These philosophic forms tend to be characteristic of the philosophies of idealism and realism. The second category consists of philosophies that deal with natural or empirical facts. The philosophies of naturalism, existentialism, and pragmatism represent this classification or overall philosophic view. From these categories further delineations of philosophic viewpoints can be made.

Many attempts have been made to classify the various philosophies. The three most fundamental schools of philosophical thought suggested by leading philosophers are idealism, realism, and pragmatism. These three most common philosophical categories are subdivided into a number of subphilosophies or philosophies representing differences from the overall classification.

These subdivisions can be described by the philosophic classifications of metaphysics, epistemology, logic, and axiology. These divisions have been briefly presented in this section. They can be applied to a number of philosophies that are classified within the basic philosophies of idealism, realism, and pragmatism.

In idealism, mind and spiritual self are considered independent of material relationships. All that exists, exists in the mind. The concepts constituting an integral part of idealism are the following:

1. Reality comes from ideas.
2. Belief in God.
3. Reality is self.
4. Man experiences mind and spirit in self.

Idealism not only has a number of subdivisions but also can be interpreted according to the four branches of philosophy previously mentioned. In the metaphysical branch, the questions about reality are found in the mind. Mind (or spirit) is basic and real to the individual. Man has a soul, which makes him higher than any other form of animal life. The entire universe is essentially the mind.

Idealism from an epistemological point of view is characterized by an emphasis on the acquisition of knowledge; namely, man must experience in order really to know. Experience must be interpreted if one is to acquire knowledge. The world is only meaningful if one makes an attempt to interpret his experience. According to idealistic epistemology, the mind creates knowledge and explains experiences. It is mind over matter; truth is orderly and systematic.

Within the philosophic branch of logic, idealism is characterized by relating knowledge and ideas. The intelligent person should be capable of establishing facts and determining what they mean. In this process the basic systems of reasoning are deductive and inductive analysis. The reasons form a premise; the results cannot go beyond the original premises.

Idealism can also be classified under the branch of axiology, which is a branch of philosophy that interprets systems of values. Idealism under axiology is characterized by an emphasis on human values. Self-realization is a serious matter. According to this philosophical position, man must have faith and belief in God; truth, beauty, and goodness are real and important and can be achieved by man. Man will be able to understand nature if he can forget himself and strive for more knowledge and wider experiences.

Idealism deals with systems of values—life, soul, and spirit. This philosophy is applied, in this section, to the four branches of philosophy previously mentioned. There are a number of philosophies that are essentially idealistic philosophies.

- *Essentialism.* Essentialism is a branch or subdivision of idealism that is more conservative than idealism. The intellectual values of man are foremost and beliefs are usually expressed in absolute terms. Knowledge and skills are important as well as their application in meeting environmental requirements. Individual self-realization is also stressed as an important goal. In man, truth and goodness set the limits for self-realization. The love of knowledge and ideals and their widespread dissemination to others are major aspects of essentialism.
- *Scholasticism.* Scholasticism is a subdivision of idealism placing importance on the Christian philosophy that transcends all people. It is both a system and method of thought. Theology involves the control of reason and thought, with revelation an important factor. Scholasticism is a subdivision of theology, traditional in its processes, social in its applications; it applies to systems of thought essentially in logic and in deductive analysis.
- *Humanitarianism.* Humanitarianism is a subdivision of idealism that has as its primary concern the welfare of man. The emphasis is on man's ability to master his destiny, with human beings being the center of focus rather than God. Efforts are directed toward social reform, alleviation of human suffering, and the general welfare of man. Love, loyalty, kindness, and honesty are personal values of importance. Religion is seen as a means of achieving the good life.
- *Aestheticism.* Aestheticism is an idealistic philosophy that places much stress on beauty. Qualities such as appreciation and understanding are important personal objectives. Beauty is truth and this is a primary aim in life. An objective as well as a logical approach to man's problems is the process of analysis.
- *Dualism.* Dualism is a form of idealism that has as its primary emphasis the contradiction between two irreducible elements, good and evil, and in some applications the separation of mind and body. These elements are in opposition to each other, but nonetheless capable of independent influences.
- *Nationalism.* Nationalism is a philosophy dealing with the desires and needs of the individual and directed toward the common good. This is a philosophy based upon race, language, religion, and geography. This philosophic position emphasizes social cooperation and is applied often as an end in itself. Patriotism is of major consequence.

The philosophy of *realism* can be reviewed and analyzed in a manner similar to that used for idealism. It can be classified within the four branches of philosophy (speculative and critical), and a number of independent philosophies can be classified under the designation of realism.

Realism is a philosophy that places heavy emphasis on empirical facts. Truth is derived from conditions and situations that exist. Reality is determined by that which man experiences; man accepts his experiential world at face value.

The metaphysical branch of philosophy raises questions about reality, and metaphysical realists have expressed differing opinions about the nature of that reality. The world is regular and orderly and is governed by the laws of physics. Man lives in this world and can make certain material changes, but his major purpose is to fit into many unchangeable settings of the environment. Science and facts serve man in his life and adjustments. The world does exist in itself apart from man's desires and knowledge. The only reality is the world.

Realism as it is related to epistemology is concerned with knowing an object as it is and as it is related to other objects. Objects are as man perceives them; man's perception is made possible through his consciousness and awareness of his surroundings.

Logic is also related to the philosophy of realism. Logical realism is based on science and experimentation. Both experimentation and logic are parts of the scientific method, which follows specific step-by-step procedures in order to make determinations of fact. The scientific method begins with hypotheses and ends with rejection or confirmation of these hypotheses.

Axiological realism follows the principle that the world is composed of actual entities that are related by physical laws. It is possible for man to understand some of the laws and this understanding is the basis, in part, for his action. Emphasis is placed on the individual rather than on the group or the universe. Axiological realism accepts things as they are and holds that through the action of man they can come to be what they should be. According to this philosophy man is considered adaptable and able to exist in many different environments. Common sense is important. An individual's experiences provide the basis for a large part of his understanding and his basis for action. Man does not have complete freedom of choice.

As with idealism, a number of philosophical viewpoints can be classified essentially as variations of realism. These viewpoints are sufficiently unique to present independent classifications and will be reviewed briefly.

- *Logical positivism,* a variant of realism, asserts that knowledge comes from application of the scientific method in endeavors directed at discovery and verification of fact. It emphasizes the need for direct measurement of a phenomenon before one can make assertions of fact about the phenomenon. Science and the scientific method are fundamental aspects of this philosophy.
- *Determinism* holds that individual behavior and natural events are predetermined. Man does not have complete freedom of will. The universe is guided by certain physical laws and man's behavior is limited by the conditions resulting from these physical laws.
- *Existentialism* places special emphasis on the experiences of man, past, present, and future. These experiences must be used to give

direction to life and to make the universe meaningful. The individual creates his own ideals and personal values and is responsible for himself. Although man is a part of the universe, he is distinguished from all other animals. The source and elements of knowledge exist in our consciousness. All existence is a state of mind. The mind is influenced by the environment and the conditions that represent the setting in which personal experiences occur.

- *Materialism* is a philosophy that treats matter as the ultimate reality in the physical world; spiritual substance is nonexistent. Everything in the universe is based on material processes and is not governed by intelligence. Everything is explainable in terms of matter. The state of man's being is limited by the physical environment and changes are determined by economic factors.
- *Empiricism* asserts that man's knowledge is derived from his experiences, not from theories about fact. Experience is the sole reality. Knowledge about existence cannot be determined *a priori;* it can come only from one's immediate experiences.
- *Naturalism* finds reality in the physical nature of the universe. All things are natural. Knowledge comes from careful observations and descriptions of nature, followed by caution in making generalizations. Values are inherent in nature. Life and happiness come from the natural order of events. In this philosophy more attention is given to the individual and his development in relation to the physical universe than to the human society. Emphasis is placed on present life.

In summary, realism is a philosophy that states that reality exists outside of the individual's consciousness. Realism, however, is not a monolithic philosophy, because there are a number of philosophical viewpoints about the nature of reality, as has been described in the preceding paragraphs.

A third major classification of philosophy is *pragmatism*, which places emphasis on and derives truth from practical results. Scientific research is not contrary to this philosophy but is an accepted aspect of it. Through research man will find a solution to his problems and will encounter experiences that are satisfying. This philosophy assumes that it is possible to find out if something is worthwhile only through experimentation and personal experiences. Truth is known through logical and physical consequences of experiences embodying the theories to be tested. It is a philosophy of learning by doing.

Pragmatism can also be classified according to the four branches of philosophy—metaphysics, epistemology, logic, and axiology.

- *Metaphysical pragmatism* states that reality exists within the system of nature. The world is characterized by activity and change and is still incomplete. Experience and the environment are the media for reality. The problem is to interpret what man finds to be natural. Man's activity must be related to past experiences.
- *Epistemological pragmatism* is concerned with the search for truth and knowledge. Knowledge comes from fact, and that which is observable and works is truth. What is proved to be right under the circumstances is also truth. Adaptation to the environment and success are bases for

truth and validity. Mind and body interact in the actions and experiences of man.

- *Logical pragmatism* attempts to establish truth through the application of the scientific method to problem solving. In problem solving man uses all available knowledge to formulate hypotheses that are tested by applying the scientific method. The definition and structure of the problem are fundamental in this philosophy.
- *Axiological pragmatism* asserts that anything that adds to life and helps man adapt to the environment is good and useful. Values must be closely related to the world in which we live. There is no supernatural; the world is as we see it and live in it. Social values are important. The highest relationship exists between the individual and society within a democracy. Beauty and aesthetic experiences are also important in this philosophy.

Pragmatism can be subdivided into pragmatic philosophies with special interpretations and with some unique differences. These are instrumentalism, natural empiricism, and operationalism.

- *Instrumentalism* is, in a sense, the same as Dewey's pragmatic naturalism. It emphasizes thought as the instrument for action. The experimental method is important in establishing truth, and thought is most basic in this process.
- *Natural empiricism* is an aspect of pragmatism that emphasizes experience as a basis for fact and not theories. Experiences are most useful when coming from the physical nature of the universe. The universe is self-explanatory and the basis for truth.
- *Operationalism* emphasizes operations as the basis for truth. If it works, it is fact. It is a belief that the meaning of a concept is established through a set of operations. Only proved operations can be accepted as fact or truth. It is the acceptance of actions that are satisfying.

Philosophy Applied to Physical Activity

Philosophy is a search for understanding and explanations about man's existence. It applies to all of life activities, including physical activity. Physical activity involves not only sports and games, but the preparation of the individual and the application of the skills he learns from the day he is born until death. It starts with the movements of an uncoordinated body in a crib and continues to the highest physical performance of which an individual is capable. The range and scope of movements are wide. Philosophical assumptions are basic to their proper application.

Philosophy is a reflection upon social ideals and provides the rationale for attitudes, practices, and general modes of human behavior. It gives direction to various types of behavior and provides explanations for behavior. Philosophy is the primary source from which practices begin. In a large and overall sense, pursuit of philosophical ideals gives meaning to one's life.

Philosophy must be applied to physical activity to provide the individual with the best possible interpretations and applications that can be made. It is unwise to engage in physical activity as a facet of one's life without having a philosophic context for the activity. It is also not enough to have a superficial knowledge of philosophy. One must thoroughly understand a philosophical position in order to apply it properly; on the other hand, one must also understand physical activity in order to judge the relevance of a philosophy and its potentials for directing physical activity.

Five formal philosophies have been selected for application to physical activity. Others could be applied but they appear to have fewer possibilities for relevance to physical activity. The selected philosophies are idealism, realism, naturalism, pragmatism, and existentialism. The application of each will be briefly reviewed.

Idealism and Physical Activity. According to idealism man is a physical being with a soul and a mind that are basically real. Reality lies essentially in the mind and spirit. The existence of matter is not denied, but the mind and the spirit determine the nature of physical things and matter. Idealism encompasses moral and spiritual standards and applies human development to man's ideas, attitudes, and insights about life activities and experiences. The application of idealism to physical activity will result in the development of the social and moral potentials of activity, elements such as sportsmanship, justice, and other values that give wholeness to man. The philosophic context for physical activity is the judgment of results, with respect not only to physical changes within the organism but to how those changes fit the individual within a social, moral, and spiritual context. The idealist believes that physical activity is essential to one's well-being. Development can come through participation in physical activities. This can be accomplished best through self-direction and self-analysis. Standards set by oneself will result in the most desirable results.

Realism and Physical Activity. Realism is predicated on the theory that material things exist independently of the mind. Realism is a philosophic correlate of science. One lives in a material world and sees it as it really is. The world remains the same after one has experienced it, and thus reality is independent of the mind. Realism is founded on fact; truth comes from conditions and situations that exist. Implicit in this doctrine is the understanding that interaction between objects must exist, if, of course, objects are related in a materialistic setting.

According to realism, physical activity is applied as a scientific medium for learning, within the context of natural laws and as a method for understanding these natural laws. The applications of physical activity are deliberate and systematic to control the environment and to generate interactive incidents that will modify behavior and attitudes.

The realist sees the mind as needing a healthy body. Vigorous activity is therefore encouraged. The approach to the selection, evaluation, and adaptation of physical activity is scientific and objective; the approach is organized and justified by the results produced. Activity is directed with experimentation and explanation. Physical activity is vigorous to develop and perfect the body, and development is planned toward goals and by sequences in participation that will achieve the goals.

Naturalism and Physical Activity. In naturalism the universe does not require a supernatural cause. Life and the physical world are the natural results of events—actions and reactions. The events are self-explanatory and self-directing; all values are judged in this context. The substances and the processes of the physical world control and determine the nature, aspirations, and activities of man. Scientific investigation and experimentation are essential to an adequate understanding of the physical world and its effects on the individual.

Under naturalism, physical activity is essential in one's life. One must meet and conquer the forces of the physical world. To do this, physical activity should be meaningful and based on enjoyment. Physical activity and participation should be in accord with the natural laws of the physical world and with the objective of the individual. Artificiality should be eliminated. Games, sports, and all physical activity should be enjoyable in order to yield optimal results in learning and development. The human intellect is fundamental in its use of physical activity for desired results in human learning and development.

Pragmatism and Physical Activity. Pragmatism emphasizes, and derives truth from, practical results. This philosophy holds that if a thing works, it is good. It encourages one to emphasize anything that is practical, efficient, and satisfying. Truth results from action; current problems have first priority, whereas the problems of tomorrow are of little concern today.

Scientific research is not contrary to pragmatism. It is an accepted aspect of it. Man in action and in research will find a solution to his problems and will encounter experiences that are satisfying. Experiences are most valuable in reaching an understanding of the ultimate nature of reality. Authoritarianism violates the fundamental tenets of pragmatism. One must be free to experiment and observe in order to judge the worth of his activities.

According to pragmatism, physical activity that is satisfying and produces the results desired is good. Whatever the objectives sought, they should be capable of achievement through physical activity. The problems of participation and achievement will be solved as they come and at the time they come. In pragmatism there is a continuous sensitivity to working patterns and their effectiveness. Those conditions that are unsatisfactory are changed within the context of practicality. Emphasis is placed on the needs, potentials, and interests of the participant. There is also concern with self-evaluation and problem solving. The search is always for efficient, practical, and satisfying personal results.

Existentialism and Physical Activity. In existentialism man looks at himself objectively. It is man's responsibility to blend all experiences that have meaning and direction into a world view that results from man's ideas and efforts. This philosophy works toward self-determination for life and social conditions that are satisfying and acceptable. The mind is all-important in existentialism, for it is the source of all knowledge. The external world does not have existence except as the mind determines it. Personal responsibility and decisions are stressed in existentialism in order to give purpose and direction to the world.

According to existentialism, the individual assumes responsibility for himself and society. Physical activity and individual participation in it fall within this context. Individual selection of and participation in physical activity are important. Physical activity will impress on the individual his responsibility, not only for himself but for others who should be involved in physical activity. The experiences coming from participation represent the basis for judgments and decisions about self and society. They will determine the scope of participation and resources provided for physical activity. Unfavorable conditions and results from participation will be the basis for any change. The individual then takes action. Self-determination in all matters of action is fundamental in this philosophy.

Relationships Between Physical Activity and Philosophy

Because physical activity provides experiences as in other social groups, it represents another medium for application of philosophy by the individual. The one major difference between this social medium and others is the intensity and closeness of personal associations, which normally are not found in most other social groups.

Closely related to physical development are other qualities of the human being that can be developed within this medium. These qualities are found in the mind, the emotions, the spirit, and the social qualities that are all a part of the total individual. If the individual participates in physical activity, then the potential exists for the development of all these qualities. Under such conditions the philosophies selected for application are closely related to physical activity. The results will be forthcoming if the philosophy is properly applied.

Guides for Idealism. Idealism can be closely correlated with physical activity. In applying idealism the point to remember is that physical activity is secondary to the principal focus, the human being. Although physical activity for the physical development of the body is important in idealism, the potentials in physical activity are of larger importance. According to the idealist, the full development of the human personality is not only highly desirable, but a most desirable preparation for participation in physical activity. Activity then becomes more than a physical process with physical results; it becomes a most favorable setting for human development.

Guides for Realism. From the perspective of the realist, man is developed through physical activity that provides a setting requiring understanding and knowledge through experimentation and analysis. Emphasis is placed on knowledge of the potentials of physical activity and its related environments (physical and social) for human development. The results come from using all elements of the setting for successful participation and human development. The scientific method is important in this philosophy and when it is applied to physical activity, man is able to apply and change the environmental forces to his advantage.

Guides for Naturalism. The naturalist sees physical activity and the setting in the physical environment as the basis for the development of the human organism. Physical activity should take place in physical nature rather than in a simulated, artificial setting. Physical activity is a natural process and man should be prepared to understand the worth of the physical environment as the proper setting for his development. Naturalism considers the human intellect as the means with which to understand the physical environment and man in relationship to it while participating in physical activity. According to this philosophical viewpoint, nature presents the best facility for human development. Physical activity in nature not only leads to an understanding of the environment, but provides a setting for physical activity that is more enjoyable than artificial settings.

Guides for Pragmatism. Pragmatism and physical activity, if success and satisfaction are objectives, are closely correlated. When physical activity is applied as sports, pragmatism is the most common philosophy. If it is successful the process one uses in participation will be considered superior. If it meets the requirements of the individual participant, then it and the activity are considered valid. If one is a pragmatist, one is interested in what is successful according to his objectives. If the objectives are met, the individual will continue the patterns. When failure comes, one seeks new information from further trials and experiences.

Guides for Existentialism. Physical activity is a personal responsibility. Existentialism is applicable and valuable for physical activity and the individual. Physical activity is indeed very personal and one must prepare according to one's abilities. No two individuals are alike. This philosophy does not exclude viewing physical activity as a total human experience. It includes all conditions and factors that will aid the individual in understanding and meeting his responsibilities for successful and satisfying experience in physical activity. It is the individual and his needs and responsibilities that represent the basis for choices and reactions to experiences. In existentialism the individual is the basis for all actions.

An Overview

Philosophical assumptions are the directing force for all human activities. This certainly includes physical activity. One must examine personal values, goals, objectives, and attitudes about oneself, about one's profession or occupation, about one's leisure life and activities, and about all the experiences in one's daily life. The objectives and values deemed important by an individual will set the pattern for participation.

Philosophy is an attempt to unify all aspects of life into a satisfying whole that will fit the individual. It is possible for one to find a philosophy that will provide a rational explanation to experiences. Man needs explanations and purpose for his actions. Philosophy can help meet this need.

Physical activity provides a potentially powerful medium for meaningful human experiences and personal development. It is fundamental to a culture. It is a part of the people and life. Physical activity is aesthetically satisfying. It is an art, a form of human movement that has grace and beauty. It is emotionally involving to the point that one can become lost in the activity. It demands all from the individual. It is also socially oriented and demanding. It is the group that plans the strategy or patterns of play that will determine success or failure. If success is the goal, the result will become known from participation. It becomes obvious to a team member that the social structure of the team is an important factor in success.

The lack of verbal expression during one's involvement in physical activity does not mean that there are no values, goals, and principles associated with that participation. One should keep in mind that philosophies may be implicit as well as explicit. Participants in physical activity are characteristically so absorbed in the activity that it seems that it is only the activity that gives direction to the individual. This does not mean a lack of individual philosophy; indeed, it may emphasize the strength of an existing implicit philosophy.

In observing human participation in sports for physical activity, one could reasonably assume that some individuals are not guided by philosophical assumptions in these endeavors. The principle of *implicit* philosophies will deny that it is possible to engage fully in any activity without holding certain philosophical ideas. The individual's actions or judgments in physical activity will reflect a set of concise principles that can be described philosophically. There are few people, indeed, who are not directed by personal wishes or desires that have their rationalization in some philosophical point of view. In a democracy the broad range of individual choices gives each person an opportunity to direct his or her life toward satisfying individual goals. Philosophical assumptions that are generally related to sports are usually implicitly held before their rationale is verbally expressed. It probably is not possible to formulate a systematic philosophy before the accumulation of adequate amounts of experience and insights into life's activities and certainly into sports participation. Philosophical ideas must develop out of experience before they can guide subsequent personal endeavors.

Philosophical inquiry is generally viewed as the highest and the most fundamental quality of human behavior. It therefore provides the basis for human actions so that they may be properly analyzed, just as it provides a basis for change if satisfactions are not gained. The potential outcomes of involvement in physical activity are so powerful that one cannot risk blind participation. Philosophy is not an end in itself, but a valuable means for furthering personal happiness.

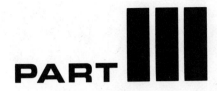

PART III

Professions

Physical activity occurs in several well-established areas, ranging from recreation to high-powered, commercially oriented sports. Consequently, physical activity has achieved an important place in society. Its significance is rapidly increasing because of its potential to achieve goals considered desirable by both society and the individual. The result has been the development of professional associations designed to serve the people according to the highest possible standards.

In the last twenty years, physical activity, both individual and professionally organized, has advanced in status. This is because we are in part increasingly aware of its potential for improving health and general well-being.

The chapters in this section are designed to review the possibilities of physical activity in the ten presently organized professions. In general, these go considerably beyond "possibilities," but some are still in the early stages of development.

What is a profession? What is the difference between a well-established profession in any culture and professions that have difficulty in sustaining operations? In a general way, a profession is a formally organized group, with its own internal controls, designed to render a public service. It must have an important contribution to make. High goals and potentials have little value unless the service meets important human needs.

The question is now, "What is the difference between a profession and the daily services rendered in such areas as supplying food and entertainment?" These services are also important. There are significant differences. It is recognized that there are certain characteristics of the more-distinguished professions that differentiate them from the less-recognized ones. The fundamental basis for the differentiation is determined by people's conception of the worth of the services that are rendered to them. How valuable and important are they?

1. A profession is distinguished by a highly specialized technique that is based on service and learning, the practices of which serve practical

ends; in the pursuit of these ends the practitioners assume a large measure of individual responsibility.[1]
2. The professional technique must be capable of communication through a highly specialized educational discipline.
3. The professional technique must be of sufficient social significance and importance to warrant the exercise of some control over it by society, the practitioners themselves, or both operating together.
4. Preparation for, and practice of, the professional technique so stimulates the practitioners that they form professional associations for improving its standards and extending its public acceptance.
5. The conduct of the practitioners is a matter of concern to the profession and results in the formulation of codes of ethics.
6. Within the profession there is a conscious recognition of a spirit of public service that places social duty as the highest goal of the profession.

The criteria prepared by Kaufman will identify the professional applications of physical activity that help to qualify it as a profession. In this section of the text ten professions are reviewed that are both independent and unique and that have utilized physical activity either partially or totally as the medium for the achievement of service goals. It is amazing to observe the flexibility and the functional power of physical activity when used in these ten professional settings to meet various societal needs and goals. For example, it is capable of serving autocratic political purposes equally as well as democratically directed goals.

There are many conditions in society that will aid or hinder the development, survival, or growth of a profession. If the services are not essential to the people or accepted as a part of their life, survival is not possible. There are at least four major factors in the development and growth of a profession: (1) the influences exerted on the profession, (2) the professional organization itself, (3) education for the profession, and (4) professional responsibilities. When these conditions are favorable, a professional organization will be able to grow through the development of acceptable standards. As a result the profession will gain greater recognition.

Because a profession is a part of a society, it may be influenced by all kinds of social forces. The conditions that affect the lives of the people will also influence the effectiveness of a profession. Some of these factors, the more closely related ones, will be reviewed and then related to each profession as they are presented in the succeeding chapters in this section.

[1] L. A. Larson et al., *Problems in Health, Physical and Recreation Education* (Englewood Cliffs, N.J.: Prentice-Hall, 1953). (Reporting study by Earl Kaufman on criteria for the evaluation of a profession.)

1. *Philosophy.* If the mores of the people are contrary to a given professional service, of course, a professional need does not exist and failure will result (for example, a professional service contrary to an existing religious order).

2. *Economics.* Without appropriate economic support for a professional service, the profession cannot be sustained. With a reduction in the quality of services rendered comes a rapid demise for a profession. There are numerous examples of groups organized around a professional service that have not succeeded.

3. *Geography and population.* The level of quantitative need for professional services is a most vital requirement for a profession. It will be noted that most youth-serving agencies (e.g., Boys Clubs) are located in metropolitan centers and in densely settled areas. A quantitative need exists in these settings. It is most unfortunate that less-populated areas often do not receive services available in urban areas because of the criterion that services be related to certain levels of quantitative need.

4. *Culture.* The culture and heritage of the people served by a profession must be consonant with the professional services it offers and they must be understood by the profession. Public relations programs are required to present what the profession can do and the worth of its professional services. This is most essential for the continuation of any professional services.

5. *Legislation.* Professions plan services within the framework of governing bodies. Laws and regulations set the structure for the profession. The legal and legislative structures encourage and support services. For the professions, laws and regulations are designed to support rather than limit their services. For the professional applications of physical activity, regulations are designed to make professional services available for those needing the benefits that can be derived from this type of endeavor. In these instances, laws and regulations are designed for public welfare and benefits.

6. *Politics.* All professions are part of the political structure of the nation. The political structure is designed to give protection, security, and freedom. Certainly in the professional applications of physical activity, the political structure is generally most supportive if the services represent useful services. Regulations and laws are minimal in this regard. Freedom of action and choice is possible with little restrictions for either individuals or groups, whether they are involved in physical recreation or highly commercialized sports.

For the professions that utilize physical activity as a medium, there are several requirements that must be met if they are to be successful. The organization itself should develop standards that apply to the administrative structure, personnel, programs, facilities and equipment, safety, ethics, and so on, of its operation. The profession must meet the requirements of a sound administrative structure.

Of major importance in any profession are the services rendered by the practitioner. For the physical activity professions, of course, these services will vary with each profession. The practitioner must be prepared to serve the public with skill, knowledge, and demonstrable results. Public satisfaction is probably the most fundamental factor in success.

Professional responsibilities are both internal and external. Internal matters are standards for ethics, security, working conditions, guidance, legal status, and professional growth of the services. External matters are those related to the public. Growth is reflected in a greater recognition and acceptance by the public. The elements that lead to acceptance are the standards of education and preparation of the practitioner with regard to services to be rendered, the quality of professional membership, the research contributions and requirements, the nature of the services rendered to the people, and the certification and licensing requirements.

Chapter **8**

Athletics and Sports

Physical activity in the form of sports and athletics is an integral part of the culture of every nation. This common heritage shared by the people of all nations has a major influence on the populace, on the nation, and on the peoples of all nations. The power of athletics and sports, as large and growing elements of today's culture, is now a highly recognized social and political force. Sports and physical activity are part of man's leisure and play a major role as a profession, involving huge financial investments.

Athletics and sports provide a medium that is very personal with minimal interpersonal restrictions. These will aid in understanding the individual, his cultural interests, skills, and way of life through the media of work, play, and leisure. It is a barometer with which to measure the individual and his cultural understanding. Sports also appear to be correlated with the socioeconomic status of a nation. In the United States, for example, they play a major leisure-time role for nearly everyone. Most Americans today are spectators in one or more of the professional sports.

The need for international as well as national understanding and good will is now greater than at any time in the history of civilization. The people of every nation must find some way to live together or face the consequences of war. Economically strong nations must assume a leading role. Certainly the United States is one of the nations that views its responsibilities on a worldwide basis. The United States, United Nations, and other governments and organizations search constantly for ways to achieve common understandings. During the past few years support has been extended to athletics and sports on an international scale. This is partially due to the role of sports in the culture of almost every nation. Sports provide one of the world's common grounds.

The increasing popularity of sports and physical activity in the United States and other nations makes it a very powerful basis for human communication. Rapidly developing international travel provides a way for people and countries to achieve cultural understanding. Sports taken in this setting, or as properly administered activity under prepared coaches, can be a potentially important social factor in improving the way of life of individuals in countries throughout the world. Such experiences will serve as the basis for national and international understandings.

Professional Status

Athletics and sports are major social and professional facets of American life. This is also true in other nations with relatively high socioeconomic levels. The statistics supporting this statement are overwhelming. Every United States city of any size has at least one golf course; all our schools have gymnasiums and many have swimming pools; finally, all communities have playgrounds, athletic fields, and other facilities for sports.

Sports permeate nearly all levels of contemporary society and involve human status, race relations, business life, and the professional world. In addition, human values ranging from gambling to moral values of the highest order are also elicited through sports. According to Boyle,[1] sports, for better or worse, give form and substance to much of American life. American newspapers frequently devote more space to sports than to such forms of entertainment and art as books, education, cinema, theater, sculpture, and painting. Front-page headlines sometimes present the results of the local team or the "big" game.

According to Boyle, sports in the United States result from some flaw in the national character. In large measure they are the end result of a number of factors: industrialization, immigration, urbanization, increased leisure and income, commercial promotion, and upper-class patronage. Boyle says that American sports are not of the common people and the frontier, but instead come from an upper-class and urban impulse.

Sports, like any other social institution, can be used for both good or evil. If they are used to show superiority of race, creed, or nationality, they will serve only as an additional source of misunderstanding and conflict. A setting does exist within sports for common understanding, respect, equality of opportunity, and reasoning through good judgment and intelligence, which, in turn, provides the requirements of a strong

[1] Robert H. Boyle, *Sport—Mirror of American Life* (Boston: Little, Brown, 1963).

profession. Sports appear to have the ingredients to serve professional objectives similar to other strong professions such as medicine and law.

Athletics and sports have numerous professional groups and associations. There is virtually no sport that does not have a professional association bringing together those associated with that sport. The associations are local, regional, national, and in many instances international. In the United States professional associations are found in football, basketball, baseball, hockey, golf, tennis, and several other sports and are subdivided into coach, player, owner, trainer, and personnel groups associated with the particular sport. There are also associations that deal with the entire scope of sports, such as the National Collegiate Athletic Association; American Association for Health, Physical Education, and Recreation; and many others. They all have a concern for regulations and standards in the conduct of their sport. It would be most difficult for individual institutions to program athletics and sports without standards and regulations set by professional associations. The degree of regulation varies considerably; some sports are closely regulated and some are only minimally regulated.

An attempt will be made in this chapter to give an overall view of the status of athletics and sports in the American culture as they represent a segment of the culture and as they compare with other associations that have been established over a number of years. The criteria for determining the strength of a profession will be used as the basis for future analysis. This review will not be generated through direct comparison but simply will include statements about athletics and sports as a profession.

Specialized Techniques. Participation and leadership in sports and athletics are distinguished by specialized techniques for the participant, coach, trainer, and other professional leaders. They are developed and learned by the participant and by professional leaders in all facets of sports and are essential for effective participation and for effective teaching on the part of the professional leader. Athletics and sports are recognized as requiring specialized skills and techniques, but in some instances their social significance is questioned.

Communications. Professional technique must be able to be communicated through a highly specialized educational discipline. Because a number of leadership roles in athletics and sports require a university degree, the preparation for professional leadership in sports and athletics is a specialized program of physical education. For the participant, educational preparation is unnecessary, as is true for many professional leadership roles, such as that of professional coaches. For sports and athletics in educational institutions, leadership preparation is usually required.

Professional Controls. The requirements of professional control for practices within a profession will reflect the status of a profession. For sports and athletics controls do exist through some professional associations (e.g., NCAA for member institutions), but professional control bodies do not occur with enough frequency for sports and athletics to be considered a profession. Controls remain institutional, through associations or conference membership (e.g., Big 10 conference, NCAA, and so on). Sports and athletics still have a great deal to achieve with respect to professional status.

Standards. A strong profession will set standards for all operational aspects within its bounds, such as training, leadership qualifications, and so on. Sports and athletics are, of course, not without standards for participation and leadership, but these standards come from local associations, institutions, or even conference memberships. This criterion has not been achieved throughout sports and athletics. Standards are set by subgroups rather than by the professional body in totality.

Codes of Ethics. A strong profession is regulated by a code of ethics applied to all phases of practice and leadership. In many sports and athletic organizations individual groups, institutions, and some membership associations have established their own code of ethics. This is not true, however, in the case of professional groups dealing with sports and athletics on a national basis, except in isolated instances. On an international level the International Olympic Federation has requirements that must be met for membership. This can, however, hardly be considered a professional association.

Public Service. Service to the public beyond the limits of mere personal gain is an important requirement for a profession. Sports and athletics are, indeed, primarily a matter of individual involvement, but they also provide services to the public. These services are provided through programs whose objective is the achievement of educational goals from sports and athletics for personal recreation and personal gain. The requirements of this criterion have yet to be fulfilled by the various professional associations in sports and athletics.

Professional Domain: Conceptual Structure

Sports and athletics permeate nearly all levels of contemporary society. There is virtually not a single person who is untouched by sports or athletics in one way or another. The interest generated by athletic contests is reflected by the fact that the sports page of our daily newspaper is second in readership only to the front-page news. Radio and television both devote major segments to sports, and millions of copies of special-interest sports magazines are sold each week. Whatever the values and goals, the effects of sports and athletics are deeply significant. As international interests and travel have grown, the effects have become worldwide.

The professional domain of physical activity is conceptually conceived (List 5). The following deals with the components of this conceptual structure.

List 5. Professional domain of physical activity as sports and athletics

1. Sociocultural structure.
   - a. Communications.
   - b. Education.
   - c. Ethnic.
   - d. Health.
   - e. History.
   - f. Human involvement.
   - g. Integration.
   - h. Mores.
   - i. Occupations.
   - j. Political categories.
   - k. Professional categories.
   - l. Recreational categories.
   - m. Security categories.
   - n. Social categories.
   - o. Traditions.

2. Personal and societal goals.
   - a. Achievement.
   - b. Biological goals.
   - c. Competition.
   - d. Health.
   - e. Individual goals.
   - f. Interaction.
   - g. Leisure.
   - h. Physical fitness.
   - i. Public goals.
   - j. Skills and mechanics.
   - k. Social goals.
   - l. Understandings.

3. Professional structure.
   - a. Associations.
   - b. Certification.
   - c. Development and growth.
   - d. Education.
   - e. Ethics.
   - f. Evaluation.
   - g. Facilities.
   - h. Finances.
   - i. Leadership.
   - j. Legislation, laws, regulations.
   - k. Organizations.
   - l. Programs.
   - m. Safety and protection.
   - n. Services.
   - o. Societal contributions.
   - p. Standards.
   - q. Training.

4. Specialization structure.
   - a. Handicapped sports.
   - b. Individual and dual sports.
   - c. Lifetime sports.
   - d. Low organization games.
   - e. Modified sports.
   - f. Play therapy.
   - g. Recreational contributions.
   - h. Team sports.

5. Program structure.
   - a. Adaptive.
   - b. Athletics.
   - c. Club sports.
   - d. Educational programs.
   - e. Extramural programs.
   - f. Games.
   - g. Intramural programs.
   - h. Preventive programs.
   - i. Recreational programs.
   - j. Rehabilitation.
   - k. Sports.
   - l. Therapeutic programs.
   - m. Vocational programs.

Sociocultural Structure. What constitutes the sociocultural domain of athletics and sports in society? Like any strong sociocultural or political force in a community, athletics and sports influence the lives and practices of almost everyone. In some way, as either spectator or participant, sports constitute a part of the life of nearly everyone. Athletics and sports have become a major part of the American culture and therefore have become an integral part in the programs of social institutions.

The largest sociocultural influence of sports is found in schools, colleges, universities, and many commercial agencies. They have become part of the educational program. The acceptance of athletes and sports by educational institutions is of primary significance in the professional domain of athletics and sports (List 5).

In addition to individual occupations, other sociocultural components affecting sports include politics, communications, education, social and religious traditions within a community, and other cultural elements that constitute a particular society. The societal setting is a powerful force in shaping the choices of sports that are used as leisure activities.

Personal and Societal Goals. The social structure in sports is in many respects a duplicate of society. Sports contain all the elements of a social order and a way of life desired by its people. Sports and athletics in the American culture carry beyond a mere physical base and contain elements of human development and understanding. The most unique of these elements, of course, is the physical component. No other social medium can make such a substantial contribution to life and health. Sports and athletics also make equally important contributions in social adjustment and development—in the broadening of the intellect through understanding the human body and the effects of physical activity, and in the environmental and emotional adjustments of the individual to himself and to society.

The goals for sports and athletics are numerous and vary with professional backgrounds and interests of the participants, institutions, and professional education programs. These can be idealistic goals or merely the goal of participation, for the sheer fun.

Sports involve the sociocultural dimension, characteristic of such social institutions as the YMCA, Boys Clubs, and so on, or the professionally planned dimension, which is developed for financial gain. In either case the goals will differ.

The following presentation is a summary of individual sports goals.

1. *Individual health.* Physical development is one of the major components of health. Vigorous sports represent the medium for physical development. Probably the major reason for sports in educational institutions is the realization that other school programs cannot accomplish the goal of physical development. In recent years, with the lack of physi-

cal work in today's society, sports and athletics have become important to nearly everyone. Physical exercise is needed to maintain normal bodily functions and to control weight and make a normal diet possible.

Fitness is required for participation in sports and athletics. For the professional athlete the major concern is his ability to perform at the level required for success. This is also a health goal, although the level of fitness will differ.

2. *Skill and physical work efficiency.* One cannot participate in sports and athletics without adequate individual skills. The more skillful the individual, the more likely it is that he will enjoy participation and will continue physical activity. For educational goals, skill in sports and athletics has increased meaning. Sports skill is important in preparing the body for all physical work by developing the highest degree of neuromuscular efficiency. Health and neuromuscular efficiency in delaying the onset of fatigue require one to learn how to apply the necessary powers of the body with the minimum expenditure of energy. Through basic instruction in efficient movement, an individual may more readily learn to adapt to other motor movements that are not necessarily directly associated with sports or athletics. One, therefore, prepares for efficient living through preservation of the body energy reserves by reducing unnecessary strain. This is another major goal for sports and athletics.

3. *Understanding the human organism.* In recent years participants in sports, especially professional leaders, have become increasingly interested in the science and medicine of sports and have been instrumental in the sports medicine discipline. One reason for this development is the recent emphasis given to physical exercise. Research in sports medicine and its varied sciences has advanced most rapidly during the past decade and a half. Knowledge and understanding of the effects of sports and physical exercise are now reasonably well developed. The importance of conditioning in achieving success is recognized by both participants and coaches. This is true in both professional and nonprofessional sports.

Knowledge in modern sports includes many aspects of the organism functioning, such as how it adapts to stress of various kinds, how it recovers from the stress of vigorous exercise, and how preparation and habits of living affect performance.

4. *Social goals.* Social goals definitely play a major role in the purposes of sports in schools, youth groups, and social agencies. With proper leadership and supervision, sports can contribute to the desired individual and group social qualities. Educational programs are therefore designed to prepare youth for leadership and citizenship.

5. *Leadership.* Preparing the individual for leadership and follower roles in democratic life is a responsibility of all social institutions. Because of the informal nature and close association of sports-oriented relationships, sports and athletics are particularly well equipped to

contribute to this citizenship goal. The athlete is constantly in either a leadership or follower role. The question, of course, is how the roles are related to performance in sports.

Democratic principles are fundamental to successful participation in sports. Such principles as respect for the human personality, equality of opportunity, and solution of problems by reason and intelligence are some of the democratic principles necessary in sports and athletics. These principles also apply to other social interactions.

6. *Human adjustment.* It has been demonstrated that successful athletes have a higher capacity for adjustment to the group than those without athletic experience. Sports and athletics under proper leadership and controls can contribute to this important human goal.

During the primary years the child can use physical activity to learn about his abilities, his traits, and how he relates to other individuals. In the attempt to find a satisfying role in life, recognition of strengths and weaknesses is extremely important.

Professional Structure. The professional domain of athletics and sports incorporates all facets essential for sports advancement and operations in society. These include leadership, professional associations, standards, ethics, and so on. The quality of any profession is determined by the social controls and standards for operation.

Those interested in sports range from the interested citizen to the professional. The citizen may serve on school boards, institutional boards of trustees, or boards of control giving professional direction to athletics and sports. Sports professionals provide some measure of quality to the conduct of athletics and sports within numerous professional institutions. The professionals are the school administrators, college and university personnel, community social and political leaders, administrators of professional sports clubs, community social agency directors, and others professionally prepared and salaried.

Professional associations are organized within each sport to regulate and promote the sport, to bargain collectively and so on (e.g., action on whether members should strike). The regulations and controls are internal for associations, which also fall under the jurisdiction of institutional regulation. These associations and institutions establish the guidelines for sports that help promote and maintain their position. With the powerful social influences of sports, the establishment of social controls is, indeed, necessary (List 5).

Specialization Structure. Sports and athletics are found in many forms. These stem from the organization and direction set for and taken by physical activity. The specialized activity forms include modified sports for a variety of age differences; sports for the handicapped; lifetime sports for development of skills that can be applied on all age levels; individual and dual sports specifically designed for a small number of people with little group organization; and sports organized for recreational participation (List 5).

Specialization in physical activity is designed to fit a specific segment of society. The sport may remain essentially the same in performance but have a quite different purpose. Tennis taught in a professional educational institution is planned to give understanding and skill that can later be utilized during leisure. Tennis for the professional athlete, however, is designed for commercial reasons and financial gain. Professional requirements for success must be on a level that represents optimal individual capacities. The athlete, to begin with, must have the basic aptitudes and physical attributes that fit his chosen sport. It is impossible to prepare a huge endomorph for a championship performance in the pole vault. Each sport has certain intrinsic requirements that must be met if the sport is to be applied by the individual on a professional level.

Sports and athletics, however, can be utilized by everyone if participation is planned for exercise, enjoyment, or competition with peers of similar aptitudes and abilities (List 5).

Program Structure. Athletics and sports attract a large segment of society. Sports have become more than mere diversion. They affect the lives of all people in some way. Sports and athletics are now more than just parts of society influenced by the culture, but they have themselves become cultural forces with such strength that society is influenced by them (List 5).

Physical activity in sports functions as an adaptation to the interests, abilities, and capacities of people. In addition to these personal restrictions, facilities and the individual environment are also major factors in sports selection. Basically, physical activity starts with the abilities and interests of people in a particular activity that require certain preliminary qualifications in coordination, balance, muscular strength, agility, and other physiological functions. These qualities are combined with a particular sport; participation then becomes enjoyable and a part of the life practice.

Age and motivation are important in sports participation. Sports can be modified to fit the individual, so that it is possible for everyone to participate. Modifications come in nearly all sports. These modifications allow individuals lacking maturity or physical ability to participate in and enjoy such sports as basketball, football, tennis, baseball, and many others.

Another major factor in sports is the emphasis, or the lack of it, on competition. Golf is a popular sport for individuals of varying abilities. For most it is a period away from professional stresses on the job and a pleasure to be in the open and walking during pleasant competition. The ability to play and the score are important, of course, but not of major consequence. This is not true for the pro golfer. He lives by the winnings he receives from playing the game. Each stroke is of major importance. The differences between the majority of pros is one or two strokes on any given day. On this level the entire person must become part of each movement on the course, so that total mental-physical harmony can be achieved. This concept represents a major difference from golf used as recreation.

Another major factor in sports is the reason for participation. Sports are part of the programs in schools, colleges, social agencies, clubs, and hospitals for individual achievement of goals important in human development. The goals are numerous and include health and fitness, skills for sports, mechanics of work, socialization, human relations, and racial integration (List 5). Sports involve participation goals such as recreational games, intramural sports, extramural or club sports, adaptive sports, and sports for the handicapped.

Sports also have to meet the adaptation needs of the physical and social environment. These include population congestion, climate, and physical terrain. Sports tend to modify themselves to fit the environment.

Programs of sports have vocational application. Coaches, physical education instructors, trainers, and rehabilitation specialists study and apply sports professionally. Programs are planned for each professional category. The curriculum is designed to give understanding and skill to the applications of physical activity and sports in the achievement of vocational and professional goals.

Professional Domain: Content Structure

The scope and conceptual structure of athletics and sports have been presented in the preceding section. It is worthwhile at this time to view the primary conceptual categories that comprise the professional foundations of sports and athletics. This is followed by a delineation of these primary categories into the subparts or concepts that constitute them. This analysis is designed to give understanding to physical activity planned as a profession within the context of athletics and sports. It is extremely difficult in the presentation of the conceptual structure of athletics and sports to separate "structure" and "content," because some content is necessary to present a given structure with reasonable understanding. The primary intent is to concentrate on both; therefore their content is separated into two sections. Initially, it seems important to understand the structure of sports and athletics before professional development can begin. The essentials of successful operations are therefore included in the structure. The design for this section calls for emphasizing content. This is accomplished by further development of the conceptual structure of athletics and sports.

Sociocultural Content. The mores of a society influence the nature and role of sports and athletics, but the influences of sports and athletics on these mores are also becoming increasingly evident. They now play a major part in the leisure life of people of all ages. The varying content of the many sports makes it possible to fit the needs and desires of people of various age, motivation, and goal levels. Participation with some children begins early in life and continues through the later years of life. There is always a sport to fit the desires of the individual.

The major requirements of sports and athletics are the skills and the physical requirements for participation. Unless it is possible to participate, there is little chance to benefit from sports, except through spectatorship. Each sport has particular requirements and therefore will also vary in possible outcomes. It is possible to group sports into categories based upon numerous common participation requirements and outcomes. Nevertheless, each sport is unique in some respect.

What is the sociocultural content of sports and athletics? The method in which the individual participates in a sport is the primary determinant of the end results. The outcomes will also differ with each sport. With participation in the appropriate sport it is possible to induce sociocultural changes in the individual and society. Negative results are also possible if sports are improperly applied and administered. Positive results have been found to have a high correlation with a number of social problems. These include the fight against racial, religious, and social prejudice. It is not inappropriate to state that blacks received one of their first major boosts toward economic and social equality through sports. This achievement was possible because of the close sociocultural contact and personal interactions made possible by sports.

The content of sports and athletics has contributed to governmental and political goals in the human resources management and integration projects in communities, in nations, and between nations. The Olympic Games contribute to the cultural understanding among the participating nations. Positive results far exceed any negative consequences.

With the need to fill increasing leisure hours now becoming a major sociocultural problem, sports have contributed significantly to the lives of people away from work. This is particularly true for the rapidly increasing retired population. The development of sports centers, camps, lodges, and recreational facilities has been so rapid during the past ten years that it would be almost impossible to keep account of this development on a national basis. This development has been made possible by the short work week and improvements in transportation.

The increasing role of sports and athletics in the communications media is evidenced by the amount of time now devoted to them in programming. Week-end sports, for example, take up a major portion of today's television time.

Personal and Societal Goal Content. Sports and athletics are of individual and societal importance in achieving personal and societal goals. Participation in sports and athletics can contribute immensely to the health, fitness, and human association patterns of the individual and group. These achievements not only extend life, through physical development and organic maintenance, but, of more importance, provide the physical resources for an energetic life. Today's demanding society requires mental and physical tolerance levels. The goal is to prepare the individual adequately for living in such a society.

Sports and athletics have biophysical and sociopsychological applications to human development. It is possible to change the human organism within these disciplines. The change can be biophysical (Chapter 4) or sociopsychological (Chapter 5). The changes, of course, will be determined by how one participates in the activity—the intensity, duration, and frequency of participation. It is possible to advance the human organism to high levels. Development can advance to the level of the individual's capacity. Each individual will differ in capacities and also differ for each individual quality. The content of sports and athletics is objective and valid in meeting individual and societal goals within the limits of physical activity.

Professional Content. Sports and athletics have been developed into numerous professions in the United States. There are as many professions (or more) as there are individual sports. In most instances there are associations for the coaches, trainers, educators, scientists, and medical personnel organized to establish policies and standards within each individual sports activity.

In the United States, a professional association does not exist encompassing all sports and athletics or their constituent parts. Professional associations number into the thousands and are all independent and self-regulating. The only common professional regulations or policies are the laws (e.g., state laws on preparation of coaches for the schools, use of drugs, and so on) and national associations for university or professional sports for its members (e.g., NCAA, NFL). There are other regional professional associations, such as the Big 10 Athletic Conference, which sets policies for the Big 10 member universities in sports and athletics.

Without professional regulations and policies, the world of sports and athletics would probably in many instances become antisocial within the culture. Gambling and bribery alone are major threats to maintaining the concept behind sports. Efforts by professional associations (e.g., the Olympic Committee) to eliminate drugs from international competition, for example, have been difficult and not completely successful. Without regulations, competition would be on an "anything-goes" basis and would soon be out of control.

The role of the profession in sports and athletics is more important than anything that is a part of these programs. The professions set directions, standards, and controls in order to gain positive physical and social benefits. These programs are "locked in" to a society or institution to provide it with internal balance. They have become integral parts of life, but they are by no means the most important influence in life. One such exception would be the professional coach, whose job and life in the community are directly connected to sports. For the average citizen, sports become an important part of leisure, but that is all. There are other components of the culture that make demands on the attention of the citizenry.

The professional association functions of sports and athletics include every element of the game, such as leadership, facilities, finances, and other elements necessary for participation and competition. Sports leadership must be properly prepared, and professional standards must therefore be established and administered. Professional guides and policies deal with ethics, preparation for each of the many facets within the sports, schedules for the protection of the athlete, medical standards for participation, safety of the participant, and standards that regulate the physical setting for participation.

It would be nearly impossible without a carefully planned survey to estimate the number of professional groups that exist in sports and athletics. Any group that has objectives, purposes, officers, and a definite program is considered to be a professional association. The influence of associations may not be of major consequence, but the group accepts their decisions and implements them. The actions of associations, then, are primarily of importance to a particular institution, sport, or local setting.

It can be safely estimated that every school, every higher educational institution, every social agency, and nearly every individual in the United States are influenced by sports and athletics in one way or another. The professional responsibilities for such influence are numerous and management is of major importance. The fulfillment of responsibilities determines the worth, acceptance, and growth of sports and athletics, whether in a local community or internationally.

In dealing with professional associations in sports and athletics, responsibilities differ, from operational to policy-determining responsibilities.

Operational Professional Associations. Operational professional associations include groups, conferences, committees, and councils that regulate institutional programs among membership institutions. They will decide on requirements for institutional membership in a conference and the requirements for keeping that membership.

The objectives of professional operational associations differ with each association. The principal purpose of these associations, however, is to conduct among membership institutions sports and athletics programs that contribute to the welfare of the participant and give institutional balance to sports and athletics within an institution. The functions of these associations include determining eligibility for participation and membership, scheduling, determining the length of the season, establishing personnel qualifications, and recruiting, in addition to the other regulations necessary for fair and favorable results.

Policy-Determining Professional Associations. Policy-determining associations are organized to review practices, provide information, and prepare statements on professional matters for the benefit of the members who have elected to become a part of the association. They do not have any *direct* control on institutional programs in sports and athletics, but they set the policies, principles, standards of operation, and standards of knowledge and education of professional people in these fields. These groups also prepare professional people for sports and athletics in all phases. This preparation is based on the premise that it will improve the worth of sports and athletics for the participant and their contributions to culture and society. Professional workers who are sincerely interested in sports and athletics will become members and contribute to the programs of these associations and other institutional programs.

Professional standards are needed for all operations in sports and athletics. In the United States a number of professional associations are actively working in sports and athletics. Some of the work of these associations is outlined in the following:

1. *Objectives.* Reports, studies, and research on the potentials of sports and athletics for developing youth and adults and its contributions to culture and society are major functions of professional associations. A profession must be judged by its professional members. The objectives to be met and the contributions to be made to individuals and society are generally planned by the associations.

2. *Personnel.* An important responsibility for a profession is to set the qualifications for personnel working in sports and athletics. The profession represents the only control upon institutional practices, which in many instances will underestimate the qualifications for leadership in sports and athletics.

3. *Programs.* Program standards are important professional responsibilities. They include not only sports and athletics but also programs for the systematic development of the participant. Standards also apply to the time schedule for sports and athletics with respect to the individual

maturation level. Each sport and physical activity has unique value in human development. The method of planning the program is therefore of great significance. The major purpose of sports and athletics is to promote individual development. Despite the concerns and accomplishments of individual institutions, this function is a professional one. Of course, differences will be found in institutions, but they must be judged in the light of the standards set by the profession.

4. *Facilities and equipment.* Standards for facilities and equipment in sports and athletics programs are professional responsibilities of the first order. Standards apply to all ages and social institutions. There is always a question of how funds should be allocated for optimal program results. Standards representing the best judgment and utilization of data based upon program results are used to provide guidance to administrators in the many social institutions utilizing sports and athletics in their institutional programs.

There are a considerable number of studies and conference proceedings that deal with the subject of facilities and equipment for sports and athletics. These will aid workers in providing facilities efficiently. The costs for sports and athletics are high.

5. *Administration.* Standards for administrative policies are important professional functions. Professional guidance will aid administrators in the many social institutions with their sports and athletic programs. Administrative policies of particular importance are salary and salary schedules; specialization requirements; classification of professional workers; safety standards for equipment, facilities, buildings, and land; legislation and regulations providing support and protection to all participants and professional workers in sports and athletics; standards of ethics for professional behavior; attitudes and working conditions for those in sports and athletics; and certainly standards for the behavior of both spectators and players.

Institutional administration and professional associations must be closely related. It is the right of every individual to choose not to become associated with a professional association, because professional associations are made up of members who elect to belong and contribute. The fundamental value of professional associations is their freedom of action and implementation, even though the failure to participate by some members hurts the profession. Decisions are made through democratic operations within the social institution and on the premise that each institution desires to improve services to the members seeking help from that institution.

Professional Preparation. In addition to a professional association's responsibility for standards in sports and athletics, it has a *second* major responsibility, that of guiding institutions in the preparation of personnel associated with or working directly for programs of sports and athletics. Institutions alone should not perform this function without first requiring professional reviews, standards, and certification of personnel. Many physical education institutions put minimal and less than minimal resources into these programs. In many instances graduates are inadequately prepared. This is particularly true in the sports and athletics facets of physical education preparation.

Preparation for sports and athletics includes various classifications of personnel preparation in content and preparation in institutional services and services to different age groups. Programs for preparation of personnel will differ, but guides for the preparation of each are necessary. Numerous professional meetings are held on professional preparation. Guides are available to individuals and institutions who seriously wish to improve personnel and institutional standards and programs. Sports and athletics preparation ranges from that for the performer who is an outstanding professional athlete to that for the M.D. and Ph.D. graduates who plan to work in colleges and universities and who have specialized responsibilities in some aspect of these programs.

Specialization Content. The flexibility of sports and athletics in meeting the interests and abilities of people is nearly beyond imagination. It ranges from the champion representing the best in a sport to sports that can be played by everyone. It represents activity for all ages from the very young to the aged who both need physical activity. It includes the normal person and those who are in wheel chairs or are paraplegic. The same sport can be modified to fit nearly everyone.

In sports the high degree of specialization in skill and physical abilities is a challenge to the participant and of deep interest to the spectator. Spectator interest is correlated to skill and physical requirements in a sport.

Program Content. Physical activities in the form of sports and athletics are planned in U.S. communities for all age groups. It would be nearly impossible to conduct a survey and determine the costs involved in planning and conducting programs of sports and athletics, but such programs are now a firmly recognized part of the economy of this country.

The difference between physical activities classified as sports and those classified as athletics lies largely in the attitude of the participant and in his professional objectives for the physical activity. In both sports and athletics the participant applies physical activity in a competitive role, either by himself or with others. In sports, physical activity may in some instances be purely for enjoyment and fun, without any other objectives. In athletics the goal is success, and success is winning. Competition between individuals and teams is usually in direct proportion to the importance given to winning.

The setting of sports is different from that of athletics. Sports involve physical activity by individuals and groups for personal motives and objectives. The reasons are numerous and include fitness, health, enjoyable leisure, and social contact.

Sports and athletics begin when a child enters school and they continue through college, university, or other post-high-school institutions. Social agencies in a community include the YMCA, Boys Clubs, churches, fraternal organizations, and service clubs; all frequently offer sports and athletics as a service to the people in the community. Business organizations have fitness programs to promote morale. Communities program sports for commercial objectives, as a business for financial gain. Colleges and universities have extensive athletic programs for their students. Athletic programs are found in most social institutions in the United States, and in many, such as professional sports, they constitute the total program. In both American public and private schools, the programs constitute a large part of the budget for personnel, facilities, and program time.

There are a number of classifications of sports and athletics. The method by which the activities are classified will be determined by their program purposes. The author has prepared eleven classifications for physical activity. This classification system is an attempt to organize sports according to their relation or application. The eleven classifications are organizational type, developmental potentials, professional applications, objectives, academic disciplines, administrative requirements, physical environment, age requirements, maturation requirements, environmental settings, and energy requirements. In each division, subclassifications differentiate the nature of the physical activity. In most instances the organizational-type classification is most generally used because it is closely related to the number of participants and facilities. This classification includes all sports and athletics and it is based on the method in which they fit the requirements of the individual and group. This is not always the primary reason for the selection of a sport, but it is one of the most important factors in meeting personal participation requirements. The "organizational-type" classifications include low organization activities and games with little structural requirements (e.g., shooting baskets), individual activities (e.g., swimming and archery), dual activities (e.g., fencing and wrestling), team activities (e.g., baseball and basketball), group activities (e.g., calisthenics and relays), aquatics (e.g., diving and swimming), conditioning exercises (e.g., weight training and jogging), and remedial activities (e.g., weight lifting and calisthenics). It is possible to list four of five thousand physical activities in these eight classifications or with some organized as sports and athletics.

Contributions to Society and the Individual

The contributions made by sports and athletics to the individual, society, and culture throughout the world are innumerable. They have the potential for human and social development that can transform the individual physically, socially, and emotionally. These transformations also apply to the group.

Sports and athletics have spread throughout communities and nations around the world at a very rapid pace in the past few years. They have helped destroy the barriers of race, religion, and social class, in many communities and among countries. The code for the participant in sports today is not one of social, political, or economic necessity; it is play for competition and fun. With proper leadership, particularly in the schools, sports can have a major effect on the individual personality.

Probably in no other setting do the principles of democracy apply with greater emphasis than in sports activities. The principle of equality of opportunity, for example, is applied almost unnoticed. One participates by ability alone; other factors are extraneous. Some of the other democratic principles applicable to sports are respect for the human personality, problem solving by reason and intelligence, self-government, cooperative action for successful and effective play, and self-discipline as the basis for responsibility. These principles are learned and practiced. The contributions of sports to the individual significantly influence today's society.

The need for physical activity for everyone has never been more important than it is today. The physical requirements of modern living have been greatly reduced, but the need for a strong physical body is greater today than at any time in our history. Stress and emotional strain all are physiological phenomena, and the costs are paid by physiological processes. These processes are affected by modern life. The increase in heart disease alone gives significant evidence of what is occurring to the individual in the modern world. The countermeasures are not escape devices such as drugs, but effective physical preparation of the human organism to minimize these stress factors. One can hardly change the nature of modern life; society and its various professions must recognize these conditions and then prepare individuals to meet the requirements of our demanding culture. Sports, athletics, and other forms of physical activity can accomplish this task.

The need for physical activity in modern life and the value of sports and athletics in meeting individual needs form the foundations for a profession. As a career, sports and athletics provide life-long opportunities. In this respect, professional status has been achieved, and there are many professional opportunities. When criteria are applied for what constitutes a profession, sports and athletics are deficient. The deficiencies primarily center around professional regulations and controls that oversee practices in all aspects of sports and athletics and that define qualifications for leadership and participation.

There are numerous groups organized around some aspect of sports. They establish and administer regulations adopted by the group. Many of these groups have well-established regulations and are regarded as a profession in most respects. These organizations have made it possible to govern sports.

Chapter 9

Culture and Leisure

Culture and leisure are closely related. Leisure in modern living cannot be studied or analyzed outside of a specific cultural context. Knowledge about a culture is essential to understanding a people and their traditions, ways of life, and leisure interests fully.

The culture contains the resources and social institutions that enable people to solve the problems posed by the total environment. It is developed by and shaped around the problems and responsibilities an individual must face as a part of a family, group, business, or society. The activities of an individual are not isolated phenomena, but are related to his associations with other individuals and groups as well as the physical setting. In this sense it appears that people are shaped by their culture. This is, in part, true, but an individual can have a significant and, in some instances, major effect on both the social and physical environments. With the present speed of travel cultural changes have become evident in spectacular and tangible ways. Cultures are both different and divergent. Some differ significantly. The leisure life of society and its pattern of daily living are significantly influenced by the culture, and individual habits and practices affect the practices of society. These changes represent adaptations by the culture. The processes, however, are in most instances relatively slow. Rapid changes come only through violent upheaval such as revolution, rebellion, and, during the twentieth century, world war, prosperity, or depression.

Kaplan [1] cites Herskovits's characterization of culture as (1) learned and constantly created; (2) made up of elements from the biological,

---

[1] Max Kaplan, *Leisure in America: A Social Inquiry* (New York: Wiley, 1960).

142

environmental, psychological, and historical "components of human existence"; (3) structured; (4) constantly changing; (5) exhibiting patterns and regularities; and (6) the instrument by which the individual adjusts to his social setting and gains the raw materials for creative expression. Kaplan summarized the principle stating that "culture is the basic conceptual tool for all the social sciences, from the daring task of comparing whole cultural systems to the humbler and more tractable research on the development of personality." Kaplan further states that understanding the nature of the whole culture is relevant to understanding leisure. The leisure activities of an individual take place within a culture, wherever and whatever it may be.

Rather than relying on individual views of the interpretation of leisure, Kaplan first summarizes and classifies possible definitions of leisure that could apply to personal interpretations and uses of leisure and second he presents the essential elements of leisure as they are organized within his structural framework. Because these interpretations are relevant in the study of leisure and physical activity, each will be reviewed.

The first interpretation involves categorizing individual views and classifying them into a viable system that would encompass all the elements necessary for an acceptable view of leisure.

> Leisure as a bulk of time, qualitatively distinct from other time, such as the evening.
> Leisure as freedom from those activities that have to be done, such as work or household chores.
> Leisure as an end, distinct from work as a means.
> Leisure as a minimum of obligation to others, to routine, even to oneself.
> Leisure as re-creation, to prepare for better work, to store up energy or knowledge.
> Leisure as self-improvement, whether in study, seeking new friends or new experiences.
> Leisure as social control, using the time of others to win them over or influence them, i.e., Roman Games, German Youth.
> Leisure as a social symbol of class position, age or success.
> Leisure as sets of attitudes or motivations, not a content.
> Leisure as physiological or emotional necessity, such as therapy or physical rest.

The second approach by Kaplan is a construct that will permit both subjective perception and objective analysis. This construct contains the elements against which both leisure and physical activity can be assessed. The elements of leisure within this construct are "(1) an antithesis to 'work' as an economic function, (2) a pleasant expectation and recollection, (3) a minimum of involuntary social-role obligations, (4) a psychological perception of freedom, (5) a close relation to values of the culture, (6) the inclusion of an entire range from inconsequence and insignificance to weightiness and importance and (7) often, but not necessarily, an activity characterized by the element of play." Kaplan states, "Leisure is none of these by itself but all together in one emphasis or another."

Culture and Leisure

The quality of a culture will, to a very large degree, be determined by the quality of the leisure activities available. These can range from unsocial practices or no practices at all to activities that enrich the lives of all, adding significantly to the cultural level of a society. Culture ranges in its effects from the individual as a single entity to the individual in a group or home situation to individuals and societies finally on a worldwide basis. The cultures in this country are determined by the people who comprise them, and these cultures can be easily observed and differentiated from cultures in other nations. There are some major differences between cultures, representing different ways of life, and varying cultural patterns may all be acceptable in their respective contexts.

In many countries around the world the sociocultural roles of physical activity, particularly those involving sports and athletics, are major and increasing in prominence. In the United States sports and athletics represent a significant element in the lives of many people, and therefore in the culture, and their influence is also increasing. As a result of the development of automation during the twentieth century and the resulting loss of physical work, people have begun to realize that leisure-time physical activity is essential for the maintenance of health, thus the increasing emphasis on participation.

The contributions of physical activity in its various forms are indeed valuable. The professional applications of physical activity are directed toward the development of the individual as a person and his relations with others. Professions are developed for the achievement of such goals. There are at least ten professions involved with the functional application of physical activity, and each contributes to leisure life and to the upgrading of the culture. Physical activity, however, must be properly applied. Its potentials in the context of culture and leisure are reported here as outcomes of properly administered physical activity.

1. *Physical activity contributes to the health of the individual and allows him to prepare for effective and positive outcomes from leisure.* A person in poor health does not have the vigor or enthusiasm to engage actively in leisure pursuits. He may do little more than sleep or rest. In such cases the individual may become discouraged and confused about life and his role in society. Certainly this setting is not conducive to a

positive, health-producing leisure program. Valuing good health is an essential part of preparation for an active leisure life that will result in higher levels of participation and further improvements in health.

A leisure life centered on sports, athletics, and physical activity has numerous contributions to make to health. The physical body can only be developed through a well-planned program of physical activity. Poor health practices are detrimental to the organism, and physical activity alone may not be enough to overcome such practices. Furthermore, the outcomes of physical activity will be severely curtailed because of lack of vigor and reduced intensity of participation.

Participation in physical activities is probably, as a total experience, one of the most positive leisure pursuits. The potential social as well as physical results are numerous, but the most basic contribution is the preparation of the participant to resist the forces of stress and fatigue. Within the bounds of physical activity, it is possible to find satisfaction and personal well-being that aid in making life rewarding.

2. *Physical activity contributes to the ability of the individual to perform effective and efficient human physical movements of all kinds, especially the sport and physical activity skills that contribute to the positive uses of leisure.* Enjoying being physically active requires that the participant achieve some degree of success, and for this physical resources and skills are needed. Of course, normal physical requirements can be met without skills in sports, but the potential results of physical activity will be greatly lessened and, more importantly, the pleasure greatly diminished without adequate sport skills.

Leisure is a time for personal enjoyment. Moreover, value is attained by selecting activities that aid in the improvement of individual personal responsibilities. The ability to participate in a sport causes the individual to plan adequate time for participation in it. In this way he will become an active user of leisure. The resulting pleasure and physical well-being prepare the individual for an active life and provide the physical resources to meet the body's daily demands. Leisure is, of course, important for enjoyment and fun, but leisure is also important for preparation for all other life activities and requirements.

One must be prepared for an active leisure life. If a person has no interests or skills, he finds little to do during the long hours on weekdays or week ends. All leisure life cannot and should not be physical in nature. A balance of many possible physical, social, and intellectual interests add to personality development and general well-being. Over a period of time, balanced leisure activities aid in maintaining the interest and enthusiasm needed to continue an active leisure life.

3. *Knowledge about the physical organism and the human personality aids in planning the wide use of leisure.* Knowledge of the human body is required to plan physical activity for leisure hours. Leisure should be a time for the body to recover and for health to be promoted. For

most favorable results, leisure should be planned in a similar manner to professional activities. Undesirable leisure practices can easily destroy health levels, but desirable activities will maintain and advance health. Physical activity should suit the individual's interests, personality, and available time. Of course, attitudes may serve as stronger motivators toward specific leisure pursuits than knowledge and understanding, but the latter are the essential requirements for obtaining desirable outcomes of leisure.

4. *Physical activity in the form of sports, athletics, and games represents a powerful medium for human socialization.* Physical activity can be highly structured and regulated as in athletics or informal with a minimum of rules and regulations in sports planned for personal fun and well-being. It can be a means of relaxation, providing a good change from highly demanding professional work.

There are many human qualities exhibited during physical activity. The informal interchange among individuals in sports activity has lasting effects. These can be good or bad, but changes will definitely occur. Because personal intensities reach extremely high levels during participation, the social effects of leisure can be powerful.

Each social being is characterized by qualities that distinguish him from all others. Certain social requirements are particularly applicable to sports participation, for example, the acceptance of discipline. Successful group interrelations require personal discipline. The desire to belong and the need for group acceptance are some of the important social motives for physical activity.

The social qualities inherent in sports can be classified into several groups. These include (a) self-discipline, (b) self-sufficiency (initiative, confidence), (c) personal regard for self and in relation to others (dignity, respect, honesty), and (d) the individual personality in daily work and leisure (interests, motivations, appreciations).

Leisure, of course, is a human need. It is necessary for balance in life and for recovery from the stress of work, but leisure used unwisely can destroy the individual both as a worker and as a human being.

5. *Physical activity in the form of sports, athletics, and games represents a medium for democratic human associations.* The establishment of democratic human associations is a desirable way of life and it is also a desirable basis for people living together in self-government. The potential of sports, athletics, and informal games to aid in the development of democratic behavior and understanding is substantial and includes all the democratic tenets of human associations. Knowledgeable and skillful leadership is required for the development of democratic attitudes and behavior through proper participation in sports, athletics, and games. What are the possibilities for the development of democratic behavior in physical activity? The basic democratic concepts can be grouped into the following categories.

a. Respect for human personality is an important tenet of democracy in all individual human relations as well as in self-government, and this quality should be an integral part of sports.
b. Equality of opportunity is a democratic tenet that is extremely important to the individual and democratic government, and it has been an important part of the desire to participate in sports and athletics.
c. The democratic tenets involving cooperation, discipline, responsibility, communication by fact and reason, and self-government are all essential ingredients in physical participation within its cultural context.

6. *Physical activity potentials are both a means and an end in rehabilitation.* Physical activity is applied in the physical rehabilitation process to prepare the individual for leisure physical activity. This process ranges from specific, formal exercises to improve human functions to the recreational applications of physical activity as sport and games. The understanding and techniques of physical rehabilitation come from several disciplines such as medicine and surgery, social sciences, psychological services, and education.

Medical and surgical rehabilitation is designed to prevent loss of conditioning; to recondition the patient whose physical powers have been reduced; to restore normal bodily functions; and to maintain human physical powers reduced through aging and general deterioration of the body by environmental forces and poor health practices.

The application of physical activity to the patient under medical treatment or following surgery must be carried out on an individual basis. Physical activity aids in the restoration of functions, but unwisely adapted can delay healing and aggravate an injury. The objective of rehabilitation is to restore the individual to normal health, and this objective will guide the choice of leisure physical activities.

Social rehabilitation is planned for those unable to make normal adjustments in society. Maladjustments may be individual or part of the family or societal context. Physical activity represents a powerful medium for the socialization of the individual. Socialization aids the process of physical participation, leading to continued improvement or development. Activity then becomes fun and social benefits result. The individual is then conditioned to want physical activity in his leisure program.

Psychological rehabilitation and social rehabilitation are closely related. Psychological rehabilitation is essentially concerned with mental traits, ranging from mental deficiencies of neural underdevelopment to organic deficiencies that render an individual incapable of meeting social requirements. Individuals with mental deficiencies caused by organic disease or hereditary problems can be aided by physical activity and physical therapy. Individuals with nonorganic deviations traceable to traumatic social experiences can be rehabilitated to normal status. Physical activity is a powerful medium for such rehabilitation. Leisure physical activity will serve to maintain individual normality by neutralizing the forces in daily life that exert negative influences on the individual.

Physical rehabilitation deals directly with physical handicaps resulting from disease, injury, or other causes. The objective is to correct the physical handicap or to provide mechanical means of support to prepare the body for normal movements or functions. Sport as physical therapy aids in rehabilitation. Physical rehabilitation can be accomplished through light, thermo-, electro-, and hydrotherapy. Preparation for and participation in physical activity will continue improvement to the limits of the handicap and aid in general rehabilitation of the individual to normal life activities.

Educational rehabilitation is designed to develop skills and understanding for normal activity in a society. Unfavorable daily living practices can negatively affect health and the ability to cope with the demands of one's job and society. This, in turn, will cause maladjustments that must be corrected. Some of the other factors that influence adjustment are attitude, dietary practices, interests, and leisure practices. These conditions can be influenced by education and educational rehabilitation, but preparation is needed to apply and participate in physical activity properly. The process is educational, but it requires knowledge of the activity itself and the values of physical participation. Proper preparation for physical activity provides the basis, and participation in physical activity continues to add to the positive development and pleasure provided by good use of leisure.

7. *Physical activity participation occurs within social and physical environments. When properly applied, physical activity represents a medium for understanding and enjoying the environment.* A major purpose of leisure is to rest, recuperate, and enjoy oneself. The environment provides the resources and the facilities. Physical activity serves as a social medium but also provides other benefits. One of the major purposes of physical education in our schools is to prepare the individual for the physical skills and requirements of adult life. The physical environment is the laboratory for the medium of physical activity. This country's mountains and lakes provide ideal facilities for leisure that contributes physically and socially to individual health and well-being. Leisure physical activity under such conditions is a constructive alternative that contributes to the expansion and enhancement of life.

8. *Physical activity is a factor in the growth and development of both youth and adults throughout life. It is therefore essential in the preparation for leisure and a positive factor in maintaining the human organism.* Physical preparation opens many additional opportunities. Leisure that includes sports adapted to individual physical potentials is constructive and enjoyable. The choices made will be motivated by physical resources, skills, and capabilities; by personal knowledge of possible results; and by availability of the social and physical environments that make sports

a rewarding experience. During the later part of life, major emphasis should be placed on leisure planning. Physical preparation and maintenance are major factors, because without physical abilities, energy and enthusiasm will be low and leisure performance will become more difficult.

9. *Physical activity contributes to the enrichment of life and thereby adds quality to life itself, particularly during leisure periods.* Years ago, man had little leisure. Physical work required most of one's time and most of one's physical energies. Rest was the needed ingredient during any free time. The reverse is now true. The work week has been significantly reduced and this trend is continuing. It would have been difficult to imagine a twenty-hour work week during the early years of this country's development, but this is now an actuality in some vocations. The large amount of free time available in today's society represents opportunities that can make living pleasant and satisfying. Physical activity should not represent the only leisure interest, but it may occupy a large part of leisure life if one includes sports spectatorship in addition to actual participation.

10. *Physical activity not only is an essential factor in maintaining human life, but also provides balance to living.* It does not seem possible to have enough leisure to meet all goals or be fully prepared for leisure. Leisure is intrinsically bound in the qualities of life and the uses to which it is put by the individual and by society. Whether leisure interests lean toward sports or travel, painting or community theater, woodworking or gardening, these new blocks of leisure time must find ways into man's life. The time must be actively used. Leisure is now available not only to the upper socioeconomic class but also to the remainder of society. In fact, a slight reversal in available leisure has been noted. The daily unskilled worker or technician today has more leisure than the professional who is actively engaged in achieving professional success.

Cultural Determinants of Leisure

Daily activity differs with each person, family, community, state, and nation. The infinite variety of activity available throughout the world is beyond imagination. Summing up the activities of an individual, family, or nation over a period of time leads to cultural classification, representing the cultural makeup of a society, from a single setting to the various national settings throughout the world.

Culture is the common way of life of the individual or group that enables one to solve problems posed by the total environment. Sociologists differ in the classification of cultural concepts or categories. They do agree on the organization of a general scheme for the major categories of these cultural concepts. These categories for characterizing the culture include speech in all forms; the physical needs of man in modern life; the knowledge, skill, and understanding required to meet ever-increasing societal pressures; religion and religious practices; the family and various other social systems; the government and all other forms of human management; and war and social conflicts of all forms. These categories are further described by sociologists as follows: (1) the elements arise from the components of human existence, (2) the elements are constantly changing, (3) the elements are structured to the nature of the individual and the group, (4) the elements exhibit patterns within life and life practices, (5) the elements are learned and put into practice, and (6) the concepts include the means by which the individual and the group adjust to a social setting. An attempt is made within this chapter and book to classify the primary categories of a culture as they are related to leisure. It should be noted that general and special cultural classifications are not significantly different.

The *influence of commercialization* represents a major cultural influence on leisure. Economic success determines to a large degree the scope and quality of individual and community leisure pursuits (List 6). The leisure activities available are largely influenced by economics. The economics of a community will determine what one is able to do during leisure, because economic levels determine what the community can do in providing resources, facilities, recreational activities, leadership, and so on.

List 6. The professional domain of physical activity in leisure

1. The influence of commercialization.
   - a. Athletics.
   - b. Automation.
   - c. Availability of resources.
   - d. Competition.
   - e. Equipment.
   - f. Facilities.
   - g. Interests.
   - h. Leadership.
   - i. Mass media.
   - j. Recreational activities.
   - k. Time and energy.
2. Social and institutional determinants.
   - a. Automation.
   - b. Church.
   - c. Communications.
   - d. Cultural mores and traditions.
   - e. Family.
   - f. Fraternal groups.
   - g. Government and politics.
   - h. Industry.
   - i. Occupations.
   - j. Peer groups.
   - k. Racial characteristics.
   - l. Schools.
   - m. Sex roles.
   - n. Social agencies.
   - o. Subcultures.
3. Personal factors.
   - a. Age characteristics.
   - b. Capacity levels.
   - c. Ego involvement.
   - d. Ethics and values.
   - e. Financial security.
   - f. Intelligence level.
   - g. Interests and hobbies.
   - h. Physical fitness.
   - i. Somatotype.
   - j. Tension and stresses.
   - k. Tolerance levels.

4. Transportation and communications.
   a. Advertising.
   b. Air.
   c. Automobile.
   d. Bicycle.
   e. Books and magazines.
   f. Motorcycle.
   g. Press.
   h. Radio.
   i. Rail.
   j. Snowmobile and sports.
   k. Television.
   l. Theater.
   m. Water.
5. The physical environment.
   a. Altitude.
   b. Climate.
   c. Geographical location.
   d. Health standards.
   e. Mountains.
   f. Pollution levels.
   g. Population explosion.
   h. Recreation resources.
   i. Survival resources.
6. Public relations.
   a. Economics.
   b. Government.
   c. Governmental agency.
   d. Government facility.
   e. Human relations.
   f. Human resources.
   g. Integration.
   h. International.
   i. Legislation.
   j. Military.

Social and institutional determinants are cultural forces influencing leisure. Social institutions direct activities to be engaged in by society and provide resources for these activities. They represent not only the resources of leisure, but also the facilities to fulfill these desirable objectives. Preparation for leisure comes to a large degree from the activities of social institutions. Their objectives are to prepare society for leisure as well as to provide for leisure program requirements. Facilities range from social clubs and churches to camps and physical recreational facilities needed to fulfill the varying societal interests.

Personal factors are generally highly correlated with leisure interests and practices. Leisure is the time when one's freedom of choice is restricted only by personal and financial limitations. Fullness of life comes largely through leisure interests and practices. One must prepare for this as one prepares for a profession. Vocational life does not provide much variety in its range of activities. Even at the highest professional levels, the degree of freedom is limited. A major portion of an individual's time is spent preparing for and practicing his chosen vocation, but preparation of leisure is generally left to chance. Individuals who learn a craft or skill or develop a hobby are prepared to gain fullness from their life. The person eager for freedom and time to continue a hobby will carry this enthusiasm over to his job and the remainder of his life. All life's activities will then benefit from this personal preparation.

Transportation and communications are important leisure determinants. Developments in transportation over the past fifteen years alone have revolutionized life in nearly all parts of the world. Traveling several hundred miles a day on modern freeways is not an uncommon event. Air transportation in the past ten to fifteen years has developed so that people can now travel throughout the world in a matter of hours. These developments give society the opportunity for leisure experiences that are deeply satisfying and personally beneficial. There are a number of resources available to the individual that will greatly enlarge his leisure interests, such as the press, television, transportation, and other modern technological developments that bring nations and cultures into close relationships with each other.

The physical environment represents the natural resources available for leisure pursuits. Preparation for the enjoyment of the physical environment is initiated by programs of schools and social agencies. Knowledge and skills are extremely important, particularly for leisure. In physical education, for example, the gymnasium, swimming pool, and athletic field represent the facilities for physical skill development. The objectives of this development are to prepare for leisure physical activities and to enjoy the natural facilities (e.g., lakes, rivers, mountains) and the many activities (e.g., swimming, boating, hiking, and camping) possible in nature.

Public relations on all governmental and societal levels affect leisure. The ways of life made available to the people in a community or nation must be carefully planned. Political and governmental agencies are created to fulfill these related goals, and public relations plays an important role in assisting in their accomplishment (List 6).

There are numerous needs in preparing for the positive application of leisure. The resources of a community or nation represent the potential available for construction of facilities and implementation of programs. Through public relations procedures laws are established allowing for the public availability of leisure facilities otherwise not fully used. The result is costs acceptable to the public. Through the efforts of governmental agencies environmental resources are made available to everyone in the community.

Leisure Within Cultures

In seeking a concept that can be useful in relating leisure to physical activity, two positions can be assumed: (1) define and relate leisure to its role in the activities that are considered leisure pursuits or (2) plan an ideal construct that includes the full range of concepts, categories, or activities that are considered to be within leisure.

Kaplan [2] interprets the first position in two ways. The first he determines by seeking responses from individuals on what they consider to be leisure or leisure pursuits and the second is a nonsophisticated classification in an attempt to organize the various views into a concrete

---

[2] Kaplan, op. cit.

classification system. Examples of the first case involve the motive for participation in an activity. The replies include relaxation, rest, getting away from work, exercise, developing fitness, and other similar motives.

The second approach, according to Kaplan, is to construct categories that avoid narrowness and permit both subjective and objective analysis. Such theoretical or professional classifications permit evaluation against situations representing normal societal modes of living or analysis against the desired outcomes of leisure and leisure activities. The "ideal construct" is presented as containing what are considered the essential elements of leisure.

1. An antithesis to work as an economic necessity.
2. A pleasant expectation or recollection.
3. A minimum involuntary social obligation.
4. A psychological perception of freedom.
5. A close relation to cultural values.
6. A full range of important to nonimportant activities.
7. Activities considered to be pleasant, fun, and play.

With this general understanding of leisure in culture, how does physical activity fit this concept as viewed through the interpretation and practices of society during leisure?

In order to view the leisure role of physical activity systematically, Kaplan's construct will be followed in the remainder of this discussion.

1. *Physical activity provides an antithesis of work.* Work per se may not be an antithesis to leisure. On the contrary, physical activity is work, but work viewed as a requirement for attaining the economic necessities of life is not generally viewed as leisure. It may, however, be very pleasurable and a more popular choice than leisure.

Leisure, however, is generally considered time away from the job. If work is sedentary, physical activity should be an integral part of leisure. If work is a professional sport, leisure choices may very well be sedentary. Physical activity in any form is a necessity for everyone. The pleasures may be the same despite different interests. Sports, however, do contain the potential for individual enjoyment as well as positive values for the physical body. Sports should therefore be an integral part of leisure life.

2. *Physical activity provides a pleasant expectation or recollection.* Enforced leisure, more commonly known as unemployment, is not pleasurable. Leisure per se is not an objective; rather it is the opportunity to enjoy activity not possible through work. Constructive leisure requires adequate planning and preparation. It is very unwise to start planning the day that one finally has leisure available, because inefficiency detracts from the enjoyment of the leisure pursuit. Sports have the potential to provide the individual with many rewarding and pleasurable memories.

3. *Physical activity provides release from social and professional obligations.* It is not possible to live in a group or in a society in isolation.

Every individual regardless of vocation has numerous social and professional obligations. The obligations of each individual in his role as a citizen must also be added. These obligations become part of our away-from-the-job life, but they are not generally considered to be leisure because they do not involve total freedom of choice. These obligations can, of course, also be pleasant.

4. *Physical activity or sports provide a psychological perception of freedom.* The perception of freedom in leisure becomes leisure. Choices are personal and individually made. Participation in sports to one individual might become an obligation, whereas to another it is freedom from any obligation.

5. *Physical activity as sports has a large role in American culture.* It is closely related and favorable to other leisure choices in society. Leisure is an end for many individuals but may also take on the role of a means. In both instances it is a part of society and all its facets help to make up the composite identity of our culture. If leisure is used without regard to moral, ethical, and intellectual standards, the cultural levels of society are reduced. Leisure practices are powerful forces.

6. *Physical activities and sports provide opportunities for a full range of personal values.* For many individuals their jobs are so important and have so many demands that leisure becomes simply a matter of rest or physical and mental recovery. The exhausted worker may not desire activity of any kind during free moments away from the job. Leisure may be planned as valuable or constructive programs or may be just a matter of doing what seems desirable at the moment. There are a number of examples of leisure practices becoming professions or economic sources of livelihood. Some artists have found their pleasurable leisure pursuit of painting in demand by the public and profitable for themselves as well.

Sports can be as routine as a spectator viewing an athletic contest when time is available, or it may be seriously planned and executed to improve skills and/or physical fitness. Leisure involves freedom of choice. If used constructively, it can add significant value to life.

7. *Physical activity and sports have the potential to provide pleasant experiences, enjoyment, and play.* Enjoyment, play, and fun are synonymous with leisure and free time. Most people look forward to leisure periods when personal choices of activities can be made. To provide balance to life, these leisure periods should be enjoyable. The deep satisfactions that can result from leisure can help in maintaining happiness and health in a world with troubles.

With the possible exception of the sports as a profession, the very word *sports* connotes fun and pleasant experience. The joy of effort and the physical results of participation are outcomes that yield deep satisfaction. These experiences should be a part of everyone's life. The many sports available today make it possible for each person to find an area where success and satisfaction are possible.

Foundations of Leisure in the Culture

Leisure is a significant part of all cultures and is growing ever larger. One occupation alone has reduced its work week from forty hours to fewer than twenty hours per week. The four-day work week is now under consideration, and it has been found to be possible for some vocations. A full month's vacation is a common practice in many professions. With free time on the increase, what are the requirements for leisure planning, preparation, and personal involvements? Knowing that leisure must fit into the framework of a given culture, what are the opportunities and responsibilities of society? What roles can physical activity in the form of sports, athletics, and games fill as part of the leisure life of the people?

Cultural forces can be very strong because the traditions and mores of a community or nation through a collective majority become the code of established practice. These forces are not easily changed, although they can be. During the past ten years, war has had a major effect on nearly everyone in the United States. The social trends in dress are always in a state of flux. Activities such as the theater or motion pictures have exercised a profound effect on American culture. This is also true in sports. The nature of these influences on and within the modern culture is reviewed in the next section of this chapter.

The Influence of Commercialization. Business has entered the sports field and made it into a major enterprise. The rapid increase in this type of enterprise has come about only during the past few years. Professional sports, as one example, is now a major business. Professional football has risen from the few local teams of the 1930's to the twenty-six-team nationwide conference that includes most of the major population centers in the United States. Basketball, baseball, and hockey are also well-established professional sports. The capital outlay and receipts of professional sports represent one of the largest investments of any business designed strictly for the leisure pursuits of society. Typical leisure investments include radio, television, and all leisure-oriented media, including sports equipment, the widespread purchase of which has resulted in sports stores springing up in every community. There are facilities such as stadiums, swimming pools, and gymnasiums in every community. The level of commercialization in sports has risen until it represents about 8 to 10 per cent of total consumer expenditures, although this is, by now, probably underestimated because of the rapid rate of increase in this field. Sports centers, camps, ski lodges, and mountain resorts find immense public demand. These commercial leisure facilities provide excellent leisure opportunities.

Social and Institutional Determinants. Only in recent years have social agencies and institutions become concerned about the leisure life of employees and the public in general. A good number of institutions have planned leisure programs for their patients or employees. The concerns of such groups include working schedules, periods for leisure, vacations, travel, and maintenance of worker morale and fitness.

The advances of physical activity and sports for leisure programs in social institutions have been most rapid during the past few years. This development is continuing and, one hopes, will result in physical activity becoming an integral part of the leisure programs of social institutions. These social institutions include the church, schools and colleges, family, communications media, fraternal groups, and other related organizations. Sport programs are today a part of the overall program of many of these institutions.

Personal Factors. Personal factors are major determinants of the amount of leisure and its utilization. The range of physical activity and sports used in leisure is as varied as the number of available physical activities. This can range from just walking to the most vigorous of sports. Factors that determine choice of activity include age, intelligence, levels of stress and tension, interests, fitness and tolerance levels, and so on. Regardless of personal abilities and skills, the individual can find some activity that will yield physically beneficial results.

Transportation and Communications. The rapid development of transportation and communication has had a major effect on leisure and increased interest in sports and physical activity participation.

The reporting of sports events on television and radio has increased the interest in sports beyond all possible projections of a decade ago. Football is taking prime time on week ends and Monday night for nearly six months of the year. The reason, of course, is public demand. Today's rapid transportation now takes millions of individuals to the country or to other nations for the week end or during annual vacation periods, resulting in a very mobile population with an increased interest in sports.

The Physical Environment. The use of natural resources and the physical environment for physical activity is now receiving major emphasis. Commercial enterprises are attempting to use the natural physical environment for pleasant recreational experiences during leisure periods. In the United States variations in climate and physical terrain make almost all kinds of physical activity available. Transportation allows an individual to reach these resources in a matter of a few hours. Special rates lower the cost of such activities, making them available to the average working man. There are opportunities for everyone to enjoy physical activity in preferred climates, whether it be skiing in the mountains or surfing in the ocean.

Public Relations. Political involvements in leisure and sports have significantly increased in recent years. Nearly all political platforms and programs stress the importance of leisure and leisure programs and resources. Government is involved in planning for future recreation facilities. The power of professional sports lobby groups is unquestioned.

Relationships of Leisure and Physical Activity

Leisure and physical activity are closely associated. One must set aside time for physical experiences unless professionally engaged in sports or athletics. Even in these instances, constant repetition of the same sport cannot be considered to utilize the full potentials of sport for personal well-being. The most vigorous activity will not produce the results that would arise from a variety of activities appropriate to leisure time and leisure resources. Physical activity should be a part of everyone's leisure pursuits, and the activities selected should be determined by individual vocations and therefore personal needs.

The principles presented in this discussion will reflect the relationships that should exist between leisure and physical activity. These are guides for the individual and for the professional worker in physical recreation or education.

Principle 1: A system of values should be developed for personal living that goes beyond materialism and egocentricity and establishes values that add fullness to life. The individual vocation, important as it is, cannot represent all of an individual's important commitments. Work cannot maintain the individual at healthy levels over a number of years. Varied experiences are needed and desired. It is necessary to develop new commitments along with those already held while maintaining respect for all human qualities.

Principle 2: In order to channel desires into specific accomplishments, these desires should be translated into goals that precisely set directions for desired achievements. Human desires when applied to daily life often become vague and without specific meaning or precise direction. Goals are necessary to establish this direction. Planning for leisure pursuits will probably remain unchanged, but programs stressing achievement will change as new experiences are encountered.

Principle 3: Preparation is essential for utilizing leisure sports. It is necessary that skills be developed to best utilize time, facilities, and per-

sonal abilities. The individual must have the skills to pursue his chosen leisure activity. A set of goals that cannot be implemented into a leisure program is of little value to the individual. The modern emphasis on lifetime sports, such as tennis, golf, and swimming, is a good example.

Principle 4: Preparation for leisure includes understanding the requirements of the body that should be met during leisure. Understanding the needs of the human organism is part of education. Because physical work can maintain fitness and health levels, it is of particular importance to understand physiological needs and exercise requirements. It is also important to understand the effects of vocational stresses and health practices as they relate to the maintenance of proper physical functions of the body.

Principle 5: It is an essential part of education to plan for the development of leisure literacy. Agreements on what constitutes a sound education vary according to the professional educator consulted. The same is true of education for leisure. Some simply say leisure is preparing to live a satisfying life. Leisure is generally considered to include education for any activity other than work. It involves both formal and informal preparation for utilizing discretionary time in a satisfying manner while developing individual talents. Leisure starts with individual values, interests, and appreciations. It is preparation in attitude and personal way of life for the achievement of satisfying outcomes. It is more closely related to finding outlets for personal desires than to meeting outside pressures and social mores. A leisure program should help the individual discover himself and should be planned to fit individual personality traits and competencies. Because education for leisure has age and maturation requirements, it must differ with individuals and fit immediate, short-range goals according to varying personal maturity levels.

Principle 6: Preparation and planning for leisure programs and schedules should follow a designed program, as if it were preparation for an individual vocation. The only difference between preparation for leisure and that for a vocation is that the individual has more freedom and his leisure choices can be very personal. Of course, there are restrictions to these choices (e.g., funds, time, or facilities) but within these limits one does have bountiful freedom. It is tragic to waste free time because of the lack of some designated plan. The losses resulting from the lack of interest or absence of leisure plans can only be depressing to the individual and have negative effects on his vocation. A major misconception is that leisure time is for doing anything one pleases. To appreciate the importance of leisure planning and education, it is necessary to look at the far-reaching consequences of inadequate preparation. Even with an absorbing vocation, the individual who does not develop a program of leisure activity cannot enjoy the potential fullness and joy of an active life.

Principle 7: In preparation for leisure, personal interests, maturation, goals, and desires should be fully explored because they do not come by chance or without direction. The individual utilization of free time depends not only upon how well prepared one is, but also upon one's attitudes, values, interests, and competencies. There are also other factors affecting leisure, such as where one lives, the availability of natural and man-made facilities, vocation, income, educational and cultural background, ecological conditions, customs, mores, transportation, community size and status, and fundamental desire of the individual to learn some activity.

Principle 8: The individual should establish a balance between work and leisure. Leisure alone is not enough to satisfy the individual's needs, nor is work, unless it has special significance. Active leisure and work together make for satisfaction and fullness of life. For those who have only leisure, freedom is meaningless. To individuals who are overworked, leisure may become equally meaningless, because they only desire sleep and rest. It is indeed unfortunate if day after day one finds nothing stimulating or significant in either work or leisure or is so exhausted from work that leisure cannot be constructive. People require the opportunity for both challenging work and a leisure life that is personal and deeply satisfying. If the leisure program includes physical activities, additional satisfactions and results can be attained.

Principle 9: If leisure is to be constructive in a community, each person should assume a responsibility for the community's leisure requirements. Providing for leisure is a social responsibility. It is not possible or desirable for each citizen to provide personally the facilities to meet his family's leisure interests. Natural resources are in the public domain, and if the citizenry does not determine their usage, few public officials will. In order to be adequate for leisure, facilities should be publicly planned and financed. There are, for example, only a few individuals who have the financial resources for a private pool. Any community can provide fields, indoor facilities, land, recreation equipment, and other facilities to meet the interests of the people.

Principle 10: The citizen is responsible for the social, moral, and behavioral status of all people in the community. The individual does not have the right to complete behavioral freedom. These rights are defined by law, tradition, and the mores of a society. The standards are set by the entire society and therefore should be observed by all the people. Of course, there are always dissenting or minority opinions. If standards are set by the majority, however, they should be observed by all members of the community until change can be achieved through democratic procedures. The antisocial activities in a community are the final responsibility of the public. Public officials act according to law, tradition, and the will of the people. Unless they have public support, they can accom-

plish little good. There are numerous examples of corrupt cities in the
United States and throughout the world. They are fully the result of
public disinterest. Fortunately, most communities are planned and administered by moral, ethical, and social standards that make each citizen
proud of his community and help him enjoy life more fully. This is an
essential requirement for leisure, because only then can one be free to
choose what he desires to do. It is necessary that individual citizens in a
community guide public choice. This is particularly true for our youth.

*Principle 11: The citizens and community have a responsibility to
provide leadership for leisure programs in a community. These responsibilities involve all echelons of government and society.* Because of the
importance of leisure programs, the role of democratic government becomes a major directing force within each community. Public institutions
should be designed, in part, to provide and prepare leaders for these programs. Only a few of the public-minded citizens will be professional and
paid leaders. The remainder will voluntarily serve in these leadership
roles. Public leadership roles are usually established by voting for desirable community standards, serving in official capacities, and assuming
leadership for the community and public.

*Principle 12: Fullness in life comes from wise and effective leisure
programs.* Work alone is not satisfactory, important as it is. Economic
security is important, but work cannot yield the fullness in living that
can come from deeply satisfying leisure experiences. Work, pleasant as
it is for many, can result in tension and stress. Boredom through constant
repetition of routine, rigidity of schedules, travel over great distances,
lack of opportunity for creativity, and constant pressure for success and
recognition can detract from individual enjoyment and fullness of life.
When man ceases to be challenged, his difficulties in attainment of personal satisfaction begin. With hobbies, sports, and hundreds of possible
leisure activities to challenge the individual, it is possible for him to gain
satisfaction and happiness in life that will make living fun and worthwhile.

An Overview

Physical activity within our culture as it is programmed in leisure has
contributions to make as a profession. Physical education must direct its
attention at making significant contributions to our culture through
physical activity and sports in leisure. This chapter not only develops
the nature of physical activity within the culture-leisure context, but also
presents the contributions physical activity can make to the individual
and thereby to society. If physical activity can effect changes in cultural
and leisure levels that are socially worthwhile and culturally significant,
then physical activity provides another professional outlet for service

to man. The analysis of physical activity as presented in this chapter gives strong support to physical activity as a cultural-leisure profession. Leisure programs involve activities that fit the culture and cultural goals. Just as cultures differ from community to community or nation to nation, so will leisure physical activity programs.

This is a multidisciplinary profession, and preparation for the various leadership and administrative functions essential to its operation involves the same components as any other service profession. The talents and the skills of the sociologist are required to understand adequately culture and leisure relationships, of the psychologist to understand the individual and his role in leisure and its various cultural settings, and of the physiologist to identify the requirements and changes possible in various leisure settings. The other disciplines, such as education, medicine, the physical sciences, physical education, recreation, and health sciences, all contribute to the requirements for professional application of physical activity through leisure. No professional worker will be fully prepared in all the preceding areas but should study physical education and recreation with equal emphasis in the social sciences and with some background in the biological and physical sciences. Such individuals would then be prepared to work in a community physical activity planning program as the single most important force in public leisure. Such a leader should be prepared to work with members of various other professions and vocations to understand leisure more fully, to plan educational programs for the preparation of leisure skills, to plan and develop leisure programs utilizing appropriate physical activity, and to maintain all standards and requirements of the profession. This would require establishment of a definitive philosophy, social agencies, programs leadership, and evaluation procedures involving the entire community and its agencies and government structure. As a result of professional involvement, it will be possible to interest people in active leisure pursuits and physical activity beneficial to both the individual and society.

Chapter 10

Dance

In this chapter, we shall analyze the nature of physical activity in dance as a profession. Our interest is focused on whether physical activity has a legitimate professional application in the dance and on the nature of the various forms of physical activity in the dance and their professional potentials. Our concern is not the dance per se; rather, it is physical activity or movement as employed in the dance, and the professional worth of physical activity within this context. In brief, does physical activity when applied in the dance have more or less value than sports, athletics, physical recreation, and other applied forms of physical activity in developing desirable human qualities?

Dance is movement, and this movement has physical requirements. The rationales for the movements, of course, go beyond the physical. Sometimes the physical base is only incidental, a by-product, and involves no direct professional considerations. However, because the movements in dance must be correctly performed to give the proper basis for interpretation, the physical, in this instance, becomes a major focus.

Both physical activity and the dance are applied commercially for reasons that deal only with the activity. The concern is not with the effects on the participant, but with an already developed ability and a performance that is of interest to the spectator. This emphasis on performance is a part of any profession, but the fundamental framework for this analysis is the individual, the group, the society, and the culture, and the influences of physical activity in the various dance forms on the physical being and on other human characteristics and abilities. The basic disciplines that provide the content for analysis are those that deal with human development and learning such as physiology and psychology.

Thus the setting for a professional analysis of physical activity in the dance is established. It will be of significance to determine whether certain human qualities can be developed from physical activity in the dance. This will determine its possible worth as an independent profession.

Professional Status of the Dance

The dance is an integral part of the culture and is important in the lives of many people. It is also a part of education, contributing to educational goals. It is a commercially organized profession for entertainment of the public. It is a creative and artistic medium for self-expression and personal creativity. It is an individual developmental medium emphasizing the physical organism.

This chapter studies the dance within the context of (1) physical activity and (2) physical activity as a possible profession or subprofession. It will include only that information needed to provide evidence toward the understanding of these two goals. In order to introduce the professional study of physical activity within the dance, we shall apply some of the criteria used to determine professional status, that is, to determine if dance is a profession or has the possibilities of becoming a profession.

1. *"A profession is distinguished by a highly specialized technique that is based on service and learning, the practices of which serve practical ends; in the pursuit of those the practitioners assume a large measure of individual responsibility."* [1] The dance is distinguished by "highly specialized techniques" that require learning, practice, ability, and other personal and professional qualifications for successful participation. All forms of the dance involve expression and communication through physical movements that are the result of highly specialized skills. Thus the dance meets this major requirement of a profession.

2. *The professional technique must be capable of communication through a highly specialized discipline.* A close relationship exists between a discipline and a profession. A discipline involves the accumulation of knowledge about a phenomenon relevant to the culture, society, or individual. The dance is a combination of many disciplines. Among these are sociology, psychology, philosophy, history, physiology, both mechanical and general physics, and education. The content results from the interpretation of the performance as communicated in the dance.

The dance viewed as a physical activity is highly complex and specialized. The human body must move with extreme precision and with physical patterns that give meaning to the performance. Interpretation is in many instances the goal, but the physical base is an absolute requirement in order to reach this end.

The physical basis for human movement involves knowledge of the human body such as is found in physiology and medicine. It requires understanding and skill in movement, both physical and mechanical. It

[1] Earl Kaufman, Jr. Ph.D. dissertation, New York University, 1948.

requires moving in relationship with others and the physical environment, as described by sociology, psychology, and the physical sciences. Physical performances are of many patterns directed by the physical activity itself and by the cultural and societal patterns established by the activity. Because of the complexity of the requirements of physical performance, the dance does need the content of knowledge from several fundamental sciences.

3. *The professional technique must have sufficient social significance and requires sufficient competence to warrant the exercise of some control over it by society, the practitioners themselves, or both operating together.* Dance starts with children in playgrounds and schools, and it reaches into highly specialized and commercially directed public performances. It is a public enterprise of major magnitude, involving controls and directions. This criterion in judging the dance as a profession is applied both by society and by the practitioners. The dance has a large and valued place in society. There are a number of subgroups or loosely organized professions around the various forms of the dance that give some supervision and direction to their many activities. Viewing the dance from the criterion of social control, current social acceptance and self-imposed regulation does justify its place as a profession.

4. *Preparation for and practice of professional techniques stimulate the practitioners to form professional associations for improving standards and extending public acceptance.* The major function of a profession is to set standards for all facets of professional work. The only truly meaningful standards come from professional members. If they set the standards, the likelihood of implementation is greatly increased. They are also qualified to set standards, which is not always true for the public.

The professional associations in the dance have made significant progress in developing professional status. The dance has a significant place in physical education associations, its educational contributions coming through physical activity in the same manner as such forms as sports and athletics. It is, of course, recognized that this is only one professional application for the dance, but it is significant.

5. *The conduct of the practitioners is a matter of concern to the profession and results in the formulation of codes of ethics.* There are numerous societies, special groups, and organized professions representing dance in its various forms that set goals for dance achievements. The standards include personal requirements for membership and professional practices, including personal ethics, skills, aptitudes, and abilities. The requirements will differ according to professional goals, for example, whether emphasis is placed on physical expression, or performance, or skills.

The cultural applications of the dance are nearly as many as the cultural classifications, ranging from bar-room performances in nude dances (with emphasis on the body for sexual expression) to national expression, as in the programs prepared in China and Russia for high-ranking visitors. Cultural presentations through the dance reflect the country's traditions, mores, religious beliefs, ways of life, whereas other presentations represent more the people themselves. These are cultural communications of the highest order. It would be most difficult to find the words to represent the traditions of a people more effectively and realistically than through the vehicle of the dance.

The professional concern in this instance is ethics. In all applications (nude dances included) professional ethical behavior is a factor. Probably the most important professional basis for success is the ethics of the practitioners.

6. *Within the profession, there is a conscious recognition of a spirit of public service that places social duty as the highest goal of the profession.* This professional standard is a requirement for all professional associations. The profession is designed for the public. If it is to be successful, it must serve the public satisfactorily. If a profession represents a significant need (medicine, law, education) of the public and renders services that the people judge as satisfactory, it will be successful and will continue to render and improve its services to the people.

There are many professional failures. Some groups are organized around a service that neither represents a cultural need nor is of significant interest. A profession also requires outstanding leadership. The cost of sustaining a profession and its services is much too high for it to continue without constant requests for services. Another important factor in success is the quality of the service. This particular standard is now under critical review by many professional groups, for example, educational groups.

During the past few years a number of teachers in local schools have organized with labor unions rather than within the education profession. This could represent the difference between education of quality or education as a daily job. It is a question of whether the practitioner's concerns are personal or professional.

Dance has a significant place in physical education and in the culture. It has organized and should continue to organize professionally to provide quality services. Individuals make up a profession; thus individuals must contribute to its establishment. There is strength in and through the group that is seldom obtainable individually. Yet the strength of the profession depends on the combined individual efforts and abilities of its members.

A profession must have an organization with regulations that define membership and practices. These regulations provide (1) influences and services to meet important needs of the people, (2) an organization with goals for service rather than personal goals and achievements, (3) the educational requirements for certification of the practitioner, (4) for all the responsibilities of the profession with commitments from each member, and (5) for ongoing and long-range goals that are consistent with changes in society.

Professional Domain: Conceptual Structure

The dance is a physical phenomenon or deals wtih physical performances. It is considerably more, however, than physical activity or the skills of human movement. It produces many of the results that come from physical activity, but it also has unique contributions to make to the development of the human being, the culture, and the society. Here we shall examine the professional possibilities of the dance in its various forms.

The dance represents a unique use of physical activity and therefore results in personal and cultural outcomes that are unique to the dance. Of course, like the other applications of physical activity, it also has common results of worth.

An attempt is made to characterize the dance by conceptualizing the professional domain of physical activity in the dance. Understanding what concepts and values fit or represent the dance as a profession is the objective. Our task is limited to the context of physical activity, and will not include other outcomes that might result from the dance.

The professional domain of the dance is conceptualized as cultural, artistic and creative, personal, and societal. These four major categories represent the potential outcomes. How the dance is presented and applied determines what outcomes will actually be achieved.

Cultural Values and Understandings. The dance has cultural worth. It can contribute to understanding among people of various backgrounds. Understanding among people is gained through traditional forms of folk, religious, ethnic, and ritual dance and is the cultural goal set for the dance itself. It reflects the people or their beliefs through the physical expressions that come from dance movements and types, yielding cultural meaning through physical performance.

The national dance is a representation of the people. The dance steps or patterns may have similarities among nations but have a national character. The dance can be an expression of the spirit of the people. In such instances, how the steps are planned is as important as what the steps are.

The national or cultural forms of dance are characterized in several ways: light and graceful (Latin), exotic charm (Oriental), force and heavy body movements (Slavic). Other emphases have included religious prayer, the hunt, the war dance, sentiment, graceful movement, and so on.

**List. 7. Conceptual structure: The professional
domain of physical activity in the dance**

1. Cultural values and understandings.
   a. Ballet.
   b. Character.
   c. Ethnic.
   d. Folk.
   e. Modern.
   f. National.
   g. Recreation.
   h. Religious.
   i. Ritual.
   j. Social.
2. Artistic and creative expression.
   a. Aesthetic.
   b. Dramaturgy.
   c. Literary.
   d. Movement exploration.
   e. Movement and skill.
   f. Music.
   g. Play.
   h. Sculpture (the body).
   i. Self-expressive aspects.
3. Personal benefits and developmental potentials.
   a. Aesthetic.
   b. Balance.
   c. Communications.
   d. Coordination.
   e. Creativity.
   f. Cultural aspects.
   g. Ego.
   h. Physical aspects.
   i. Posture.
   j. Rhythm.
   k. Self-realization.
   l. Social aspects.
   m. Spatial aspects.
   n. Timing.
4. Societal values and benefits.
   a. Aesthetic aspects.
   b. Artistic and creative aspects.
   c. Communications.
   d. Cultural aspects.
   e. Education.
   f. Human relations.
   g. Integration.
   h. Personal and interpersonal aspects.
   i. Professional aspects.
   j. Social aspects.
   k. Therapeutic values.

Culturally, the dance literature is extensive and has depth of meaning. It has profound relations to religion. It has deep ties with the intellect. In this respect the dance is also a language. The use of the physical body as an instrument of communication is applied by those who dance seriously, expressing emotions and feelings.

The cultural value of the dance, of course, is determined by what it can do for the people. The dance can be both very feminine and very masculine. How it is physically applied will determine the qualities developed.

The cultural potentials in the dance are determined by the dance itself. Each form of the dance will have its development in the cultural component to be emphasized. These include folk (national characteristics), modern (human development and expression), ethnic (racial differences and customs), religious (prayer and religious traditions and beliefs), recreation (movements expressing the emotions and feelings), ritual (religious ceremonies and observances), social (customs and current social practices), character (distinguishing human characteristics and traits), ballet (artistic, dramatic expression), and national (the mores of the people) forms of the dance.

The dance makes many significant cultural contributions, and these are based on the medium of movement or physical activity. Of course, the mind and the emotions cannot be separated from the physical components of performance, and they are necessary to express fully the cultural facets. It is fair to say that the professional domain of physical activity in the dance is supported by the cultural emphasis, potentials, and contributions that can be made by the various forms of the dance.

Artistic and Creative Expression. The dance is an art form, a means of self-expression, a method of communicating. It utilizes human movements to convey feelings and thoughts; it is movement with interpretive content. This may consist of one's most cherished ideas, ideals, hopes, and insights. The movements of the dance are rhythmic expressions of one's nature, culture, and aspirations and may be considered both artistic and creative.

In the dance the eyes and gestures are the means of communicating content. Words are inadequate for full communication; the dancer utilizes all his physical, emotional, and mental faculties in the presentation. In the dance the muscles, the senses, and the mind are rhythmically integrated into meaningful creativity. The body becomes an instrument of communication and therefore must be trained to respond to impulses accurately, skillfully, and with the grace that represents ideas artistically.

The dance can be developed within the patterns of play. Play itself can be a dance form. It expresses ideas. It results from emotions and mental images that must have expression. The content can be any thought communicated through play. Play is the most frequent application of physical activity, and the movements in play represent the patterns found in many dance forms.

Dance forms can be found in dramaturgy (drama representing cultural events and history) and in representations of the human body as sculpture. Dance expresses the beauty of the body and its grace in movement.

The creative and artistic role of music in the dance is difficult to delineate. Music and dance go together, and creativity is increased by their combination.

The professional domain of physical activity in the dance is found in its artistic and creative potential. Some individuals can communicate their feelings best through physical movement. It would be difficult to identify an application of physical activity that does not have some creative and artistic content. This content can apply to the human mind, body, emotions, and social expressions.

Personal Benefits and Developmental Potentials. The personal benefits resulting from the dance are physical and social as well as emotional and intellectual. The application of the dance by the leader and the participant determines what the results will be. In human development both the processes of leadership and participation as well as the physical participation itself are essential for the developmental contributions that dance can make.

In addition to the physical results, the social, emotional, and intellectual qualities are of particular significance in the dance. The dance is different from other physical activities in that emphasis is centered on expression and creative and artistic ideas. The physical plays a subordinate role after the skill and movement patterns have been learned and developed. Of course, physical patterns must be appropriate to the intellectual conceptualization to ensure that the ideas are properly presented.

There are additional personal qualities that can come from the dance. It is a sociocultural phenomenon, and sociocultural qualities can be cultivated through participation; such qualities range from those found in personal relationships to those that apply in the society and culture.

The dance contributes to aesthetics. It gives beauty to physical performance through its setting, personal expression, and movement; the dance itself is a beautiful performance by dancers with grace, beautiful bodies, and skills. It includes all concepts that have deep meaning in a performance.

It is in personal development and adjustment that the professional domain of physical activity in the dance is most significant. Personal qualities are found that are important to the individual, society, and culture. The dance as physical activity also has significant professional potentials stemming from the physical elements in the dance. The physical performance is, indeed, a large portion of nearly all forms of the dance, and is, by far, the major reason for the dance.

Societal Values and Benefits. The dance through the process of physical performance contributes to the development of society and the culture. It is reported by some dance writers that the social outcomes that can result from the dance are only slightly less than the physical qualities. Both are major forces and elements in the dance.

The dance is individual and personal. It deals with the person as a social being and with his development. Through it he is taught to be courteous, respectful, sympathetic, and other such social values as are important in human associations. These qualities are important if the dance is to be an acceptable and a contributing part of the culture.

The dance can be used in the development of better social beings by providing appropriate experiences. Both in its formal and informal forms the dance can be used as a social laboratory. Some of the concepts that can be achieved through appropriate forms of the dance are moral responsibility (self-discipline), common consent (resolution of conflict), respect for excellence (mind, character, and creative ability), pursuit of happiness (individual opportunities within society), and spiritual enrichment (experiences that transcend materialistic aspects of life).

There are additional societal values and contributions that can be made through the dance (List 7). Communicating within a society adds to the possibility of social integration. Emphasis on the mores and traditions of the people may result in changes in life patterns that improve social practices. The social potentials of creativity and art are qualities important to society. They are part of the dance, and the dance is part of educational programs in schools, colleges, and social agencies. It is used to achieve educational goals and, in part, designed to improve the community and community life.

The possible contributions of the dance to the social order makes it a social component with strong professional potential. This is true also of physical activity as the medium for the dance. It, again, is difficult as well as undesirable to separate the physical from the social components in dance. It is, however, possible to define the qualities that can come from dance. A profession stems from the people and as such must make worthwhile service contributions to the people. The dance does have social potential.

In summary, it is the purpose of this section on the conceptual structure of the dance within its professional domain to review the dance within the context of physical activity. The attempt is to judge the dance as a physical activity and to conceptualize the qualities or values developed through participation. This analysis, then, representing the professional domain of physical activity in the dance is similar to the analysis of physical activity in athletics, but the professional goals are quite different.

Professional Content in the Dance

The purpose of this section is to review and present the knowledge and skill content of the dance from two points of reference. The first is the content of physical activity for development as it is applied within this physical context. The second is the professional potential of the dance within the context of physical activity, determining its professional worth and placing it within the applied professions of physical activity.

A profession, to be worthy and successful, must serve the people and its service must meet vital needs. The contributions that dance-physical activity can make are classified into four major categories of concepts and values.

Cultural Content of Values and Understandings. The content of the dance as applied in physical activity is significant culturally, representing the mores of a society and certain human and societal cultural qualities. Professional content should also meet the needs for health, well-being, adjustment, and personal development.

The dance provides an opportunity for *creative expression*. It is both an evaluation and a representation of the culture. Expression in the dance ranges from crude physical expressions to the most highly skilled performances.

The dance itself represents a *history of traditions and the culture*. People have used dance in different ways through the centuries, and the records of each period show the culture of that age. It is a most effective means of transmitting and understanding the history of cultural interests and developments.

The dance is a part of *religious ceremonies* in many cultures. In the progress of man ritual has become part of religion. Among the great religions of the world, dance has played an important part. The dance reflects the daily life, the drama, the philosophies, and the religions of the people. The dance reflects human feelings of devotion, loyalty, and tenderness.

The *modern dance*, as one example of the dance in physical activity, represents modern life and its individualism, mode of living, freedom, and worldliness. This is a period that emphasizes the role of the individual.

The dance, in its cultural role, is a *communal-recreational* form. The dance is a part of the marriage ceremony and the various social expressions of marriage. It is a personal form of expression, designed for achievement of personal worth and not necessarily for entertainment of others. The dance is part of the social life of a community. It contributes to the personal well-being and the feeling of contentment necessary to sustain one in daily living.

The *ethnic dance* is a representation of class structure as well as the general structure of society itself. In some countries, such as Japan, restrictions were at one time placed on the dance, and the social class that could participate in it was also restricted. Tribal life is reflected by the dance, which mirrors common emotions and provides a way to explain life and various feelings graphically.

The *American social dance* is also a physical expression of the dancer. There are many forms, and they change from period to period, helping to mark the changes in generations. Social dance is formed from a blending of many cultures, because Americans are blends of many cultures, but the dance is American, and the performers show that they too are very much American. It does reflect the American culture.

The literature contains and supports the cultural nature of the dance and its physical expression. With the firm cultural role of the dance established in societies throughout the world, its professional status has also become an integral part of the various professions that serve the people and their needs. Cultural needs are not as readily recognized as medical or educational ones; but for the society to develop and provide a setting for optimal personal and social development, dance must be represented in every culture in every community and nation.

Artistic and Creative Content. Dance content is creative, and it is artistic because of its many patterns of physical activity. The dance is a combination of movements that provide for an infinite number of creative expressions and presentations, and it remains one of the few physical forms to provide the depth of interpretation evident in music, literature, and other artistic productions.

The dance is *art and is artistic* in its content and patterns of human movement. The artist can find creative freedom in the dance for communicating personal feelings. Certain communication must be regarded as art, and the presentation of the dance in many forms qualifies as art. The dancer communicates by expression in the dance the same way an artist does through his art.

The dance must not be considered subservient to music; rather, it should be presented along with music. Music must be suited to the dance when it is the dance that is the primary means of expression. In dance that is planned for artistic expression, all the parts must fit together to create a successful performance.

The dance, in its physical performance, involves *exploration, discovery, and invention* of movement and expression. It is a means, in itself, for personal expressions of feelings and is therefore a way to relate to the environment in a unique and personal fashion. The motivation of the dancer leads to unique and varied means of physical expression.

The dance is an *aesthetic* presentation involving the appreciation of the dance as an art and its performance as a thing of beauty. It is the beautiful patterns of movement within the dance that best represent its aesthetic values. It is the physical patterns reflecting interacting movements or forces that provide the beauty. The movements are rhythmic, and the dance presents the various human movements that are uniquely possible in space.

The dance is a medium for performers and professionals who have interest in *creative research*. The opportunities the dance provides for creative research, imagination in action, and new experiences in thought and performance appear to be unlimited.

The dance is *drama*. It is possible through physical movements to portray joy, sorrow, love, hate, and the many elements of human expression that are found in drama. Accomplishing this entirely through movement, without benefit of words, requires artistic talent of the first order.

The dance, as an art, is a medium for the appreciation of *sculpture of the human body.* The shape and form of the body must be an integral part of the dance. The professional dancer meets these requirements through long practice. If the dancer's body is not perfectly developed, the dance is not as effective.

It can be reasonably concluded that the dance can make major contributions to the arts and to artistic talents and interests. The dance as an art requires the full resources of the human personality and mental abilities within the context of physical movement. The absence of any of these major qualifications will reduce the quality of the dance as an art.

Personal Developmental Content. The dance is one of the leading physical activities for the development of the human organism. Its physical content is extensive, requiring highly skilled movements. In some dance performances the physical and physiological requirements lead to physical exhaustion. Study of the dance results in the symmetrical development of the physical body into a pleasing figure that lends a large part of the artistic worth to the dance for both the performer and the spectator.

The dance develops *kinesthetic awareness and neuromuscular coordination* that are necessary for its performance. Performance and consistent training result in the development of the elemental traits of balance, steadiness, agility, rhythm, accuracy, and flexibility that are essential for total body coordination in physical movements. The sensorimotor development and spatial judgments in movement also play large parts in physical performances of the dance. They are the basis for the development of kinesthetic ability, leading to skillful and beautiful performances. The dance makes major contributions, in comparison with other physical activities, to the perfection of these physical abilities.

The dance is an *environmentally related activity* that enables the dancer to communicate with others through physical movement. The setting includes social and cultural components of the environment.

The dance has significant *fitness* content, particularly through its vigorous performances. Aesthetically, the dance also requires a physical body with symmetry, coordination, and skill. These qualities go with and add to the dance. It has the potential to develop attractive and physically fit bodies.

The requirements in the dance are the *neuromuscular skills of movement.* The dance is a physical performance. The first requirement is the ability to move in the exact patterns that represent a particular dance design. Skill is the most fundamental requirement in the dance. Dance requires aptitude to achieve high performance levels, and it requires practice by the hour on a schedule with few breaks. Social dances change from time to time, and skills must be learned and developed to the level of personal satisfaction. Skill, however, is required in all movements of the body. In the dance the requirements are particularly high.

The dance contributes significantly to the *symmetry* of the human body. The physical movements in the dance involve neuromuscular patterns. The patterns are infinite, and they lead to the development of body symmetry. The physical appearance of the dancer is a large part of the dance. Achieving fitness for a specific physical activity results in a corresponding change in one's appearance. Some physical activities do not require the symmetry that goes with the dance. One example is the weight lifter, whose muscle mass is an asset.

Societal Developmental Content. The dance is a large part of any society and culture. It is found in many forms from social dancing to professional performances and is enjoyed by people of nearly all social stratas. Physical activity in the dance is a source of personal enjoyment. It is also a source of appreciation for the spectator when performances are highly skillful and artistically performed. The dance has many contributions to make to society and the culture.

The dance *contributes to social integration.* The acceptance of self in relationships can be achieved through the dance. In a social group the dance serves as an integrating force, providing enjoyable social leisure and a close setting for human understanding.

The dance, for the young in particular, provides the beginning of *motor development through play.* The desire to play is inherent in children. The dance in play is a way for the child to express feelings, emotions, and the strong desire for physical movement. Because the dance is a natural activity for the child, it provides an excellent setting for the teacher to develop motor patterns that will lead to nearly all types of sports patterns at a later period of development. Because the motivation is strong, the opportunities for significant development during this period are provided for both the teacher and the child.

The dance is a *cultural and aesthetic* facet of society, providing a medium for development of social qualities. It emphasizes the beautiful, and is an appropriate way to represent the traditions of society.

The dance is a medium for *human relations and personal communications.* It is a most personal activity, a way for the individual to express feelings, thoughts, and physical abilities. In instances of language differences, it makes it possible to communicate attitudes, feelings, and thoughts. Language for many is not always the most expressive form of communication, and religious ritual is also effectively expressed in the dance.

Artistic and creative contributions are potentially large in the dance. The movements in any form of the dance can be creative. They require rhythmic skills, and it is possible to develop personal patterns in a dance. Dance can be learned by anyone who has the desire, the insight, and willingness to practice. Creativity can be expressed most vividly in the movements of the dance.

Social, professional, and educational opportunities are found in the dance. Dance can comprise a large part of the individual's social life, and for many it is a profession. The dance, finally, has the power to develop one to meet educational goals of schools and social agencies. It is a natural medium that requires the coordination of the mind and the emotions and can therefore result in personal development.

Professional Potentials in the Dance

A brief review will be presented on the dance as an applied profession for physical activity. The chapter itself gives the scope and content of physical activity as accomplished through the dance.

1. *The dance is a physical performance phenomenon.* The human worth and the societal values in the dance come from the dance performance. It is physical movement used to express ideas, feelings, love, hate, and those elements that represent communication between individuals and within a society. As an applied profession or as a dance profession, the dance meets the professional requirements of planning programs for the public to achieve personally and culturally those values and qualities that are important and worthwhile.

2. *The dance is a medium for physically developing the human organism.* One of the prime reasons for physical exercise or physical activity is to develop the body. Life cannot be sustained without physical activity, and its quality can be improved with proper physical activity. The dance provides the full range of activity from highly coordinated to vigorous physical performance and yields excellent physical results. The professional value of this contribution is indeed considerable.

3. *The dance through the physical patterns of its various forms leads to understanding the physical body and the organism.* The dance must be implemented through physical performances. The physical resources and capacities must be known and developed by the performer to fit the dance itself and the various patterns needed for proper performance. One learns about the body by preparing for the dance, what it can do and how it can be developed.

4. *The dance as a physical performance phenomenon represents a setting for close human relations and associations.* Preparation for democratic human relations is a major role of physical activity in sports, games, and athletics. It is equally, if not more powerfully, applied in the dance. Respect for the human personality, equality of opportunity, and resolution of issues by the use of reason and intelligence are some of the democratic values that can come from the dance.

5. *The dance provides opportunities for social development and integration.* Physical activity is planned by many social and educational institutions as a setting for social development and integration. This has long occurred in physical education and sports, with positive results. The socialization of the individual through the dance is equally possible. Self-respect, respect for others, self-sufficiency, and positive social action are important personal and social qualities. The dance under proper leadership and with enthusiastic participation can result in these desirable social qualities. In this respect it is a most valuable application of physical activity as a profession.

6. *The dance plays a major part in the culture and has significant intercultural worth.* The need for cultural and intercultural development is more important today than at any time in history. In recent years the people of the world have become closely and personally associated. Sports have become international over the past few years. The dance in its national characteristics has also become part of schools in each country and part of international festivals. Professions designed to improve the people and the culture find important human content in physical activity, especially physical activity as experienced in the dance, and the dance is being increasingly utilized as a basis for the solution of international and intercultural problems.

Chapter 11

Education

The world in the final quarter of the twentieth century provides a setting that differs significantly from that of the first quarter of this century. It does not take a historian to tell us the world has changed markedly in the last fifty years. We have always lived in a changing society and a kaleidoscopic world, but until the past fifteen or twenty years the pace of change was not nearly as rapid as it is today. The causes of this increased pace must begin with man's passion—war. The United States has been deeply involved in four major armed conflicts during the twentieth century. The latest, Vietnam, has cost this country billions of dollars, nearly 50,000 American lives, almost an equal number of disabled veterans, and political conflicts that will continue long into the future. This price has been high and has had a major effect on life in this country.

Other factors have caused changes in today's society. The rapid advances in transportation have had and will continue to have major influences on our culture. Travel throughout the world is at the level reached within the United States in the 1950's and 1960's. Low-rate tour groups by the hundreds leave the United States daily for all parts of the world. It now is possible for almost anyone to travel abroad. This potential for education on a worldwide basis has never before been known in the history of mankind.

Despite its share of poverty-class citizens, the United States remains the wealthiest country on earth. For most, wages, salaries, and commercial profits have made this an affluent society. For the most part, Americans have the economic resources for a full and rich life. Beyond just meeting daily needs, we can now afford to enjoy such leisure pursuits as boating, camping, tennis, golf, winter sports, and a myriad of other recreational activities. Our societal mobility, at this time, includes almost everyone; we are a nation "on the move."

There are still other conditions that lead to a changed life-style today. The average life span has increased from thirty to forty years during the late nineteenth century to the current average of seventy to eighty years. The population reflects this trend and is now heavily weighted by middle-aged and older people. The retired population is large and increasing each year. Fortunately, most of this country's retired citizenry are able to manage with Social Security and present medical services through Medicare, in addition to perhaps modest retirement allowances. The emphasis is now on improving conditions for these people in every possible area, and the costs for this will be substantial.

Another factor worthy of note has been the shift of the population from rural areas to the urban centers and cities. The number of farms and small rural towns is rapidly decreasing. Farming today requires a substantial financial outlay and considerably more land to put this traditional enterprise on a firm economic footing. The result has not threatened this country in direct ways because modern technology has made it possible to produce considerably more food with fewer farms and workers.

It is not possible to view education and educational planning without a thorough understanding of the forces acting upon the people. What effects have these changes in society had on people? What are the implications for the individual living in a community or in the world as it now exists? The personal implications of modern life have caused changes and problems for both the individual and society. These, along with the factors that cause the changes, must be understood to start the process of education. Education is the only public enterprise charged with preparing the people for life and society as it should be by systematic design. We shall in the following pages discuss some of the conditions of modern life.

Living today causes *emotional and physical stresses* that differ from those of past decades. The pace today is a rapid one. The isolated, small community still exists, but its numbers have dwindled rapidly and its role has also greatly changed. Our outstanding highway system, millions of automobiles, consolidated industry, consolidated schools, and so on, have all been constructed with the idea that travel to these central locations would be logical and economic. This trend has helped make the large urban centers larger and still growing and the smaller rural centers smaller and ever dwindling. Many small communities have disappeared. All of this adds to personal pressure from urban living that is vastly different from what was known in isolated, rural settings.

Despite unprecedented knowledge about health, *abuse to personal health* is increasing. The drains today on the human organism are many. These include disease; physical defects; constant tension and stress; lack of proper sleep or rest; poor diet; overindulgences of food, alcohol, and smoking; accidents; use of nonprescription medications and drugs; poor human relations; unwise or complete absence of exercise and chronic fatigue. Of course, these conditions do not apply to everyone, nor are they restricted to present times. Elements of this history, however, do apply to the vast majority. This results in reduced work ability, irritability, and unhappiness because of inability to live fully at the limits of one's capacity.

The individual does not have adequate protection to meet the *hazards of modern life* and the environment. Automobile accidents alone kill hundreds of persons each day. These figures soar on week ends, especially on long holiday week ends. Home accidents also injure 5 million persons per year, kill another 30,000, and cripple about 100,000 more. Most accidents could be avoided. The causes of accidents are many and varied and include emotional upset or instability, hostility, frustrations and aggression. A person's emotional state sometimes overrides his intellectual control. Reasoning and the thinking processes may be forgotten under stress.

The *lack of exercise* or physical activity is increasing. Exercise is basic for life. Without it the individual will lose functional power, and deterioration will result. A simple exercise program can provide the individual with vitality to progress considerably beyond the needs of daily life and really enjoy living. There is no need for a healthy person to feel fatigued or unable to meet the simple requirements of daily living. Lack of exercise produces physical inefficiency. The sluggish individual does not have efficient reasoning power. Sluggishness in turn leads to less physical activity, which usually causes further decline. Any activity short of regular exercise must be considered as selling one's own body short and therefore having a negative influence on other human factors. In the world today, with its constant stresses, the need for systematic physical activity is greater than ever before.

In spite of modern labor-saving devices, more free time, and abundance of recreation resources, people today exhibit *fewer personal relationships and concerns* and *boredom* often is the rule rather than the exception. Unhappiness, tension, and social rejection hinder personal development, and can lead to poor health, slow development, and, for some, personal destruction. Boredom results from the difficulty in breaking from the daily routine. Motivation for new learning and new experiences becomes lacking. With the resources of the world today, however, boredom and unhappiness need not be the state of the majority of the population.

Now, before looking at the topic of education as such, a brief review must be made of the positive conditions existing in the modern world that can significantly advance the cause of the individual and collectively improve our societies and cultures. These conditions must also be recognized as resources that can enrich education. Changes can be made by students in today's schools if they are properly prepared and cognizant of realistic world conditions. Solutions to problems come from this setting.

Modern resources in recent years have provided ample opportunity for people seeking higher education. With the interest and motivation to search for knowledge, these resources, in large measure, become countermeasures in combating dissatisfaction in education.

1. *Food for proper nutrition is available to all people of the world.* Of course, there are people living in poverty, ignorance, and hunger. The reasons are primarily social, governmental, and international jurisdictional difficulties that fail to provide for nutritional needs of the people. The overabundance of nutritional resources in many countries is often stored, or efforts are made to cut production. This occurs in the face of the great need for surplus foodstuffs in less-fortunate countries. This condition cannot be ignored in any country because it represents the fundamental basis for any educational program. Education is designed to prepare one for a satisfying and rewarding life. This condition must have high priority.

2. *Institutions for learning and for the development of vocational skills are in abundance in the United States and in most countries of the world.* Many institutions for the preparation of a satisfying vocational profession are available in the United States and in most countries in the world. These institutions range from schools that place emphasis on skills to institutions of higher learning dealing with the complex problems in a society. In each instance, job opportunities are available with sufficient incomes to provide for family needs. Life in a society developed through high levels of science and technology requires formal preparation for nearly all vocations. The early days of apprenticeship are now, for the most part, over. Personal preparation is within the reach of all, but it requires motivation and training.

3. *Provisions for leisure and recreation are now found in most communities in the United States and throughout the world.* With the rapid increase in leisure, it is important that communities provide recreation resources that cannot be personally provided. Such resources are especially essential for children and youth. Wholesome and enjoyable play is as important for youth as are the requirements of exercise and nutrition. For the child fun is the basis not only for proper social and emotional development, but also for physiological adjustment. On the adult level it is essential that a change from routine, providing enjoyment and personal satisfaction, become a part of adult life. In the United States one need not be bored, because there are recreational pursuits to fit all interests, skills, and abilities.

4. *Opportunities for work and economic security can be provided for nearly all people.* Of course, a small percentage of the nation's population does not have the skills or the abilities to be gainfully employed.

Those who are fortunate enough to have the personal resources required for work must help provide satisfying work activities for those less fortunate who cannot meet their economic needs. This is the case in the United States and in most countries in the world. For the individual who has goals and ambition, it is possible to find a vocation or work that provides for personal economic needs. It is recognized that a large percentage of the people now live on a poverty level in the United States, but the poverty level does provide food, shelter, and a life that can be pleasant and even happy. Opportunities, however, to raise oneself from this level are open to all with personal motivation and some type of basic qualifications. It must be recognized that qualifications for skilled occupations can be developed. Education is most basic in this respect, and must view its programs from this important social need.

5. *Personal fitness and health are possible for nearly everyone.* Disease strikes thousands of people each year and leaves many disabled. Some others are born with physical and mental handicaps. For nearly everyone, however, it is possible to improve health and fitness status levels and provide an improved basis for meeting daily demands. Resources to evaluate physical fitness levels can be found in the home, but public assistance and resources are also plentiful. The individual, however, must use the medical resources available and participate in physical activity offered in order to maintain physiological functions. Those who are physically fit have considerable physiological protection against accident or infectious disease. This is also a major reference point for educational programs. Understanding the physical body and its needs is a fundamental objective of human knowledge. One must also be made aware of how to achieve fitness and health goals. Care of the body must be part of the knowledge and goals of all individuals.

Professional Status of Education

The plan for this section is to review the current status of education as a profession. This analysis will deal with education as one of the professional enterprises of society rendering service to the people. This presentation will serve as the framework for the application of physical activity as an educational profession and as a part of the total professional program of education.

Physical activity in the United States has from the outset been a part of the educational programs in schools, colleges, and universities. In some instances it has contributed significantly to the total goals for education, and in others it has served as an adjunct to the school's educational goals. This review will show physical activity as it is today. We shall also attempt to show just how physical activity fits into educational programs as now planned.

Finally, in this section some basic criteria will be applied to the educational-physical activity relationship in order to view the professional potentials of both. The emphasis in such a probe must be placed on the potentials of physical activity as an educational profession.

Foundations for Education. Education is the heart of any society. It serves to improve life and the social order. The educational process starts with conditions as they are, and moves forward toward goals, both individual and societal, of conditions as they should be. It is one of the most constructive forces in a society, an instrument by which people may pull themselves up and improve their way of life.

The basic needs and values of the individual must have first priority. Study of philosophy is not the most constructive approach for a starving individual. Possibly, then, education should begin with instruction on how to reach a level of economic security, with the vocational goal a major aim for education. This example applies to other basic needs such as health, social and physical environmental conditions, professional and vocational opportunities and requirements, social and family life practices, cultural interests and resources, recreational facilities, quality levels of services, and so on. This would certainly appear to be a starting point for any program of education, including potential programs of physical activity.

The basic human values of the individual and society can be easily recognized and identified. *Health* is a major requirement for all. The role of education in achieving good health is far larger than the profession of medicine itself. Knowledge about the organism and health is complicated. Good health must become a part of a systematic learning process and its procedures practiced. Knowledge, skills, and attitudes must be developed as a basis for achievement of this goal.

The individual's mental facilities must be developed to be able to *think and reason critically.* Educational programs to achieve this goal constitute a major need of society.

Moral and ethical values are basic for the satisfaction of the individual and society. Like many other social values, behavior is primarily a family and parental responsibility. Skills, attitudes, and practices, however, must be established in the intellectual environment of the school. The assumption that a good mind will always produce acceptable behavior is a fallacy; the contrary is too often found.

The individual and society must be prepared for a life of *responsibility for self and others.* This is one of the most basic values for survival and for higher ideals of cooperative community living. Civic knowledge and social participation are important parts of education for all citizens. They are also universal objectives. The preparation for applications of the democratic processes, in both theory and practice, is a basic part of learning and a major goal of all education.

The ability to *communicate* is essential in developing interdependency to a level of mutuality and on to a higher level of exchange for the enrichment of all. Unless individuals and nations learn to communicate, the development of interdependency is not possible. Without free, clear, and reasonable communications a true meeting of cultures does not occur. Communication should include all aspects of life of the people in each culture. This is a most basic need or value for all people and can only be accomplished through planned and systematic programs.

All individuals and nations must be prepared in all aspects of *security* —economic, social, political, and intercultural. Personal security is a need for all people, and one must prepare for it. Security can be tested by practice and evaluation. These are also important roles for education.

Fullness in life is another basic need. One must be prepared for living beyond daily needs. Achievements in service, arts, music, literature, and other cultural facets come from preparation for goals that go beyond daily work. Of course, the discussion of professions must include the cultural aspects of life. The great cultural achievements throughout history have come from dedicated artists who have made great personal sacrifices in order to cultivate their skills. Sculpture, painting, and literature are included among the historical achievements of many nations. The study of the cultural achievements of a nation is a basis for understanding its people and culture. Aspirations, insights, and emotions are most fully expressed through a nation's cultural achievements. These are foundations for mutual appreciation, intercultural understanding, and acceptance.

Physical Activity in Education. Physical activity as physical education is designed for the individual and society as a professional service to advance toward more acceptable and desirable levels of living. The goals are the same as those for education. The difference is that the medium for achievement is physical activity, and the results come only from the potential of physical activity in meeting the total goal of education. Physical education, in this respect, has both common and unique contributions to make.

Like all educational objectives, plans for the educational applications of physical activity must start with basic values and needs. It is interesting to note that physical activity in its educational role contributes to the basic values of our total educational picture. Contributions in human development are enjoyed by all, and in some cases this role is a major one. The contributions of physical education go beyond basic needs, but these will be developed in the next section of this chapter, on the professional domain of physical activity in education.

Just as it is a responsibility for education, advancing the *health status of the individual and society* is also a major responsibility of physical education. The development of the organism through appropriate use of physical activity is a fundamental requirement for all people. It is also an important goal for education, with the major contribution toward achievement made through physical activity and in the preparation for physical activity through living practices.

Knowledge and critical analysis are stated as a major goal for education. They are also a major goal for physical education. Physical activity requires more than skills or the knowledge of how to perform. It requires the preparation of the organism for performance. Physical activity applied toward achievement of knowledge and understanding is within the context of the social and physical environments. These environments can be used for positive results through understanding each within the potentials of physical activity.

As in education, physical education contributes to personal resources for the *constructive use of leisure*. During a period with less physical activity demanded by our occupations, physical activity in its leisure-recreational roles can contribute to this important goal. The aids to growth, development, and fitness that can be provided through physical activity and educational preparation are an important consideration.

Security through the development of abilities and skills essential for life is another objective of education. Physical activity as physical education contributes significantly to this objective. Success and fortune as experienced through physical activity contribute to self-actualization. Security grows from realization of potentialities and fulfillment of requirements by planned personal development. Confidence in self and personal resources is important for the individual. It is a major role for both education and physical education.

Preparing the individual for *a life of variety and differences* is another major objective for education. Physical education contributes to this goal. Race, religion, ethnic origin, occupation, economic status, and nationality are differences that can be integrated in and understood through physical activity as physical education. In sports it is ability that counts; just as it should be in life. Education and, more specifically, physical education prepare individuals to develop their abilities. Ethnic origin is only a starting point; it is the human abilities, capacities, and resources that will determine what the individual can achieve with appropriate educational preparation.

It was stated in the preceding section that *communication* abilities are a goal for education. Education is the only institution in the community charged with the systematic development of communication skills. Participation in physical activity for physical education or simply for its own sake is a communicative process. Personal actions and interactions in physical activity are communication systems as seen between teammates. Differences must be recognized, accepted, and resolved.

Education and physical education prepare the individual for a life of *personal and societal responsibility* in all of its economic, social, and political aspects. The scope is self-action in society on a worldwide scale. The interassociation of knowledge within physical activity is a process that contributes toward this goal. Participation in sports and physical activity creates human bonds and fellowships that are important ingredients for responsibility. Discipline, cooperation, ethical behavior, courage, self-reliance, and initiative are only some of the qualities that can be developed through participation in sports with proper leadership.

Education has the overall charge of preparing one for *fullness of life, balance of interests, and citizenship.* The medium of physical activity can contribute to this goal. The primary responsibility for all facets of education is intellectual. The human mind must be prepared to solve complex problems in order to advance the life of the people to acceptable social levels. Preparation for a life of fullness and citizenship requires skills and positive qualities. These include desirable practices during the eight hours a day when one is free to make personal choices. Free time is increasing, not decreasing, and it is important that everyone develop interests and skills that provide for constructive personal use of time. Education must provide more than a liberal background or a professional preparation for a vocation. Physical activity as sports is rapidly increasing in its role of providing for fullness in individual life programs.

Professional Status of Physical Activity as Education

A profession becomes a profession only through its service to people. If the services are in demand and if the requirements for the practitioner are sufficiently specialized, the basis for a profession is fundamentally established. The status of the profession is determined by these two factors. For example, medicine is considered an established profession. Education is also considered a profession, but it does not have the same sort of requirements as those now established in medicine. Physical activity in its educational role falls short of professional standards in medicine, and some of the educational practices in physical activity fall short of the general standards of education as currently delineated by educational institutions. In order to distinguish the nature of physical activity as a current educational profession, a brief review will be presented based upon some criteria that will aid in this analysis.

1. *The professional requirement of specialized techniques is a major basis for a profession.* The acceptance and the success of a profession are in direct proportion to the needs of the people for services and the complexity of learning and achievement in rendering the service by the practitioner.

Physical activity in physical education does require highly specialized skills and techniques and does meet this criterion of a profession. The conclusion must be based, then, on the quality of the services as judged by the people for whom they are rendered. There are practitioners in physical activity that rendered services without university preparation, such as coaches in professional sports. To this extent, as a strictly classified educational service, the position of physical activity as education is weakened significantly.

2. *To be recognized as a profession, the technique and preparation are communicated through a highly specialized educational discipline or disciplines.* To gain recognition and status as a profession, preparation for services must reach deeply into the content of science or other disciplines. In many instances, skills for practice or communication of the profession are needed in preparing its services. The degree of these requirements will determine the status of the profession.

For physical activity as education, a number of content disciplines are needed for preparation of services. Knowledge is required for an understanding of the human organism that represents a portion of the content of physical education. This knowledge can be gained from the disciplines of physiology, psychology, sociology, the physical sciences, medicine, and philosophy. The services of physical education deal with human development. Knowledge and skills in the use of physical activity are therefore fundamental for the development of the techniques and procedures used by the practitioner. To this extent, physical education does meet the requirements of a profession. What is needed is a set of requirements for the practice of physical education that will not permit assignments by unqualified individuals. Physical education does have its professional potential, but the quality needed for practice has not been entirely recognized by the public or by the practicing members themselves.

3. *The professional practices must be of significant social significance to warrant controls by the public and by the profession.* The need for quality of professional services by society is the basis for professional and public controls. Controls are necessary in establishing vital services. This is particularly so if the quality of the services performed by a practitioner is the deciding factor in determining the results of the service. In such instances standards or controls are set by the profession. It is additional evidence of the worth of a profession if it plans safeguards and standards to protect the public.

Teachers, coaches, and other school and university personnel in physical education must meet standards for teacher certification. Schools and colleges must be accredited in order to render services to the public. To this extent physical education meets this criterion. Again, it is its acceptance and recognition by the public or the users of the services that establish the quality of the profession and its professional status among other professions.

4. *A profession consists of practitioners who establish professional associations to improve standards for professional practices.* Dedication

to high professional standards by its practitioners is a significant characteristic of a profession. Self-controls and regulations are the most desirable basis for any profession. Setting and enforcing standards of practice
will serve to improve services and, as a result, the status of the profession. It would be most difficult for the public to set and enforce standards
without the support of professional members, but public evaluation of
services, with the idea of improving services from a cooperative profession, will strengthen the organization.

A number of professional organizations use the medium of physical
activity for educational programs. These include teachers, coaches, trainers, professional educators, and others. In each instance the professional
organizations have meetings to review practices and, in some instances,
to recommend standards. The process of establishing and enforcing standards in physical education takes too long and is ineffective. The choice
is made, in most instances, by the practitioner. Professional physical education associations have had some effectiveness in setting standards for
personnel, but these professional organizations have been ineffective in
putting into practice needed standards necessary to become an established and recognized profession.

5. *Professions have codes of ethics as bases for practices.* Violation
of codes causes personal review and possible discipline. In some professions, license to practice may be withdrawn. Codes of ethics are essential
for professional services of critical necessity to the public, which must
have full confidence in the practitioner and the services rendered.

In education and physical education, various professional organizations establish codes of ethics. The enforcement of codes, however, is
ineffective and has resulted in nearly complete freedom to establish
personal codes. Of course, moral indiscretions are sometimes disciplined
by the law and the employer through dismissal and job rejections.

Personnel in physical education are regulated, in most instances, by
the codes of ethics of the institution. The regulations of the institution
are the bases for disciplinary action against ethical violation. Education
and physical education have not yet attained a position of desirable
control over ethics and practices for the profession.

6. *Professions place social service and duty as their highest goal.*
The public is the evaluator of a profession and its services. A strong profession views this responsibility with concern. Unaccepted practices are
reviewed by the profession and corrections are made. Such self-regulation
represents the heart of the profession and affects its status as judged by
the public.

Education and physical education are, of course, designed for the
public and stem from social concerns. Social duty and service is the
basis for both. The effective school is determined by the results of educational programs as judged through the actions of the recipients of
these programs. The production of good communities and citizens is a

social responsibility of all educational programs. Physical education regards this social service role highly and, in most instances, reaches acceptable professional levels of performance.

Professional Domain: Conceptual Educational Structure of Physical Activity

What is the professional domain of physical activity in its educational role? Does physical activity have significant and valuable educational content? Does it have the qualities to meet important needs of the individual and the public? If the potentials are simply frills and not essential for the individual or the public, physical activity as an educational profession will not succeed in its design to render meaningful services to the public. If, on the other hand, the services are necessary, professional growth through these services will result. A review is presented on the human qualities that can be developed through the proper use of physical activity. In this instance the context is education in service to the people in order to provide preparation for life and all its requirements. Of course, the limits of its effectiveness are set by the potentials of education in working toward this goal (List 8).

List 8. The professional domain of physical activity in education

1. Societal aspects.
   a. Achievable goals.
   b. Adaptation to environment.
   c. Cultural mores and traditions.
   d. Enjoyment.
   e. Freedom from overstress.
   f. Knowledge of environment.
   g. Personal initiative.
   h. Satisfying environment.
   i. Security: personal and economic.
   j. Self-government.
   k. Self-reliance.
   l. Societal participation.
2. Human relations.
   a. Attitudes.
   b. Citizenship responsibility.
   c. Courage.
   d. Cultural background.
   e. Group adjustment.
   f. Integration.
   g. Integrity.
   h. Loyalty.
   i. Maturation.
   j. Perception.
   k. Propriety.
   l. Security.
   m. Self-realization.
   n. Social control.
3. Leisure.
   a. Automation.
   b. Commercialization influences.
   c. Communications.
   d. Curriculum programs.
   e. Democratic government.
   f. Environmental characteristics.
   g. Ethics and values.
   h. Family and peer interests.
   i. Influence of mass media.
   j. Institutions (social).
   k. Skills.
   l. Transportation.
4. Vocational aspects.
   a. Cooperation.
   b. Discipline.
   c. Economic factors.
   d. Employment.

e. Equality.
f. Human personality.
g. Positive actions.
5. Individual and social health.
  a. Adaptive and therapeutic aspects.
  b. Body symmetry.
  c. Disease prevention.
  d. Fitness.
  e. Health maintenance.
  f. Intensity of exercise.

h. Responsibility.
i. Self-government.

g. Longevity.
h. Mental and social aspects.
i. Muscular and C-V development.
j. Neuromuscular coordination.
k. Weight control.

The educational potentials of physical activity are classified into five groups or categories according to the human qualities developed. These include preparation for society; development of knowledge, understanding, and skills in human relations; preparation for constructive leisure; preparation for the advancement and protection of individual and social health; and preparation of the individual for a satisfying and economically secure vocation. These categories of educational qualities represent the professional domain or potentials of physical activity in education.

Societal Aspects. The social qualities of physical activity include the individual in both his association with society as a whole on local and world levels and personal preparation for self-satisfaction in relationship with others.

Physical activity in an educational and professional context contributes to the goals of society. Society is more than a government of the people; it is where one lives, what one does to make a living, and how one is able to enjoy life. Physical activity in its role as recreation, sports, and athletics and as a personal medium for enjoyment, fitness, and well-being is important in preparation for a society that has positive values and is a desirable place for its people. Although society is the setting for one's vocational life, it provides much more than economic security. Physical activity as an educational phenomenon does provide opportunities for vocations, but its contributions go considerably beyond this limited scope. It contributes to personal security, to intimate understanding of others and of the physical environment, to personal adaptation or development of a way of life, to relaxation and fitness to sustain one in social relationships and the stresses of life; and it provides other qualities that the individual can only achieve through the educational applications of physical activity.

One of the major reasons for educational agencies is the development of a society that represents the highest levels of living. Educational programs are designed toward this goal. The programs include all aspects of life, and physical activity is one of the most important facets. Society through the development of the individual has much to gain from well-conceived and functioning physical activity programs.

Human Relations. Another important goal for education is to prepare one to live together with other individuals, the family, the local community, the nation, and peoples in other countries throughout the world. The elimination of war would mean the eradication of one of man's major antisocial activities. Human relations, positively developed, stem from understanding of religion, race, color, mores, national traditions, and ways of life. Physical activity, as applied in education, can add immeasurably to preparing the individual in human understandings. The color bias is rapidly being eliminated in sports. In most cases the athlete today is judged on his ability, not his color.

Physical activity as sports, athletics, and physical recreation is one of the most informal media in education, thus providing an ideal setting for development of the qualities necessary for close personal relationships. The adjustment of the individual to a group, the integration of group members, and the responsibility of the individual to the group are some of the human values important in human relations. Physical activity probably has more potential for achievement of human relations goals than any of the other media in education, and physical activity can make one of its largest educational contributions in this area.

Leisure. The educational role of physical activity in leisure preparation is a significant one. The reasons for this are many, but two are of major importance. First is the realization that the lack of physical work and the stressful nature of today's occupations put the modern citizen into a vulnerable position because of this inactivity and stress. Of equal importance is the sociocultural recognition of and emphasis on sports, athletics, and physical activity as an important part of life. Particularly in the American culture, tremendous importance has been placed on education's responsibility to prepare people for leisure.

The philosophic foundations for American education, and education in many other countries, are developed from the goal of providing preparation for a satisfying and successful life. The role for education, therefore, must be more than preparing for a vocation or a profession. This is of particular significance when the vocation begins taking less time and leisure periods are greatly increased. Without a doubt, this responsibility for leisure has become a major goal for education in all its social roles and institutions, and physical activity in sports and athletics has been found to be particularly valuable. In this respect, physical education is a firm part of the programs in educational institutions.

Vocational Aspects. The role of physical activity in vocations consists of three major categories. The first category represents the human qualities that can be achieved through consistent participation in physical activity. Such qualities are important parts of the lives of professional workers. They work essentially with people, and the values coming from physical activity will aid in their associations. The second category is the sociocultural values that come from physical activity and provide a setting for the various vocations in a society. Vocational and professional workers in communities with underdeveloped citizenship will have particular difficulties. The third category represents the numerous opportunities for the use of physical activity in all its forms as a vocation or a profession, for example, direct participation in the activity such as in professional sports or professional work that require high-level preparation such as sports medicine.

Individual and Social Health. Health and its development and maintenance not only are a responsibility of science and medicine, but also are included in the role of education. It is unfortunate that the importance of educational health goals is so often ignored by the individual until medical help becomes necessary. Educational institutions have the responsibility of preparing the individual to develop and maintain good health. One should not wait until the damage has been done, because then it may be too late.

The role of education through physical activity is, in large measure, one of disease prevention. Many diseases can be prevented if the individual has the knowledge and the desire to apply that knowledge in his daily living. One of the major goals of education in the United States and many countries is health for all. A major drive is now on to improve the physical fitness of all citizens. It is now well established that a physically fit organism not only performs work of all kinds with less stress, but also shows good physiological functioning of the body processes, a strong preventive factor. Without physical fitness, the organism is in constant trouble and certainly not in good health. The educational role applies also to social health, or the health of the people as a whole. The community and home environments are major factors in individual health in a social setting. The role of education in disseminating knowledge pertaining to science and medicine is a major one. Education has a major responsibility in this regard, and physical activity can make major contributions toward this goal.

Professional Domain: Educational Content of Physical Activity

The educational domain within physical activity is conceptualized in the preceding section. The following presentation is an elaboration of these concepts as the potential educational content of physical activity. These statements indicate what can be accomplished by physical activity under acceptable professional leadership and operational conditions.

Societal Content. Physical activity provides opportunities for the development of *democratic behavior and skills* through participational relationships. Sports provide a social setting that is intense and invokes the deep interest and sensitivity of the individual. The democratic concepts of respect, equality of opportunity, self-government, and responsibility can all be developed through proper application of sports.

Physical activity provides opportunities for the development of *desirable social behavior* in the setting of physical participation. The leadership must, however, set the standards for participation. Social behavior in competition must be patterned in terms of desired social goals.

Learning opportunities are provided in physical activity. Learning about oneself, others, and the environment is a major aim for educational programs, and physical activity provides numerous learning experiences that can be applied in other life situations. Thinking and reasoning abilities developed through participation are basic to success in personal and professional life.

Moral and personal behavior traits are part of sports and physical activity. Another important goal for education is the personal development of the individual to fit the established requirements of good citizenship. The ethical behavior of the individual is fundamental in any society. It is of particular importance in sports because of the wide acceptance and status of sports in our society. The moral behavior of athletes has tremendous influence, and athletes are a large part of any social order. The strength and importance of sports in society can make significant contributions toward achieving this important educational goal.

Social integration and adjustment is another major goal of education. Contributions can be made both directly and indirectly by acceptable applications of sports and physical activity. Maintenance of desirable traditions and acceptable mores of a community is an important educational goal. Sports reflect traditions and are conducted within traditional settings. With proper direction the desirable traditions of education can be advanced through sports. The current international emphasis on sports makes this goal of particular value.

Human Relations Content. Education also has the responsibility to teach standards of acceptable conduct within the society. The group, as in sports, must function by rules and regulations that provide the basis for the individual to relate democratically to others. This is a major component in the development of human relations. Learning to contribute to a group involves respect, self-discipline, and cooperation based on reason and intelligence.

Interpersonal interactions in sports and physical activity provide experiences that are important in the development of acceptable human relations. Life in the community, nation, or world setting is a mixture of all cultures, races, creeds, colors, and ethnic origins and includes major differences in living habits and practices. The goal for education in establishing acceptable human relations is not to strive for common practices, but to understand and appreciate differences. The ability to accept persons different from oneself is not easily achieved, and helping one to learn this constitutes a fundamental reason for educational institutions. Physical activity can serve as a major facet of education working toward this end.

Attitudes and personal behavior are important qualities within the educational goals of acceptable and desirable human relations. Unacceptable attitudes and personal behavior are deterrents to successful participation in sports and athletics. Attitudes and personal behavior can be modified to fit the requirements of sports, and the personal motivation for participation and success aids in the achievement of this goal. It is one of the important reasons for educational programs in communities, because these qualities are parts of all educational programs. They are even more important to the life of a community than they are to sports participation.

Social motivation and adjustment are purposes of educational programs to which sports, athletics, and physical activity participation can contribute significantly. Sports and athletics represent media that involve intense personal relationships. Associations developed are nearly as free as the will of the individual. Little personal latitude for reserve is found in competition. The closeness of human beings adds to maturity and the adjustment of one to another and the group. Group goals become individual goals on a good team. This is the fundamental basis for success. This medium is thus most important to educational programs.

Leisure Content. During the last decade, leisure has increased significantly, which, in turn, increases the role and responsibility of education in preparing individuals for it. In this connection, physical activity as sports, athletics, and games is a major part of leisure preparation programs.

Abundant space, facilities, and leadership are available to encourage leisure activities of all kinds, but the major portion is directly associated with physical activity. In the United States, sports facilities represent a large part of the budgets of educational institutions and communities. Modern educational philosophy recognizes the potentials of leisure in accomplishing desired educational goals. It is a responsibility of education not only to prepare one for leisure, but also to provide leisure facilities and programs that will advance and sustain human qualities most desirable for good citizenship.

Modern emphasis on physical activity has caused major changes in how leisure is used by society. This is a concern of education and physical activity as well. A large portion of each individual's time, particularly in the United States, is devoted to sports. This includes not only time spent as a participant but also that spent as a spectator. Educational philosophy recognized that it is necessary to develop and sustain the physical well-being of society. This is due, to a large degree, to loss of caloric output because of automation and the lack of physical work. Physical activity is unique in its ability to fulfill this goal.

Education for personal living is increasingly becoming a concern. The goal of American education is more than the mastery of professional skills; personal behavior and individual qualities are of major consequence within the profession. This includes the fitness of the individual, which allows him to sustain difficult and stressful tasks. In sports and athletics one gains physical prowess that adds to the vigor of the individual performing professional tasks. It also serves as the basis for maintaining health that might deteriorate under vigorous professional work. The educational applications of physical activity can add significantly to the individual and to the goals of education.

Leisure programs give balance to the more formal programs of education. Balance for its own sake is not a goal for education, but when it broadly prepares one for the world, that is another matter. Leisure now consumes more of our time than work. It would be unfortunate to devote the entire program to the occupational or professional levels of education and fail to prepare the individual for leisure. This factor is recognized by nearly all educators. Physical activity has become a large part of educational leisure programs because of the growing need for activity in our sedentary culture. The content of educational programs is becoming increasingly leisure oriented, thus giving recognition to the importance of preparation for our nonwork time.

Rapid improvements in transportation have had major effects on leisure activities. National and international sports are commonplace, and teams are now scheduled to be in New York one day and Los Angeles the next. International activity is increasing rapidly in nearly all types of sports. Educational goals have changed during the past few years because of the changes made possible through travel. Education recognizes that the intermingling of people of all nations is a major force for international understanding, and is an important goal for education.

Vocational Content. The vocational and professional career opportunities in physical activity and its applications as sports, athletics, and other forms represent a considerable segment of the total work opportunities in a community. Physical activity is recognized as a combination of disciplines and professions. Preparation for opportunities is necessary and most educational institutions have instituted professional programs for leadership preparation.

Physical activity in its educational roles contains a *body of knowledge* that must be learned for professional leadership. The degree of specialization is high and classified into many subgroups based on the knowledge and skills needed for leadership. Suitable educational programs are now available in most universities and colleges in the United States. Leadership is now available with a high level of specialized training for professional programs dealing with the various applications of physical activity.

Physical activity and sports serve in a *supplementary vocational role* in society. Regardless of one's vocation or profession, physical activity is desirable for meeting the stresses of one's job. In addition, the social potentials of such sports as golf, tennis, and swimming relieve worries about daily tasks and give refreshment from work. Physical activity adds to the social well-being of the individual, both personally and professionally.

Wholeness in vocational and professional preparation is now viewed as *philosophically essential*. The job today is more than a set of isolated skills. It is nearly impossible to separate oneself from society or the culture even though one might wish to do so. Professions are designed to serve people and society, and one must understand society fully if it is to be served.

Physical activity in its various applications now represents *career opportunities* equal to those in other long-established professions. Career opportunities in physical activity are practically a twentieth-century development in the United States and other countries. For example, professional sports are now one of the most economically successful professions in the United States. Baseball, football, basketball, and hockey are, indeed, economically successful; and they are parts of programs in nearly all cities large enough to support attendance. Many participants find after their playing career has ended that career opportunities open up for them as coaches, trainers, or administrators. For those who are interested and have the aptitude careers in physical activity are available. Athletes all begin skill preparation for participation during their early youth. This is true in the United States and most other countries because physical activity is part of school programs.

Individual and Social Health Content. Individual health is a major educational goal. The contributions that can be made through physical activity to health are rapidly being discovered through research. Modern living, with rich diets, makes exercise a requirement to maintain physiological functions at acceptable levels. Studies in the social, biological, and medical disciplines indicate that people *must seek and participate in physical activity* in order to sustain health under modern living conditions. Considerable research has been conducted during the past fifteen to twenty years on the effects of physical activity. The role of education is to achieve an understanding of fitness and health and then to provide the educational resources to help people achieve these goals.

Participation in physical activity to achieve health and fitness should be *pleasurable*. Sports have become a part of social life in nearly all world cultures.

One must be *prepared* to participate in physical activity in order to achieve improved health and fitness. Effective participation in physical activity requires skills and practice. The individual must be prepared for participation to gain benefits from the activity. Good health and fitness come from vigorous participation, but enjoyment stems mainly from satisfactory performance. School programs must prepare one for physical activity.

A major educational goal is the *adjustment* of the individual to self and others. Physical activity can aid in accomplishing this goal. Social and physical adjustment to one's environment is a basic requirement in life, and the informal nature of sports makes them ideal for achievement of this goal.

Social health and cultural interests and activities should be *planned* as integrated goals for education. Health is one of the most essential ingredients for a satisfying life. The many unhappy and unpleasant settings in the world must be improved; a large part of the responsibility for this belongs to education.

Physical Activity: An Educational Profession

Of the ten professional applications of physical activity examined in Part II physical activity within the educational context is probably the most firmly established. Hardly a school exists in the United States that does not include physical education as part of its curriculum. In most instances the instructional or basic program is required, but sports, intramural and athletic periods, or school volunteer programs are open to all students. Educators have noted the value of physical activity, and belief in its contributions has increased in strength during the past ten to fifteen years, largely because of the increasing needs of the people for physical activity. The contributions to the goals of education are more than theoretical; they are part of realistic programs whose worth is demonstrated each day.

There can be little doubt about the value of physical activity planned as physical education. The professional structure, functions, and philosophic bases are well established. The professional structure is rapidly improving, and subprofessional groups are forming. All of this tends to indicate the validity of the professional application of physical activity.

Chapter 12

Health

"There are those who create knowledge and those who apply it. The former, in search for truth, endeavor to define reality with precision. The latter hope to elicit the need for new knowledge. Those who investigate foresee the benefits for mankind of the results of their studies. Those who apply them enjoy the well-being derived, but dream of the new frontiers further research could attain."[1] Both of these efforts are part of the never-ending services that society provides for man. They represent a growing relationship between disciplinary and professional applications of knowledge. The role of those on the frontier of knowledge discovery is to understand and illuminate various phenomenona; at the same time, others must apply this knowledge to meet human needs.

Research to study human needs and the fulfillment of those needs require special effort. A close relationship between research and its application is ideal. Such a relationship is certainly essential in the health field, possibly more than in any other area.

The development of the health potentialities is probably the most important reason for physical activity. This is true in each of the ten professional applications made in this section of the text (Part III). The importance of good health is probably emphasized more today than at any other period in history.

Individual health, of course, has a physical base. The body is a biological organism, and its level of total performance is usually set as the health level of the individual. Health goes beyond the scope of merely ridding society of disease or of sustaining life. It is a dynamic phenomenon and must be maintained to counterbalance physical work, leisure activities, and normal physiological bodily functions, all of which place tremendous stress upon the body. Another dimension to today's health problem is that of the dietary habits of today's society, particularly in the United States, which have resulted in a ballooning weight-control

---

[1] J. Lederberg, "Health in the World of Tomorrow." Pan American Health Organization, Sanitary Bureau, WHO, p. 1.

crisis. Individual health is also a social, emotional, and personal matter, because it affects the very life breath of the individual. Personal interests and habits are the basis for achieved health levels and contribute to one's health potential. Emotional reactions to stresses or environmental conditions also help to determine the individual's health level.

Environmental conditions, both physical and social, are major factors in the health picture of the average individual. The mores of a society influence the individual. Personal habits, such as diet, alcohol, drugs, and personal hygiene, have both beneficial and harmful effects on health. Today the physical environment itself is an increasingly important factor in the health picture. Air and water pollution, sanitation, noise, slums, and other substandard living conditions, and other environmental conditions beyond the individual's control have cut deeply into individual health.

In a recent text [2] the author reviewed the personal factors that reflect levels of individual health. These are the end results of physical activity potentials and their components that are presented in this chapter on the professional domain of physical activity. These components represent guidelines for basic and professional programs used by all health agencies to gain desired end results, which in this instance are attainable especially through physical activity.

1. *Disease* is a major personal health problem and physical activity can aid both in its prevention and control and in recovery from it. The contribution of physical activity to developing a strong, vigorous, organism helps the individual combat the negative effects of disease. It also contributes to the recovery and rebuilding to the status of normal bodily functioning. In each instance environmental protection is the most essential factor in attempts to prepare the individual for highest possible positive results from physical activity.

2. *Physical defects* may be both structural and functional. Both have the potentialities for correction and both many times can be prevented. The term *structural defects* refers to the loss of body parts; modifications in function to compensate for body deviations represent *functional defects*. The former may be corrected in part by prosthetic devices; the latter in many instances require corrective exercises or programs through physical education.

Physical activity is important to all individuals as a deterrent for malfunctions caused by physical deviations or defects. Obesity, for example, can arise from inactivity, which, in turn, leads to a number of further complications, including high blood pressure, decreased work capacity, and heart disease. Maintaining total body fitness through physical activity leads to the maximization and continuation of normal body functions, the basis for good health and physical vigor.

[2] L. A. Larson, *Curriculum Foundations and Standards for Physical Education* (Englewood Cliffs, N.J.: Prentice-Hall, 1970), pp. 77–83.

3. *Organic vigor* is evidenced by the ability to maintain normal bodily functioning while resisting the organic and inorganic forces that act as catabolic agents to the human body. Simply remaining free from disease or physical defects does not constitute good health. Man must be led toward the realization of what for him really does constitute good health, the nature of which will differ with age and maturation level. The sooner this process is instituted following birth, the less relearning will be required.

Progressive development, in close coordination with the maturation schedule, will result in a strong physical body capable of combating the stresses of various environmental forces. Good health is also the basis for a vibrant personality.

An individual in good physical health achieved through physical development beyond daily work requirements will be able to meet excessive stresses of both work and play with little more than temporary adjustments. This adaptability will add to the individual's personal development and allow him to cope with adverse situations.

4. *Weight control and symmetry* are primary health factors and are both extremely influential in determining efficiency and adaptability for action. Cumulative fatigue, decreased work capacity, and other by-products of overweight will lower the vitality of the body and result in a decreased health level as well as a marked decrease in life span because of related heart and circulatory ailments.

Proper diet is essential for maintaining the food resources needed for the body to achieve optimal benefit from physical activity. This is not only important in maintaining normal weight but is also of major importance in maintaining the normal bodily requirements necessary to perform and sustain exercise as well as the requirements needed to reach physical developmental goals.

A symmetrical body not only is aesthetically pleasing, but lacks such deviations as poor posture and poor segmental relationships, which characterize the asymmetrical individual. Bad posture is the beginning of the process leading to maladjustments that could eventually result in physical deformities.

5. *Fatigue* is a measure of health. A healthy individual is able to live a vigorous life, both socially and professionally, with only noticeable temporary fatigue. Good health allows the tired individual to recuperate fully with adequate rest. At the highest fitness level, an individual can maintain an extremely vigorous life. Prompt recuperation reflects the optimal human resource attainable through good health.

Constant fatigue will gradually influence the normal functions of the body until an abnormal condition is reached. In some instances, damage may result that is so serious that it makes a return to normal difficult or impossible.

The basis for all of man's actions is the physical body. A strong body developed through consistent and appropriate physical activity will sustain normal physiological functions, barring disease, through a full span of life. Moreover, that life span will be appreciably extended.

Health: Professional Status

In this section we will try to establish an understanding of the scope of health and its professional potentials. This analysis will deal with health as a requirement for all people and with the health services needed by society to sustain personal health levels and goals. The various services rendered and their specializations will determine the number of professions that can be sustained through such services.

The review will be presented in three parts: (1) the foundations for health as a profession or professions in service to society, (2) the role of physical activity in meeting health goals of society, and (3) the professional status of health in its various roles in society.

Professional Foundations. The foundation for health as a profession lies in the knowledge that health is a condition of the human organism that is influenced by all physical, emotional, social, and intellectual actions of the organism. Health is also influenced by all our environmental conditions, from living conditions in the home to the air we breathe. Every condition exerts a certain influence upon the organism, some extremely significant and others with little or no effect. The scope of health needs and the worth of services that will maintain adequate health levels provide the basis for professional services of various specializations. This is the basis for professional organizations that develop around specialized services.

In its largest context, individual health includes the *mental abilities, resources, and adjustments* needed in daily life. Mental health is reflected in one's ability to assume responsibility, make decisions, solve problems, find satisfaction in work and leisure, and find fulfilling social contact. Mental health can be measured by reactions to vocational success, achievements in meeting personal goals, reactions resulting from failures, and ability to survive and sustain positive goals under severely depressing situations. Maintaining a positive attitude toward changing societal conditions, personal relationships, and professional conditions is a strong indication of desirable mental health. The positive spinoff from an unsatisfactory or unpleasant situation is often the base from which is built a stronger self-image and reflects good mental health. Amplification of the negative aspects of health or basing judgments on it will do little to improve the condition or the mental health status of the individual.

The primary context for the professional foundations of health lies in the knowledge that health has its fundamental basis *in the physical organism*. Good physical health is a state of the organism in which physical resources exceed the daily needs of the individual. The individual may experience temporary fatigue, of course, but seldom is fatigue chronic.

Viewing health in its broadest context, the emotional status of the individual reflects his views about the *problems, conditions, and associations* that occur daily. A person in good emotional health is able to solve problems reasonably and intelligently; personal feelings are not then the basis for the resolution of fact-oriented problems. Emotional health is developed by and based on love, affection, and acceptance by those whom one respects and admires. Insecurity is certainly incompatible with acceptable emotional health, whereas security is an extremely positive factor.

Another major component of health, viewed in its broadest scope, is *intellectual health*. Good health allows one to reason and apply mental abilities to resolve daily problems. The individual bases his life-style on facts or judgments that have been carefully analyzed. At its highest level, intellectual health allows the individual to perform successfully in all of life's many facets. It is the ability to find facts or judgments that satisfactorily resolve issues to the full agreement of all. Mental health is extremely variable and can only be determined on a relative basis.

Physical Foundations. Physical activity makes a major contribution toward the achievement of optimal health and in most instances is the primary reason for fitness and health. Good health has many requirements. *Freedom from worry* is an important goal for individual health. In this connection, physical activity serves as both a preventive and rehabilitative measure when it is precisely applied to fit the condition or defect. Good health also means *freedom from defects*. The *symmetry of the body* for segmental balance is an important factor in human movement and physical work. An organism in peak health is *vigorous and strong, has abundant endurance, and possesses an extended threshold of fatigue.*

The physical activity and health relationships that have been previously reviewed in this text will be presented in more detail later. The objective for this review is simply to accentuate the point in dealing with the health of an individual: the physical status of the body is the primary factor. Physical activity or exercise is the only means the physical body has to develop or sustain a level of health that provides the basis for active living. A person through minimum physical activity such as walking to meet daily activity needs can, of course, survive, but survival is only the minimum level of professional and social activity. In addition, the resources are barely adequate to prevent the effects of aging and the effects of disease.

Professional Status. Health is the primary concern of numerous professional areas and organizations. One of these areas is designated *health education.* There are organized professional groups in health education on the national, state, regional, and local political levels. These groups meet to guide and direct health education through professional standards and objectives.

In physical education many professional activities are concerned with the health goals possible through physical activity. This part of the professional function is part of the greater overall health profession.

Public health is developed by health specialists in this field through the effective use of well-conceived professional goals and programs. It is probably the largest professional group concerned with the overall health of society. In public health, standards are set and administered covering all phases of health with societal importance, from disease to hygienic practices. Controls set by public health organizations serve a vital public interest.

Mental health organizations have become increasingly predominant in serving the health-related needs of individuals with regard to mental and emotional health. The professional groups working in this area of the health field also deal with such areas of mental health as mental illness, personality behavior, and other maladjustments that may lead to unacceptable behavior.

The professional scope of groups organized around mental health problems is extensive. The members of these groups employ highly specialized techniques to deal with these problems. It is only through the professional efforts of these specialists that problems can be resolved and desirable mental health levels reached.

There are other professional groups dealing with health matters. Sports medicine is a profession that deals with the health problems of sports and athletics. Coaches and trainers are particularly concerned about the health of the athlete. Many of these groups have other professional goals, but in most the health of the individual is of primary concern. Specialists are then needed to deal with these problems.

Professional Domain: The Conceptual
Structure of Health in Physical Activity

The concern of this chapter (and text) is to analyze physical activity to determine its various potentials. What are the professional potentials of physical activity? The facts and judgments needed are based on what contributions physical activity can make to the individual and to a society or culture if it is to become a part of the life of the people. The worth of physical activity in its service to the people will determine the success of professionally organized specialists (List 9). Its needs and values will be planned by individuals and organized professions.

Educational Domain. The principle that one is master of his own destiny is, indeed, a viable one for individual health. If one would daily practice the guidelines now available as a result of research in his daily living and practices, most health problems could be avoided. Many health problems, including communicable diseases, come from neglect or violation of health practices known to be desirable.

List 9. Conceptual structure: The professional domain of physical activity in health

1. Educational domain.
   a. Balanced sleep, work, and leisure.
   b. Cultural goals.
   c. Disease prevention.
   d. Drugs.
   e. Economic status.
   f. Environments.
   g. Health knowledge and skills.
   h. Individual and group needs.
   i. Injury prevention.
   j. Mass media influences.
   k. Mores and traditions.
   l. Nutrition.
   m. Occupations.
   n. Professional leadership.
   o. Rehabilitation.
   p. Sanitation.
   q. Weight control.
2. Growth and development domain.
   a. Age and aging.
   b. Air/noise pollution.
   c. Basal metabolic rate.
   d. Body composition.
   e. Body systems development.
   f. Bone mineralization.
   g. Educational levels.
   h. Effects of inactivity.
   i. Energy needs.
   j. Environmental conditions.
   k. Family life.
   l. Fitness.
   m. Health practices.
   n. Maturation.
   o. Mental and emotional conditions.
   p. Nutrition and diet.
   q. Occupational factors.
   r. Personal health.
   s. Protection and prevention.
   t. Racial, ethnic differences.
   u. Socioeconomic status.
   v. Tensions and stresses.
3. Psychological domain.
   a. Acceptance of self and others.
   b. Adaptability.
   c. Alertness.
   d. Alleviation of anxiety.
   e. Aptitude.
   f. Attitude.
   g. Creativity.
   h. Democratic character structure.
   i. Goal achievement and success.
   j. Hormonal factors.
   k. Interests.
   l. Maturation.
   m. Mental retardation.
   n. Motivation.
   o. Obesity.
   p. Perception.
   q. Personality.
   r. Problem solving.
   s. Rehabilitation.
   t. Roles and values.
   u. Security.
   v. Stress tolerance.
   w. Therapeutic values.
   x. Tolerance.

4. Sociocultural domain.
   a. Accident prevention.
   b. Adjustment.
   c. Alcohol abuse.
   d. Behavior.
   e. Concept and value
      development.
   f. Drug abuse and control.
   g. Education.
   h. Individual/social
      development.
   i. Leisure and play influences.
   j. Leisure values.
   k. Mores and traditions.
   l. Occupation.
   m. Safety awareness.
   n. Social contact and family.
   o. Social interests.
   p. Smoking and health.
   q. Social class.

5. Physical domain.
   a. Aging.
   b. Cathartic effects.
   c. Disease prevention.
   d. Fatigue reduction.
   e. Fitness and health.
   f. Injury prevention.
   g. Living efficiency.
   h. Longevity.
   i. Movement capacities.
   j. Physical/mental health.
   k. Sleep, rest, relaxation.
   l. Symmetry of body.
   m. Therapeutic and
      rehabilitative values.
   n. Weight control.

A health education program includes many requirements and elements (List 9). The educational component itself is one of five major categories that are part of the professional domain of physical activity in health. The concern is the health content of physical activity, not the many additional elements that are part of health but that do not result from the use of physical activity in gaining health objectives. For example, many diseases are not directly related to individual physical activity practices. In reviewing the educational concepts in physical activity for health purposes, however, the worth of physical activity in achieving individual health goals is recognized in the total health education program.

The preparation of the individual for achieving good health is planned through educational programs of institutions, agencies, and various media in the community. Probably the most vital responsibility is the *preparation of professional leaders.* These professional programs require professional knowledge and techniques.

The preparation of the individual for desirable *hygienic practices* is a major component of health education. This component includes nutrition, rest, leisure, work, sanitation, drugs, and all living conditions that affect health levels.

Health education responsibilities to society include the processes for *rehabilitation, disease prevention, protection from accidents or injury.* Failure to meet health education responsibilities to society is of major concern.

Health education programs must be planned by institutions in *local cultural, economic, or environmental settings;* the traditions of the people must always be kept in mind. The education programs will vary under such differing conditions.

Health education is a very *personal matter*. Weight control is a major problem for many individuals and is closely related to their dietary practices. The care of the body is one of the most important life functions of every individual who desires the maintenance of good health. The *physical appearance* of an individual is a personal matter that is incorporated within a health education program.

Growth and Development Domain. The nature and rate of growth and development of the individual constitute another major responsibility of health through physical activity. Providing a setting for the optimal growth of the individual organism also provides for potentials in human development. Physical activity has a primary contribution to make toward this health goal. Growing is aided by physical activity if and only if all other factors influencing growth provide for the most favorable possible results from physical activity.

Living conditions, food practices, hygiene, stresses, and prevention of disease and injury are all factors that are closely related to the growth patterns and development of the child. Development must accompany growth patterns, but when the growing years are over, development then becomes a major factor. The conditions that aid proper growth are also the conditions that aid proper development.

Physical activity makes major contributions to growth and development. *Fitness, body systems development, maturation rate, and health conditions* are all elements in growth and development that are aided by consistent and proper physical activity or exercise. Growth and development need physical activity, and during the early growing years physical activity should make up a major part of the child's day.

The growth and development requirements of health differ from individual to individual. *Mores, racial differences, traditions, and nationality differences* are all differing conditions for growth and development. The peoples of the world differ in physical structure, development, and life-style requirements. These differences affect the requirements for programs contributing to growth and development, including physical activity.

Socioeconomic status, educational level, occupation, and age are also factors to be considered in viewing growth and development standards and programs. The very concept of physical activity is related to these conditions. Positive contributions can be made only when programs are planned within these contexts.

Psychological Domain. The psychological domain in physical activity is of major importance. Psychological forces are closely related to performance in physical activity, and performance can influence the psychological characteristics of the individual and the group. The results contribute to the mental and emotional health of both the individual and the group.

Attitude, maturation, goal achievements, interests, aptitudes, and tolerance are all psychological factors of physical performance that are influenced by participation. They are also important factors in the health of the individual and the group.

Mental alertness, creativity, adaptability, perception, and stress and the individual's controls, roles, and values are psychological elements within physical activity that influence performance and health levels. These factors are also factors in mental health that originate with physical activity and are prominent parts of performance.

The psychological factors of human relations play primary roles in physical activity participation. Democratic human values, personality characteristics, and acceptance of self and others are qualities of human association that are paramount in physical activity and sports participation. Success is to a large measure due to these psychological forces. The level of success can become a measure of the mental health of the individual or group. Certainly they reflect most of the important qualities of the human personality.

The individual's standards of physical appearance are also psychological in nature. *Obesity, poor posture, unacceptable body symmetry, poor body hygiene, and mental instability* are undesirable individual characteristics that are important in physical activity and in gaining desirable health results from physical activity.

It is now well established through the observation of coaches and sports scientists that the physical component alone is not the basis for successful participation and achievement in sports and physical activity. Favorable internal psychological conditions will primarily determine the intensity, duration, and frequency of participation. These forces will yield optimal results if they are on a favorable level, and these results not only will aid performance but will give additional quality to most of these psychological variables. All these factors contribute to the favorable health status of the individual.

Sociocultural Domain. The sociocultural domain of physical activity is closely related to participation and is a factor that adds to the quality of health of the individual and the group.

Social adjustment, interests, social behavior, family life, leisure practices, and social and cultural interests are all sociocultural concepts that add to the quality of life and to the quality of participation in sports and physical activity. The health status of the individual, the family, the group, and the community is also closely related to these sociocultural concepts. Properly planned physical activity contributes to these qualities.

The social practices and behavior of the individual and the group are factors in physical participation and social health. *Drug and alcohol abuse and lack of awareness of safety standards* are conditions that can destroy health and reduce levels of physical activity. These effects, although generally unfavorable, are strong forces and their abuse is not uncommon in sports and in the lives of individuals in today's society.

Traditions, mores, occupations, educational levels, and leisure values are important sociocultural concepts for an individual within the framework of physical participation and his own particular health status. Physical activity contributes to these sociocultural concepts and adds value to the individual and his life in the family and community. This adds to his positive health status.

Personal abuses such as unwise use of alcohol and other drugs reduce the ability of the individual participant and the health values that result from physical participation are also negated.

Physical Domain. The physical results achieved through physical activity are the major reason for physical activity and sports. One of the other primary reasons for physical activity is the health value that results from participation. Physical activity is unique in this regard because no other medium will produce the results that can be attained from physical activity. Health is a physical phenomenon and must be developed and maintained by constant physical utilization of the body.

Reduction of fatigue levels, improvement of fitness and health, and improvement of work and leisure skills are some of the benefits of physical activity. Improvement of these personal qualities increases the work efficiency of the organism, which, in turn, adds to the health status of the individual.

The therapeutic and rehabilitative potentials of physical activity are by-products of the proper use of physical activity. It is possible to maintain normal human functions through proper application of physical activity and health practices, and physical activity has the ability to return the organism to a normal or nearly normal functional level following injury. Of course, the structural effects of any injury set certain limits.

The *effects of aging and disease control and prevention* can be favorably influenced by physical activity. A healthy individual is one who is well conditioned and remains so throughout his life. Such an individual is able to remain physically active even through the later years of his life. This is a most functional definition of health. An individual in normal or above-normal physical condition has improved resistance to all types of stresses that tend to destroy or reduce his general health level.

Professional Domain: Health Content
in Physical Activity

The conceptual structure of physical activity in health has been presented in the preceding section. Its purpose was not only to review the concepts in physical activity that are factors in participation but also to review the concepts that contribute to the health status of the individual and the group as represented by the family, civic group, and community.

The purpose of this section is to extend the conceptual ideas of physical activity and health to statements that represent more completely the *content* in physical activity that is representative of its health potentials.

Educational Content. Physical content is important to the health levels of society. Because reaching a desirable health level is so vital to each person, the health content in physical activity must be made a part of all formal and informal educational programs. *The health education content of physical activity must be a part of all educational programs* designed for any age or group of people.

Physical fitness is a major component in health. The fitness goal can be achieved through programs of physical activity found in formal exercise or highly organized sports and athletics. Physical activity programs should be designed for all age groups from youth through the late years of adult life. Physical activity must also go beyond mere job requirements, except for the professional, whose occupation stems from physical activity and performances.

Caloric balance needed for attainment of desirable health goals must be coupled with physical activity in order to determine the proper balance of activity and food intake. Maintenance of acceptable body weight and body symmetry cannot be accomplished by diet alone. It is difficult to plan a balanced diet and proper caloric intake without the aid of exercise.

Physical activity to achieve and maintain health for body efficiency and increased work capacity must always be a part of everyone's life. When exercise ceases, regression begins in body functions. The beginning of this regression is so rapid that one barely realizes the effects until an attempt is made to return to original physical work habits or activities. *One must exercise daily.*

One must be aware of health and exercise fads. Education of the public is needed to ensure the avoidance of unfortunate experiences by people who accept unsupported claims. Scientific evidence is now available to give support to programs of physical activity in achieving desired health goals. Such facts should be sought out before individual programs are begun. In the cases of both health and exercise, the programs are precise and highly specific in their results. Generalization in either case is unwise.

The value to health of properly designed physical activity in achieving physical rehabilitation and prevention of physical injury has been demonstrated by sports physicians, trainers, coaches, and professionals associated with sports medicine. It is possible to prepare for leading a normal life through a rehabilitation process for those who have been injured or have congenital physical defects. In instances where complete rehabilitation is not achieved natural compensation is made through the enlargement or increased specialization of other body functions that will permit satisfactory adaptation by the individual.

The use of drugs in sports is extremely undesirable and professionals in sports medicine and science have found little value in drugs designed to aid performance. Numerous experiments have been conducted on drugs designed to increase power or endurance in sports. In each case, the results have shown very minor positive effects. In most cases no favorable influences were detected in performance. The professional associations of both medicine and athletics have taken strong positions against the use of drugs on both scientific and ethical grounds and have considered it to be an unprofessional practice, in addition to being contrary to the personal welfare of the athlete. Strength and stamina are achieved by conditioning through physical activity, which is the only way to prepare for participation and achievement of desirable health results.

The prophylactic effects of physical activity also have positive effects on alleviating the effects of tension on the individual. Tension has the effect of elevating bodily functions from their normal level. Physical activity in these instances can serve as an agent for relaxing the organism, and if continued, can greatly reduce and eventually eliminate all undesirable effects of tension. For the professional worker subjected to stress, physical activity is very important to good health and represents an extremely desirable daily activity. Some physical activity is needed on a daily and weekly basis, although a long-range program is also needed.

Health and cultural mores are closely related, particularly through the dissimilarities that exist within each setting. The practices and community-family life of societies differ significantly throughout the world among different cultures. These traditions come to have deep roots with the people whose generations of common customs and heritage have helped establish a rewarding life-style. These customs should not necessarily be changed except to educate the people about more desirable health practices within the framework of the established culture; there should be no intent to change the culture. Programs of physical activity and sports, therefore, will differ, depending on the cultural background.

Growth and Development Content. Physical activity is related particularly to growth and development. Under completely sedentary conditions both the growth and development of the organism are severely hampered. Under proper living conditions and with proper physical activity the organism will reach its optimal growth and developmental potentials. The conditions must be set by the individual. It is clearly a question of what results are desired. The requirements for proper growth and development are high and the individual must have a strong desire to succeed.

Both growth and functional power are improved with physical activity during the growing years. It is most gratifying that the child can be stimulated during growing years through physical activity. The child wants the physical play. Activity must be frequent because it is exactly what is needed. The adult can do little about this except to ensure the child plenty of play time. The physical development and skills lost during this period will never be regained once the growing period is completed.

Inactivity during the growing years is most undesirable. Although the nature of the growth effects of physical activity is not clearly known, observations of children can only lead one to conclude that it is important for young people to be physically active. The potential functional powers and habits of adulthood are, to a large measure, established at this time. In addition to physical growth, the informal nature of play adds to the social and emotional development of the child. Physical development is, of course, increased when the child participates in physical activity.

Proper nutrition is paramount during the growing years. Nutrition is important in itself, but the value of proper nutrition is particularly evident for a physically active child. Proper nutrition adds to the growth and developmental results of physical activity and, of course, to the physical health condition of the child. To remain active, the child must have an adequate energy supply, which is provided by food, particularly in planned, balanced diets.

Growing, aging, and physical development are closely related and are all influenced by physical activity. Proper early development that continues throughout a lifetime will aid the individual in maintaining the physical resources needed during the particular periods of life. Habits can be developed early that will continue throughout a lifetime. This is particularly true if the habits are pleasant and satisfying to the child. In this way humans have considerable influence over their own physical destiny.

Family and social life are strongly associated with the growth and development of the organism. Traditions and ways of life differ in many cultures. Family and social lives are also different. Many cultures have a number of desirable traditions. Growth and development references indicate that variances in family life within cultures should be encouraged. This is particularly true if these practices are supported by scientific growth and development evidence. Some cultural practices, of course, should be discouraged on the same scientific basis.

Physical activity for each individual has specific requirements. The human body is extremely complex and individuals differ immensely in body build, personality, and temperament. There are hardly two individuals that are physically similar. Physical activity therefore must be individually designed. If exercise results are only for personal well-being, precision in planning is, of course, less necessary.

Protection, care, and treatment of the organism are essential for optimal growth and development. The losses from unacceptable health practices can be quite damaging to an individual. The care of the human body is important at all times in life but is of particular importance during the early years. Injury alone is the cause of staggering physical losses. Deaths from accidents number many thousands each year.

Psychological Content. During the two or three decades following World War II, numerous studies, reviews, research, and publications have dealt with the psychological content of sports and physical activity. At present, considerable content exists in sports and physical activity that will influence the individual or group through psychological traits, characteristics, and behavior. This includes the effect of physical activity on human emotions, the evidence for which is now extensive.

Physical activity and sports result in physiological adjustments by the individual. The release from tensions aids circulation and blood pressure. Normal physiological functioning then becomes possible. Abnormal temporary conditions will become standardized if relief is not provided. Physical activity in this instance serves as a relaxant and helps the organism to achieve a more favorable physiological state.

Physical activity that is accompanied with desirable *nutrition, rest, sleep, and hygienic practices* provides the basis for relaxation and has *positive effects on the psychological status of the individual.*

Psychological factors of motivation, desire, interest, attitude, and adaptability are all positive factors in physical activity and sports participation. If positive personal views have been established, participation is favored and the results will be more physically and psychologically favorable. The psychological concepts that favor participation will be improved along with the physical components. The individual then is oriented toward accomplishments that will continue to strengthen him physically and psychologically. If activity is continued these effects will benefit the individual throughout normal life, even into the very late years of life. Physical activity then becomes a major part of the individual's life.

The psychological therapeutic effects of physical activity have been recognized as an aid to individual improvement. The maintenance of mental normality, aid in mental rehabilitation, and aid to the mentally retarded are all psychological conditions that can be improved by the proper planning and programming of sports and physical activity. Physical activity in this instance has both corrective and therapeutic effects.

Creativity, goal achievement, perception, and democratic human relations are all psychological qualities that are important in maintaining mental and emotional health. All can be improved by proper participation in sports and physical activity. However, participation in physical activity must be on a positive basis.

The alleviation of anxiety, maintenance of a positive set of human values, and progression toward achievement for the purpose of strengthening human security are some psychological factors that are extremely important to human mental and emotional stability. All of these factors are found in sports and physical activity. The results of proper participation can be identical to those of any activity in life that maintains the mental health of the individual. The dynamic, emotional nature of sports allows these effects to be more developmentally positive than social and life situations, which are less demanding.

Sociocultural Content. Special emphasis has been given to the sociology of sports during the past fifteen to twenty years. During the early years of the twentieth century sports dealt with the character and personality traits of the individual. Recently, however, physical education literature has dealt extensively with applied sociology. Much of this work is not experimentally planned, but a number of recent studies have been conducted under controlled experimental conditions.

Physical activity, sports, and the culture have been topics for review for a considerable period of time. The rapidly growing programs of sports and athletics in most countries make this overall program a very large part of today's culture. More complete reviews are made of sports and culture in Chapters 1 and 9. The presentation is made in a series of statements in order to summarize the sociocultural content in physical activity in its many forms of sport and other professional applications.

Individual adjustments to society and culture are feasible in physical activity and sports. The many competitive opportunities in physical activity provide an ideal setting for the understanding of all the differences in race, religion, education, philosophy, and numerous other qualities that exist among people. The intimate nature of physical activity competition puts the individual in a cooperative relationship with his teammates. Under desirable leadership these associations can result in satisfying experiences for each individual. Adjustments to others and the group are then provided.

Personal habits, practices, social interests, and leisure activities all have positive potential for the individual. Sports and physical activity require physical participation that maintains the physical body and reduces the effects of personal habits that may have unfavorable effects on the body. Of more importance, negative personal habits, such as use of drugs or smoking, reduce the enjoyment of participation, which in turn provides an incentive to reduce or eliminate these undesirable health practices.

The sociocultural stress in sedentary settings must find release not only through rest but also through action and particularly physical activity. During less modern times, physical work was a part of man's daily life. This is often not so today. The machine has taken over much of man's physical work. In nearly all occupations, physical work has been reduced or eliminated. Consequently, there must be an activity substitute, because the organism cannot survive without physical activity. It is now necessary for everyone to participate in strenuous physical activity daily. Sports and physical activity must be found to fit each individual's skills, interests, and time.

Traditions, mores, and ways of life can be improved by properly planned and directed physical activity programs. Interests and skills vary within many cultures. Physical activity programs should fit the culture and remain responsive to it. Through deep interest in sports, traditions are strengthened and sociocultural ties are improved. This contributes to social integration and adds to the social and physical health of the group and the individual. Physical activity programs must *fit equally all vocations and professions* in a community because of the changing requirements and needs of each classification. The wide range of physical activities and numerous sports allows selection to be made that provides a proper and enjoyable activity for everyone.

The preparation of the individual for acceptable sociocultural roles is a major function of education. Physical activity and sports, through their primary societal role, can add significantly to the sociocultural education of the individual. The community setting, leadership, and supervision must be provided to foster the necessary social environment, for the forces of society are influential and can be negative in many cases.

Physical Content. The reason for physical activity is primarily the physical development of the individual. Some people take part in physical activity in sports solely for the enjoyment it provides. It is a pleasure to participate in sports, but the physical content of a sport also has many values. The content consists of the activity itself, its physical requirements, and how one participates in the activity. Little effort in participation will produce meager results. The physical content may range from activities requiring very little physical effort in participation to activities with high requirements. The content cannot produce any more than the participation requirements and the intensity of participation by the individual.

Physical activity adds to the quality of health throughout the individual's lifetime and adds to the individual's effectiveness over a longer period of time. Physical activity is a necessary ingredient in maintaining the fitness and health status of the individual. Health is not only freedom from disease but also the ability to work without fatigue. It is the ability to sustain life on an active level. When physical activity is pleasurable, regular, and frequent, the results contribute to the physical efficiency of the organism. Competitive sports provide incentives for more strenuous participation, and if they are enjoyable, the results will have added significance.

Health is the prevention of disease and injury and rehabilitation of the physical body to a normal level. Physical activity is a necessity in meeting these goals. An organism in acceptable physical condition can avoid injury inflicted through disease or physical injury. Physical activity then becomes a means of protection.

Physical *degeneration,* particularly during the later adult years, *is most rapid without consistent physical activity.* Aging often entails the increasing inability of an individual to meet daily needs. Physical activity, barring degenerative disease, will maintain the work capability level of the individual into the later years of life. Without physical activity the effects of aging are considerably more rapid.

Physical activity has therapeutic value. Physical activity is used in physical and mental therapy. It is used to restore normal bodily functioning to the organism and to provide therapy to the individual who is under arduous work requirements. Activity through pleasurable sports will reduce the effects of tension and also provide far-reaching therapeutic value in sustaining the individual mentally, emotionally, and physically when work requirements exceed his physical limits.

The optimal value of physical activity can be achieved only with acceptable individual living practices. Physical exercise combined with unfavorable environmental conditions such as poor diet, unsanitary living conditions, excessive alcohol or drug intake, or insufficient rest will lessen chances for attaining optimal levels of performance. In fact, participation itself will generally be less vigorous and therefore yield more meager results. One must participate with enthusiasm to achieve desired standards.

In our modern world, the reasons for physical activity in all its forms are becoming increasingly clear. Little doubt exists that in today's world, we need more physical activity than did our ancestors.

Physical Activity: A Health Profession

A profession cannot develop or grow without providing a vital service. It must fulfill a need that is essential to people's well-being. Health, of course, is desired by nearly everyone. Physical activity in itself and in sports can provide relief for and development of the individual differing greatly from his professional life; in addition, it has the potential for providing fun and excitement.

It has been noted in this chapter and in other chapters of this text that nearly all professional applications (ten in this section of the text) of physical activity improve physical fitness or deal with some aspect of health rehabilitation. This fact is basic to nearly all reasons for participation in physical activity.

In reviewing this chapter, it is noted that five categories of health concepts or qualities are possible in physical activity. Each category represents qualities that are, if properly achieved, extremely valuable for each individual. It is noted also that physical activity without plans or goals and without consistent and intense activity cannot result in significant achievements. It is possible that physical activity achieves no results beyond refreshment from and change in daily routines. Physical activity has a high degree of specificity. Physical activity must be selected on the basis of the kind of performance necessary to achieve the health goals desired.

Chapter 13

Institutions

The purpose of Part III in this text is to review the professional possibilities of all physical activity forms that are or can be used by a culture in service to society. By definition, a profession serves society. It must fulfill an essential social need and must be organized to render services of the highest possible quality. Therefore, institutions in a culture can hardly be omitted when discussing physical activity as sport, athletics, or recreation. Numerous institutions use physical activity in a cultural or societal context to achieve institutional goals. Physical activity then takes on professional roles within an institution.

What is an institution? There are many views. They range from the concept that it is a social group of little importance to the concept that it represents the strength of a culture. If we accept that institutions represent the strength of a culture, then we must also recognize that institutions are people. From this view, an institution is an entity that incorporates the social group and the individual as necessary parts of its program.

The line between a social group and an institution is a thin one. A sports team could be an example of a social group, whereas a religion might provide an example of a well-established institution. There are differences, however, and we can describe them. Social groups exist apart from institutions, but there are no institutions that lack social groups within their structural hierarchy. An institution is a social entity incorporating a group or groups as integral parts of its organization. The institution is distinguished from the social group, although not always precisely, by its procedures, by customs, natural tools, organization, and central aims. Institutions are not always the result of deliberate planning, although this is often the case. Professional football, for example, began as a local sport for the enjoyment of the participant. It is now a well-defined, well-established institution in the United States with a powerful influence on society.

Institutions are born in response to a need. Those institutions that meet societal needs with high-quality services are successful and contribute to the strength and cultural makeup of society. Institutions in the broadest sense, from a small social group to a large educational institution, represent the basic social structure of any society, local or worldwide.

Institutions are, for the most part, programs with goals. They endeavor to make life more pleasant and satisfying; however, if the goals are too idealistic and too distant from the daily needs of individuals, they cannot survive. The fact is, however, that people affect institutions more directly than the institutions themselves affect the practices of society. This question of influence is, of course, a two-way affair.

Any service institution must make service its primary objective, but it cannot afford to be too far removed from what society demands. The institution of education is a good example. Educational programs differ in each community according to the characteristics of the community.

Common concern held by both state and national governments has resulted in laws and customs that give an overall characteristic to educational programs. Financial aid is also a very strong motivator. People accepting this aid must also accept the regulations that go with it.

Institutions can be socially positive or negative. For example, religion is an institution with many subparts or subinstitutions that respond to the needs of people for faith in some force that will give them strength to meet the difficult problems in life. Crime is also a strong institution, in some instances with a number of subgroups organized on a worldwide scale. These two institutions are strong but with entirely different structures and purposes. The influence of each will be determined by the collective effort of the numerous social groups seeking to interest society in their services. Fortunately, there are more institutions that are constructive than destructive. There are several examples, however, of social institutions that live outside or just within the law through antisocial regulations that are permitted by local authorities. Fortunately, there are not many of these antisocial institutions.

There are other societal groups that influence people but cannot be classified as institutions. Examples of these groups are the crowds and mobs that have become a sign of today's social unrest. They can be strong. The technical difference between these groups and an institution is the failure of the noninstitutional groups to organize for systematic, long-term action. These groups are, instead, simply unified, to carry out some simple action for totally selfish motives. These groups many times operate outside the law or outside of normal social behavior.

People in any society are associated with numerous institutions. An individual's first introduction to an institution begins with the family unit, an institution of the highest order. Throughout life one's associations grow. The school, church, government, social club, recreation group, and athletic club are other institutions with which the individual comes into contact as he matures. All are organized systematically but independently in the community to serve society. Whenever there is a need it usually results in the development of an institution to meet it. The institution may be a socially oriented club meeting individual needs or it may be organized to render services to the people in the community. Institutions may be noncommercial or commercial. In either case, if their services are socially desirable, institutions offering these services should be supported.

Institutions vary in strength and influence. In some instances, individuals are so strongly influenced by a single institution (e.g., the church) that their entire lives become centered around it. Other individuals can be associated with so many institutions that they cannot be identified with any particular one.

There are many individuals whose lives become institutionalized because of their vocation or profession. They spend the majority of their time in a single institution. Of course, they have contact with other institutions, but the influence such contacts exert is incidental. Some live their professions almost completely. They see the same people each day and spend years with the same circle of friends. These may be the only associations these individuals have, because their contacts may be limited strictly to associates within the particular institution. Some individuals, on the other hand, may avoid their work associates during their leisure hours because of the long and intense associations at work.

Well-established, successful institutions are goal-directed and have systematic procedures for goal achievement. The working structure, goals, and employees making up an institution will establish the integrity of that institution. With dedicated employees, institutions will continue to flourish. Even with the most desirable goals, however, institutions may fail simply because of their employees. There are numerous examples of failure by institutions because employees lack motivation to achieve institutional goals. If people come to institutions for help and fail to gain satisfaction, the institution cannot survive even if the services are rendered to a varying group within large metropolitan areas, for institutional failure becomes rapidly known within any community.

This is, in summary, a general introduction to the nature of institutions. It is easy to see that an institution can have wide-ranging effects and can become a subdivision of society as a whole. It consists of groups of individuals established with their common customs, laws, regulations, and tools and organized around a central purpose. The main elements constituting an institution are social groups, establishments, customs, natural tools, organization, and a central aim.

With this background, physical activity will be considered to determine its professional validity as an institution or combination of several institutions in its many applications in society. These applications range from informal sports clubs to professional sports with their intense formal structure and organization. From the reference of institutions as herein presented, the range of the institutional context includes nearly everyone in a community.

Professional Status of Institutions

In this section we will review the professional status of the institution in society today and its potential as a profession. This review is designed to be brief and simply to set the stage for a review of the professional institutional potentials of physical activity in its various forms, such as sports, athletics, and physical activity. It is not the intent of this review to present institutions as they are now found. Rather, we will consider the nature of a profession and how it fits into the context of present institutions. The role of physical activity can then be studied to determine where it fits into the institutional picture.

We can evaluate the nature of institutions in a professional setting by using five criteria. These criteria should give sufficient understanding to institutions as professions and set the stage for the study of physical activity. These criteria are presented in the following paragraphs.

1. *Institutional cultural values.* There is a direct relationship between the devotion of a man to an institution and his feelings concerning institutional values. The cultural values he and other members of society hold are important, for it is impossible for institutions to be a part of society and also be opposed to the cultural values of its people. The strength, longevity, and influence of an institution are determined by its ability to meet its needs.

A culture does not develop out of a vacuum. The quality of a culture is determined almost entirely by the quality of the leadership and the institutions within that society. Probably the most dynamic and influential institutions are the schools, colleges and universities, and educational agencies. The influence of these institutions begins when the child is very young and continues through life, even to adult participation in an educationally sponsored activity. Such influence is indeed characteristic of a strong profession.

It is also typical that as the result of the influences of a strong institution the culture assumes the best features of that institution. This, of course, is as it should be and demonstrates the measure of success the institution has achieved as a profession. For example, a community served by religion soon is able to witness the churches of that community becoming a major influence in the life of the community.

Institutional membership comes through society or the individual community. The role played by these two sociological groups in institutional success is a result of practices closely correlating with the goals of the institution. This close correlation of goals is the finest quality of an institution and it is the most effective way to institute change.

Cultures become large-scale settings to meet the needs of man at all levels and in all its aspects. In fact, it would generally be most desirable if a culture could serve itself without institutional involvement. This is, however, impossible. For example, schools are a necessity because parents can no longer take the time to perform this function, nor are they qualified to do so.

2. *Institutional goals.* The integrity of an institution and certainly its professional status stem largely from the goals toward which the institution is oriented. The success of institutional programs then hinges on the ability to influence each individual in the culture and gain support for institutional goals through programs designed for and practiced by society as a whole. This is another true test of a profession.

Successful institutions have their own goals and programs to achieve them. The purposes of an institution may be common to other similar institutions, although they may also have unique qualities distinguishing them from other institutions.

It is difficult for a profession in institutional form to measure the success of its efforts. The people it serves may be influenced by other individuals to a greater degree and with greater effects than ordinarily can be known.

In most instances, the most stable institution is one that is chartered. A charter lends a firm structure to an institution. It gives the institution the legal basis for establishing programs and the direction needed to provide proper administration to the personnel and all other operational requirements. Most well-established institutions are chartered.

Institutions need to assist individuals with problems that they cannot solve without help. In most cases the assistance required is highly specialized, and the services must reflect this. The more common the problems, the larger the number of institutions that become established to solve them. One example is the large number of health clubs resulting from the increase in overweight and fitness problems among the American people.

3. *Services and needs.* The heart of an institution in its professional context lies in the services it renders and the needs of society for these services. The success of an institution as a profession is directly related to the needs of society for these services, particularly if they are highly specialized.

The vocation of automobile mechanic today is the dominant vocation for repairing the means of conveyance of the day. Certainly there is a great need for auto repair today, but whether these services can be classified as "highly specialized" is open to question. Certainly auto repair will never attain the unquestioned status of a profession that medicine enjoys, for example.

4. *Institutional structure.* Institutions must have structure in order to function.

The elements of institutional structure are the substance or components of the institution itself. This substance is the basis for institutional services. The church in its institutional context has the substance of man's beliefs. This substance becomes the church and all its components and practices. The success of the church will be determined by its following and by its actions. Education and the school provide another example. The substances that provide the basis for services to man are knowledge and skill. There is a strong need for these services by the individual in order to make a satisfactory adjustment to culture and society.

An institution must function within the structure set by its goals and services. It begins as a group of individuals with the knowledge and skills necessary to work toward the accomplishment of a central goal. One institution may produce individuals with knowledge and skill (e.g., schools and colleges), whereas another may involve a sport with a wide public following (e.g., professional football). Both have the services and institutional structure to function effectively in the public interest. These are successful institutions and can meet professional requirements, although, when compared with other professions, the degree to which they meet such requirements varies.

Institutions and their structures must be able to survive; that is, they must be stable. This ability to survive can involve a period as long as the services are needed; this period can extend beyond any one generation of individuals and institutional personnel. Institutions and their professional status must therefore be larger and more durable than their personnel. The army is an example. The role served by one soldier can be served by another. No one is indispensable in the institutional scheme. This is necessary for any institution to survive. If changes were made in personnel without an institutional structure and a central purpose to fall back on, that institution could not survive from generation to generation.

5. *Institutions and change.* Probably one of the most important requirements of an institution or profession is the ability to change with the changing needs of society. If these changes are undesirable, the programs of institutions must meet the changes with their own changes in emphasis. Program flexibility is an important characteristic of a good institution if it hopes to serve society with programs to meet all desirable goals.

Institutions develop in response to a need. In a dynamic society, needs change, and the only constant becomes the inevitability of change. Institutions must be alert to changing social conditions if they are to serve society. Much that happens to an individual on a daily basis involves problems with which the individual needs help. War, unemployment, increased cost of living, changes in dress and design, special opportunities for travel, and many other elements of modern life have caused changes in the needs of the individual and society. Over just the past few years, the emphasis on suburban living and the development of self-contained apartment communities have caused significant social changes within society. Downtown areas, with their shopping districts, social and professional clubs, and cultural centers, are having difficulty surviving and many components of these areas are moving to the suburbs along with the people. If institutions do not recognize social changes such as these, their death is inevitable and only a matter of a short period of time.

Professional Domain: The Conceptual Structure of Institutions of Physical Activity

It is the purpose of this section to view physical activity as an institution, as an integral part of society and the culture of its people.

The professional domain of physical activity is a conceptualization (List 10). The role of physical activity as a professional institution is broken up into eight major categories. The institutional roles for physical activity are numerous and vital to the lives of the people in a community. The institutional roles range from pure fun and recreation to maintenance of the physical powers of the body in order to sustain life itself.

Educational Domain. Physical activity plays a major role in educational institutions. In this analysis educational institutions will be considered to range from small social groups with educational goals to universities with required programs of physical education for all students and extensive physical recreation, sports, and athletics programs for those highly skilled individuals with special interests and aptitudes for participation in a specific sport (List 10).

List 10. Conceptual structure: The professional domain of physical activity in institutions

1. Educational domain.
   a. Accident prevention.
   b. Adaptive aspects.
   c. Fitness.
   d. Health.
   e. Human development.
   f. Human growth.
   g. Human organism.
   h. Integration.
   i. Knowledge and understanding.
   j. Leisure.
   k. Living practices.
   l. Play.
   m. Recreation.
   n. Rehabilitation.
   o. Safety awareness.
   p. Skill development.
   q. Social adjustment.
   r. Vocations.

2. Religious domain.
    a. Aims and goals.
    b. Community growth.
    c. Cooperative relationships.
    d. Family enjoyment.
    e. Unifying force.
    f. Wholesome entertainment.
    g. Identification with church.
    h. Leadership.
    i. Moral and ethical behavior.
    j. Programs, institutional.
3. Health and welfare domain.
    a. Adaptive aspects.
    b. Anxiety reduction.
    c. Cathartic effects.
    d. Corrective aspects.
    e. Drugs.
    f. Emotional well-being.
    g. Exercise programs.
    h. Prevention of disease.
    i. Rehabilitative aspects.
    j. Security.
    k. Social aspects.
    l. Stress tolerance.
    m. Therapeutic aspects.
4. Sport clubs and social organizations.
    a. Camaraderie.
    b. Club spirit.
    c. Competition and cooperation.
    d. Entertainment.
    e. Financial gain.
    f. Fitness.
    g. Leisure and recreation.
    h. Pleasure goals.
    i. Service.
    j. Social values.
    k. Traditions and mores.
5. Penal and correctional domain.
    a. Aggression reduction.
    b. Alleviation of boredom.
    c. Character formation.
    d. Democratic understanding.
    e. Disciplinary function.
    f. Human relations.
    g. Integration.
    h. Recreation.
    i. Rehabilitation.
    j. Skill development.
    k. Socialization.
6. Industrial and commercial domain.
    a. Achievement motivation.
    b. Anxiety reduction.
    c. Community relations.
    d. Entertainment.
    e. Exercise programs.
    f. Fatigue reduction.
    g. Job satisfaction.
    h. Motivation.
    i. Recreation.
    j. Safety awareness.
    k. Security.
    l. Socialization.
    m. Stress tolerance.
    n. Welfare.
    o. Work efficiency.
7. Governmental and political domain.
    a. Cooperation and competition.
    b. Cultural benefits.
    c. Democratic values.
    d. Human relations.
    e. Integration.
    f. International relations.
    g. National allegiance.
    h. National fitness programs.
    i. Political uses and abuses.
    j. Societal and political goals.
    k. Traditions and mores.
8. Military domain.
    a. Achievement motivation.
    b. Character development.
    c. Cohesive force.
    d. Discipline.
    e. Fitness.
    f. Human relations.
    g. Integration.
    h. Leisure and recreation.
    i. Mental awareness.
    j. Preparation for war.
    k. Safety awareness and accident prevention.
    l. Well-being.

The educational goals of physical activity are very numerous and diverse in most educational institutions. Probably the most common goal is the *development of skills and other physical requirements* for participation. Schools, colleges, and social agencies have trained instructors that aid the participant in learning and developing skills in the many physical activities available for everyone. They also teach the individual or team how to prepare physically for participation. This educational preparation provides the individual or group the skill and ability to participate in physical activity during leisure or a scheduled recreation period. This function is, indeed, a beneficial institutional service to society and certainly has a deep influence on the culture of a community.

Knowledge and understanding of the human organism within the context of physical activity is another major goal of educational institutions. Imparting adequate knowledge about the nature of organic functions and the influence of physical activity and exercise in our current society are important goals. This function is emphasized more in today's society than during the past because of the absence of physical work in modern occupations.

The role of today's educational institutions also includes the *protection of the individual* through instruction in safety, health practices, personal hygiene, physical fitness for work and leisure, and other practices that protect the individual from his environment (List 10).

Most educational institutions include as part of their programs instruction on functions and on the general *adaptations* needed.

Understanding the growth and development of the child and adult is an important function of schools, colleges, and many other related agencies in the community. Physical activity influences normal physical growth and plays an essential role in human physical development.

Preparation of the individual for leisure life is a rapidly growing educational area. The role now played by sports, athletics, and physical recreation has increased tremendously in the last few years, and the individual must be educationally prepared to participate in such leisure activities.

In summary, institutions associated with physical activity are deeply involved in the educational preparation of the individual. Physical activity, indeed, becomes an institutional service to the community.

Religious Domain. The moral development and social preparation of people are institutional responsibilities of all communities. Sports and athletics have always had a part in achieving these goals (List 10).

The goals of *religious institutions have changed* during the past several decades. The church is deeply concerned with the leisure life of society and in this concern sports and athletics have come to play a major role in church programs. Athletic leagues and conferences are now a part of church community programs. Their goal is to help develop strong moral character in today's youth. Churches also want to help the youth of the church with programs most interesting to them. These programs are also important in providing desirable leadership for the youth of the community.

The church as an institution is becoming an increasingly vital part of the community. Sports and athletics have helped to achieve this goal. Churches are attempting to serve as a unifying force to bring people together to institute improvements within the community. Programs, including sports, are designed for wholesome entertainment and personal activity that aid individual and community growth. The aim of such activities is to make the church, like the school, a vital force in the life of a community.

Churches are becoming family centers through their efforts in family programs. Their programs now extend considerably beyond religious instruction and programs. It is the desire of the church to make religion a part of daily living, not simply to impart religious beliefs and convictions devoid of any relationship to the activities of man.

Health and Welfare Domain. The institutions of a community must, and generally do, assume responsibility for the community as a whole. They are concerned with the health and welfare of society. Physical activity can do much to improve the health and welfare of the individual.

The individual must be free from stress and insecurity. Physical activity can help the individual achieve this state. Physical recreation and play not only improve the organism and its bodily functions but also give relief from organic stress and tension.

The individual must be free from disease and the fear of disease and must be emotionally adjusted to meet daily living conditions. Physical activities provide basic strength for the body so that it can ward off many disorders and they lend emotional stability to the individual who consistently participates in them. Properly designed physical activity also has corrective and rehabilitative powers.

Physical activity as a part of institutional programs can make significant contributions to the health and welfare of society. Physical activity is a needed service, and these services apply to nearly everyone in a community.

Sport Clubs and Social Organizations. The professional domain of physical activity in the form of sport clubs and social groups is as far-ranging as the sport activities it includes. Nearly every community, small and large, in the United States has been caught up in this wave until now it is worldwide.

The desire of people for companionship and socialization is strong; combined with the desire for sports participation, it makes the sport club a natural development in today's society. This trend is rapidly increasing in the United States. Socialization and physical activity provide an ideal setting for achieving professional goals within a community (List 10).

Sport clubs also provide competition and physical activity for individual fitness, which interests most people in the community. Sport clubs provide people with wholesome opportunities for leisure and recreation. These clubs are organized around nearly all sports known to man, which include some 300 sports or games practiced or played in various parts of the world.

Penal and Correctional Domain. Sports and athletics have become a major part of the programs of penal and correctional institutions. The current emphasis on rehabilitation and preparation of inmates for a normal and socially acceptable life in the community has been responsible for the substantial increase of sports in correctional programs. Sports contribute toward the achievement of this essential objective.

The primary goals for physical activity are *socialization, character formation, and democratic human relations,* which help the individual fit into a social group and prepare him as a desirable citizen and human being. Leadership is provided in order to use sports for these goals. The role of participation in sports plays a large part in how the experience is enjoyed by the participant.

Sports also give a desirable outlet for *aggression, provide an understanding of discipline, and integrate racially and socioeconomically within the social competitive group.*

Another important element of the sports program is to provide interests and goals that will *eliminate boredom and provide the individual* with an active life within the requirements of penal institutions. The opposite approach, followed by penal institutions of the old philosophy, is to confine the prisoner and completely restrict him in every way. The philosophy today in most institutions emphasizes *constructive rehabilitation.* Penal life now attempts to prepare the individual for a vocation and tries to develop social skills to meet the demands of a full life in society. The development of sport skills is of major importance within this emphasis.

Industrial and Commercial Domain. Sports and athletics in industry and for commercial enterprises have increased most rapidly during the past two decades. Commercial football is the most recent example. Developments in industrial physical activity have been equally rapid.

Commercial development comes from a desire for *financial investments and gain.* Many commercial sports do not provide significant financial profits, but they do give both satisfaction to their owners and tax benefits. These are essentially the chief motivating factors for commercial sports, although there is also a strong desire to provide a community with *entertainment* that is beneficial to community life (List 10).

In industry, physical activity serves as *recreation* for providing socialization among employees and for improving *work efficiency*. Motivating factors for industrial recreation also include *reduction in anxieties*. Institutions recognize their responsibility for helping the employee maintain good personal mental and physical health; these programs are aimed at fulfilling that responsibility. *Community good will* is also a factor; sports and athletics sponsored by industry help gain this too.

Government and Political Domain. Governments and political systems are designed for the management of people. Sports and athletics provide a medium that helps achieve this goal. The importance of sports in achieving the goals of *human relations, democratic goals and ideals, and integration of society* is known by political leaders and governments throughout the world and therefore receives their support.

The need for improved international relations has also resulted in government emphasis on sport programs. The importance of the Olympic Games, for example, is becoming increasingly a political concern in the United States. In many other countries, organization and preparation for the Games are under the supervision of the government (List 10).

The government has been accepting more responsibility for the *health, welfare, and physical fitness* of society than it once did. Sports and athletics, consequently, have found greater governmental support. The government derives many benefits by supporting sports and athletics. The support of national traditions, *improvement in cultural interests and practices, integration and cooperation of society* with government, and *achievement of political goals* are only some of the reasons it supports these programs.

Military Domain. Since World War I the military has emphasized sports and athletics as part of its military preparation. *Discipline, human relations, and personal well-being* are major factors involved in preparing individuals for military service. Sports and athletics have contributed toward achieving these goals. Individuals in military service need to be *physically and mentally fit*. Sports help achieve this fitness.

Probably one of the most important contributions of sports is in promoting the *desirable use of leisure*. In this regard, program schedules for interservice sports competition are planned as part of the total military program.

The military must always be *ready for war*. Such factors as societal *integration, motivation for combat, and mental alertness* are major components of preparedness. Sports and athletics aid the military leadership, in gaining these goals. *Safety* under stress conditions is also an important part of military training programs, and its achievement is also helped by sports and athletics.

Professional Domain: The Physical Activity
Content Structure in Institutions

The preceding section presents the scope of physical activity within an institutional context and analyzes it conceptually to serve as the basis for judgment on the institution as part of the professional domain of a society or culture. This section will deal with the *content* of physical activity. Again we aim to judge the professional worth of physical activity within an institution rather than the professional nature of the institution itself.

Educational Content. Educational programs are institutionally planned, designed, and administered. Education is an institutional phenomenon of the first order. As a societal institution, it provides a program planned specifically for society. Physical activity in its educational role helps achieve institutional and educational objectives.

The program content of educational institutions of various classifications includes sports and athletics to help achieve educational goals. These include *self-realization, human relations, individual acceptance of group ideals, emotional development,* and so on. Provision is made in school-scheduled programs to develop skills and prepare youth for a life of physical activity. It is recognized that one's daily activity must include some planned physical activity.

The objectives of education in institutions for both youth and adults are also the objectives for physical activity in all its adaptive forms, including sports, athletics, recreation, and so on. These goals include *skills, human development, social skills and awareness, democratic relations, and personal adjustment.* These goals coordinate with the total academic program of educational institutions and also serve as guides for physical activity.

Educational programs include the activities needed to prepare the individual for *modern citizenship.* Education is the only institution charged directly with this responsibility.

Religious Content. Religious philosophies and programs are experiencing major changes. The goal of religion today is to reach people in their daily life and to start the spiritual experience there. More and more, then, churches are called on to deal with the social problems of society and to apply religious and ethical principles. This is a distinct change from the earlier philosophies of religion, which individuals could not seem to understand and certainly did not practice.

Churches are concerned with the leisure life of the people. It is recognized that physical recreation as a means of leisure should be emphasized by churches. Many churches now have gymnasiums and other sports facilities to help them provide sports programs under church auspices. They now recognize that the highest ideals of life, to a large degree, must be practiced and lived in the setting of play and leisure. Many churches now employ recreation leaders to lead appropriate programs for the congregation of the church, as well as the general community, which is also encouraged to participate.

Probably no institution in the community has changed its philosophy more toward sports and athletics as churches and various religion-based organizations. This change has come in the past few decades for most religions. Theoretical religious philosophies are now simply principles that can be applied to daily life. Certainly sports and athletics play a major role in this new concept on the part of the church.

Health and Welfare Content. The health and welfare of society constitute an institutional matter of the first order. The institution must be established as a solid professional organization in order to serve society properly.

The mental and physical health of the people is a responsibility of institutions established by the government and the people.

It is recognized by health and welfare institutions that *sports, athletics, and other forms of physical activity* are important to the life of the people because they improve health and increase the enjoyment of leisure.

Rehabilitation and preventive medicine institutions are increasingly using physical activity as part of their treatment. Experiences during World War II greatly increased the rehabilitative use of physical activity in correcting individual maladies and aiding the individual to return to duty. The value of the recreational use of physical activity in mental and emotional rehabilitation is also recognized.

Therapeutic and adaptative physical activities have major roles in combating the incidence of poor posture and muscular tension, which are predominant among a significant portion of the school population and become a major problem with increasing age. These programs are professionally planned in both public and private institutions.

In recent years, *physical activities for the mentally handicapped* have been emphasized. Improvements have been significant in motor movement, and improvement has also been noted in the ability of the individual to communicate, associate with other people, and support his own life needs each day.

Also in recent years, health and welfare institutions have combated such health-destroying practices as the abuse of drugs, alcohol, and smoking. This has placed heavy responsibilities on these institutions. Drug abuse alone has increased to frightening levels during the past decade. With increased information about the health dangers of drug abuse and smoking, these practices recently seem to be on the decline.

Sport Clubs and Social Organizations Content. The number of sport clubs and social groups associated with sports is very large. A social group can be two or three people. If these individuals plan activities, such as hiking trips, they become a social group. These groups may be organized into highly structured institutions that deal with a single sport, and these institutions are as numerous as the communities large enough to organize and support such a sport.

Social organizations and sport clubs are not always the result of deliberate planning. They result from the interests and the initiative of people and facilitate social companionship centered around a sport of mutual interest.

Sports are used for institutional purposes. The sports program will bring interested people to the institution where they will participate together. This will serve society and aid the institution in achieving goals to which it is committed.

The family is a social organization and certainly an institution in the community. In many cases the family is also a sport club, in that the leisure life of the family is often centered around sports participation, either as individuals or as a group. Family camping and outings are increasing because of fast, easy transportation and rapidly growing campgrounds and recreational areas.

Governments at all political levels have supported and developed facilities for recreational sports and athletics. These are the strong, formally organized institutions in the community that can implement sports programs by financing facilities, leadership, and operational expenses. Hardly a community exists that has not made provisions for the physical recreation of its people. A strong recreational program is a major professional service rendered to the people by their governments.

Sport clubs and sports organizations provide people with opportunities to release tension that goes with their jobs. Provisions are made for hiking, fishing, sailing, boating, and hunting programs by community institutions in order to provide the help people need to maintain a healthy, active life.

Sports institutions are planned for youth to aid in their personal development, which includes not only physical qualities but also social and moral values. The primary aim of formally organized institutions is not only the sport itself, important to youth as it may be, but also the desirable human qualities that can be developed through participation and the leadership of coaches and other sport leaders.

A major purpose of sport clubs is socialization centered around an activity that provides a common interest. In this respect the club is a social institution that provides a medium for pleasant associations among its members. When reviewing the professional service potential of clubs as institutions, it must be noted that the sport club is probably the most dynamic and vital influence on the interests of many people in a community and that is now growing rapidly.

Content in Penal and Correctional Institutions. The philosophies governing penal and correctional institutions have changed considerably during the past two or three decades. Generally, correctional institutions no longer deal exclusively in punishment for criminal acts or other antisocial behavior. They attempt now to rehabilitate the individual.

Sports and athletics in penal institutions are programming activities that are satisfying to prisoners. These activities provide a positive experience for the inmates, who are able to view life in the penal institution as a positive attempt to help them toward the goal of acceptable behavior. There are considerably more successes from these physical activity programs than failures.

Sports and athletics can have favorable psychological effects on inmates. Success in sports demands that one plan his strategy within the rules. This is an extremely desirable experience for many individuals who have lived outside the rules of society. Learning discipline alone is of major importance to most inmates. The decisions of sports officials concerning the rules are rigid and participation will not continue unless they are accepted. Most will abide by these decisions because they want the game to go on.

The importance of maintaining physical fitness through physical activity and reducing inactivity is an important goal for a penal institution. Preparation for civilian life in society is also a process of preparing the prisoner physically with the requirements to meet the stress involved in becoming a part of society again.

Sports are also used in penal institutions to elevate the social class values of the inmates. The achievement of this goal requires strong leadership because sports can be reduced to class values of the lowest order. In fact, antisocial acts can be perpetuated through sports. With positive leadership, positive values are possible.

Advancing the human relations values of prisoners is an important goal of penal institutions. The potentials in sports are significant for the achievement of this objective. For successful rehabilitation one must leave a penal institution with attitudes toward his fellow citizens that are constructive.

Content in Industrial and Commercial Institutions. The use of sports and athletics in employee programs has increased rapidly during the past years. These programs are designed with the purpose of developing employee well-being and morale. Hardly a large industry today is without a sports team supported by that industry. On a commercial basis, athletics has had a phenomenal increase since World War II. Major conferences in all sports are now commercialized wherever there is public interest. They are adequately maintained by public support.

Part of the reason for industrial sports programs is to maintain the fitness of the employees. This is also considered by industry as a citizenship obligation to the people of the community. Industry seeks the good will of the people. The possible boredom of employees because of routine assembly-line work is another reason for physical recreation programs. Vigor and enjoyable sports help maintain employee morale.

Industry is also interested in the whole family and the total community in their programs for employees. Industry's support for recreation programs for families and for facilities for the community is most generous. Individual and family *security* is viewed seriously as it relates to the worker's life and welfare on his job. The employee's alertness and the maintenance of his physical resources are important to industry.

In all respects, industrial and commercial sports represent institutions in service to the public with the highest value. They represent a desirable form of leisure and participation in them contributes to the health and welfare of the individual and society.

Content in Governmental and Political Institutions. Governments of both democratic and autocratic nations have made large sports investments for their people. In either form of government, these programs can be used politically to rally the people to the government and its goals. In autocratic nations these goals include following the principles of the government; in the democratic nations they include achievement of a life that is happy and satisfying.

Governments are assuming a large leadership role in national sports programs. Their goals are to improve democratic governments or other forms of political management and to serve the people by improvements in health and fitness. National physical fitness programs have been developed and supported by the U.S. government.

Governments have recognized the value of sports in improving international relations. International sports competition is now planned in nearly all sports wth a public following. The Olympic Games are supported by the governments in most nations of the world.

It has long been recognized that sports can help achieve better understanding between members of different races and socioeconomic groups. The racial problem in the United States has been considerably improved by sports. In fact, no fixed racial barriers exist in professional sports.

Governments and political systems are institutions in service to society. This includes a responsibility to help fulfill those needs that cannot be met through individual effort. Health, welfare, and fitness are national concerns because they affect national survival as well as individual survival. Governments therefore will support sports programs to help keep the nation strong and vigorous. This is, indeed, a professional service to society by political institutions.

Content in Military Institutions. The military services include sports and athletics as part of their programs. Leadership has been provided to plan and supervise sports in all its various forms. Interservice sports competition is now common. The goals of this competition are improved fitness and morale.

Military programs have served as testing grounds for physical fitness programs. The ability of the individual soldier in combat, both physically and mentally, is an extremely good way of judging levels of fitness.

Military morale is important and therefore the reduction of personnel differences is important. Social class, race, and religious differences represent the full range of individual variations in a nation. Sports can help in reducing these differences.

Sports in military leisure programs fulfill an important need. Leisure for military personnel must be planned, for the number of personnel is large and the facilities for entertainment and leisure are limited.

Physical Activity: An Institutional Profession

Early in this chapter a profession was defined as any organized group having a central purpose and organized to render service to the group itself or service to society in general. Because physical activity includes a wide range of activities from hiking clubs to commercial sports, its institutions include nearly all the people in a nation. Nearly everyone is institutionally involved in some form of physical activity.

Institutions are formed by accident or by design within a community. Government as an institution was planned and organized by formal design. People deal with the specifics of a government and its operation. Government is, indeed, a formal and essential institution in service to society. Without strong governments individual survival would hardly be possible. In this context, it is noted that physical activity in nearly all its forms plays a major role in advancing the objectives of government.

Institutions are also informal in planning, design, and structure. The bowling group in a particular community that meets at scheduled times, the tennis club, and the hiking group are all social institutions in a community. They meet for social reasons, of course, but also find that sports represents an excellent educational and cultural setting. These are institutions that serve people professionally in a community, meeting what they consider to be a vital need.

Physical activity does have a valid basis as a profession as it is identified within the institutional context. It renders an important professional service. If institutions of physical activity were withdrawn from the community, the gap would be large and needs for physical activity would be unmet. It would be difficult to imagine what would happen in such a situation. Certainly boredom and leisure without physical activity would lead to conditions that would be difficult to manage within a society.

Chapter 14

Preventive Medicine

Preventive medicine attempts to deal with the whole man; it considers all intellectual, emotional, physical, genetic, and chemical components of the individual in order to detect early deteriorative trends and thereby take early corrective action. A considerable number of the ills of man can be prevented. Moreover, prevention of disease and bodily injury is substantially cheaper than cure or treatment of the effects of physical injury or disease. Of considerably more significance is the simple fact that in today's society, in which man possesses sophisticated knowledge about the body, the individual can by his own efforts prevent many of his physical ills if he is willing to do so. In some cases it is merely a matter of recognizing the causal factors of the disease and taking the appropriate steps toward prevention. In spite of numerous radio and TV programs on health, there are only a few groups in the United States today that are equipped to apply preventive measures for the advancement of personal health levels. In some countries, however, preventive medicine has achieved considerable attention.

The advancement of personal health and the prevention of disease encompass an area as broad as the field of medicine itself. Preventive medicine does not deal with any particular organ, function, or system of the body or with any particular age group or sex. Preventive medicine covers the entire population and involves all scientific and medical disciplines. The individual is very much at the center of the detection process and must take steps to prevent the probable occurrence of disease or ill health. In this respect, man is master of his own destiny.

Most people in ill health or faced with the stark realities of premature death recognize good health as a basic human need. The healthy individual, however, frequently gives little thought to health. The individual in good health often takes it for granted. This is, of course, most

235

unfortunate. Health cannot be considered to be a right or an endowment.

The ideal setting for workers in preventive medicine is one in which people believe that health has to be developed daily and that, once acquired, it must be maintained. The maintenance of normal physiological functions and the care of the body through acceptable daily health practices will reduce illness and poor health more than any medical remedy.

The question to be resolved, then, is what are the basic and most important values in life? In one survey these values were reported as (1) to stay alive, (2) to be well, and (3) to know the principles of maintenance of good health. If one has achieved these three goals, it is possible to expect a long and happy life. Preventive medical institutions for a society with these values would include the health services available to the people and, of course, educational programs for all. Preventive medicine should emphasize staying well and, when this proves impossible, finding a cure. Emphasis on the former is considerably more helpful to the individual and much less expensive.

Preventive medicine has its roots in the health of each individual; health-related decisions must be made each day. Science and medicine must prepare society to make choices in favor of good health. Preventive medicine is truly a profession and it greatly promotes the advancement of the individual's life to its full genetic potential.

The communications media have been used in recent years to help society avoid illness and early death. Programs on anticigarette smoking have been very successful in significantly reducing the amount of smoking per individual and many have completely stopped as the result of recent knowledge of the ill effects of smoking.

Preventive medicine, then, is the science of preserving health by means of remedial activities and regulation of daily practices that maximize health. The scope of preventive medicine includes anything that affects the human body, such as eating, working, resting, exercising, tension, the environment, and so on.

Epidemiology is the branch of medicine dealing with society and the causes of disease and ill health. This science provides the data that can be utilized in the prevention of disease.

Professional Status of Preventive Medicine

Preventive medicine is one of several branches of medicine. It differs from other specializations in that it deals with the whole human being and with his total social and physical environment. In addition, preventive medicine deals with other sciences that are associated with man and that have some effect on his understanding of health and his choice of daily health practices. Psychology is an example of such a related science.

Physiology is the base science in preventive medicine, although not all its implications are considered to lie solely within the province of medicine.

Let us now review the professional nature of preventive medicine so that we can provide a formal setting for a more complete review in the following sections of this text.

Goals. The basic goal of preventive medicine is the maintenance of the whole-man concept for health. This includes the establishment of (1) physical, mental, and emotional health and (2) practices that will advance and maintain a desirable level of health. Preventive medicine views disease as a distinctive force and, even though corrected, damaging to the human organism. Disease and illness under this concept may leave scars that will limit activity and reduce health levels.

One criterion applied in judging the status of a profession or discipline is its objectives. It is also judged by whether the goals can be accomplished by techniques available to the professional worker. In all these respects preventive medicine, through its accomplishments, has achieved professional status.

Agencies. Specialized service agencies must be quite numerous in order to render services on the basis of need. It is probably safe to say that the scope of institutions outlined in Chapter 13 will also serve as a classification for service agencies in preventive medicine. Because institutions that employ people are concerned about their employees' health status, physical activity is one of numerous health agencies dealing with preventive medicine.

A review of the agencies associated with preventive medicine must begin with medicine itself. The goal of the medical profession is to prevent disease and injury and to help overcome them when they occur. There are many branches of medicine that are closely allied with preventive medicine but fall outside its direct jurisdiction. Ideally, preventive medicine is designed to avoid any type of medical treatment.

The professional institution domain of physical activity agencies such as sports and athletics is reviewed in Chapter 13. In each classification physical activity is planned for the welfare of the individual and the group. This overall purpose is highly compatible with the goals of preventive medicine.

Reference should be made to Chapter 13 to view the roles of various institutions and agencies in preventive medicine. These are education, religion, health and welfare, sport clubs and social organizations, penal and correctional institutions, industrial and commercial institutions, governmental and political institutions and agencies, and the military. Although this classification of roles was made for discussing physical activity, it can be readily applied to preventive medicine. Of course, within the context of preventive medicine the classification will differ in categorical headings and in emphasis on content. For example, public health agencies vary in kinds and classification and deal largely with the prevention of disease as the basis for maintaining individual health.

In broad terms the agencies of preventive medicine fall into one or more of the following categories: physicians and their practices; hospitals; medical schools; community, public, and private health agencies; universities, schools, and social agencies; research foundations; mass media; professional journals and research publications; and philanthropic agencies and foundations.

Programs. The programs of preventive medicine are planned with agencies and institutions listed in the preceding paragraph. The role of these agencies is increasing in the area of preventive services. People are encouraged to seek the services of agencies as soon as they detect signs of possible disease or ill health in order to prevent damage to the organism. This phase of medicine is rapidly increasing.

The physician too is devoting more time to the preventive aspects of disease and illness. He now emphasizes, even more than he used to, regular medical examinations, X-rays, the effects of drugs and smoking and other practices on health, and so on.

People are now encouraged to undergo full medical testing at hospitals before disease strikes. One example is that of hospitalizing the individual who is obese in order to reduce weight properly, but of more importance is the education of the patient on the proper method of maintaining normal weight.

Programs in medical schools have been considerably broadened in the past few years. Preventive medicine has been added as part of the content of medical education so that prospective physicians can deal with disease and illness prevention. The basic sciences are becoming an increasingly important part of the medical school program, particularly in preventive medicine. Preparing the physician for leadership in preventive medicine places emphasis on the basic sciences and the selection for training of those individuals qualified to work effectively with the public. In preventive medicine the attitude of the leader is important. Knowledge and skill alone will not change people's undesirable habits.

Programs for the protection of the citizen are planned by numerous public and private health agencies. The United States Public Health Service is the most prominent of these agencies in this country. It provides leadership and technical assistance to states and local communities in the development of public health programs. In cooperation with state and local health departments the Public Health Service develops and tests new methods for the prevention and control of disease.

There are numerous other programs and agencies to help society. The National Institute of Health provides services and research to various centers throughout the country. There are many centers, including the Children's Bureau, with several divisions and subdivisions in state organizations. The program of the institute emphasizes disease and disease control rather than prevention as purported by the institutions of sports and physical activity.

Universities and colleges are very much concerned with the process of helping individuals improve their basic health levels. One way of carrying out this essential role is by preparing leaders to work with the public. Research on disease, disease control, and physical development and its relationship to disease control are among the major contributions made by this field in recent years.

There are many research foundations, not only in the United States but internationally, that are committed to the support of research and programs in preventive medicine. Without these foundations, both public and private, research and implementation programs would be quite minimal. There are also numerous philanthropic organizations that give generous support to research and programs in the preventive medicine field.

Historically, the mass media have been generous in allocating program time to preventive medicine, and they continue to be generous. Of course, some time is purchased on a commercial basis (for example, by companies producing disease-controlling drugs), but programs on cigarette smoking, drugs, alcohol, and other enemies of good health are common.

Techniques. Workers, associations, agencies, institutions, and other groups and individuals concerned with preventive medicine have applied various techniques effectively in individual health. The most prominent technique is, of course, research. The discipline of preventive medicine is indeed a new one. In the nineteenth century and before man often did not live more than thirty to fifty years, regardless of medical services available. With the advances in medical knowledge in the last several decades it now appears that a life span of 100 years will not become uncommon in the next several decades. Much of the credit must go to efforts on disease control and related programs of preventive medicine.

In addition to research, during recent years public discussion on disease prevention has significantly increased in the United States. Scarcely a community exists today that does not schedule programs through community agencies on some problem dealing with the health of society. The effects of these programs indicate that at this time society has knowledge that, if applied, could prevent many of the diseases known to man.

The technique of advertising is used most extensively now to aid in the preventive medicine campaign. Scarcely a public service publication comes out that does not have ads or reviews dealing with the problem of health from the point of view of preventive medicine. The result is that people have a greater sensitivity to the pitfalls of poor health practices.

For the past several decades, a significant emphasis has been placed on physical activity as the most fundamental force in preventive medicine. Programs of physical activity and regular exercise are rapidly increasing in schools and agencies throughout the United States. The greatest emphasis is no longer on the youth in our schools, but rather on adults, where obesity and lack of conditioning result in increased incidence of heart disease. Some type of jogging program, for example, is today found in almost all communities. Jogging through the parks and streets of New York and our other major cities during off hours is a common practice of a large segment of our adult society. These individuals are concerned about the effects of the stress of urban living and modern business professions. They wish to reduce or eliminate the harmful effects of a sedentary, stressful occupation through physical fitness.

Leadership. There are an increasing number of leaders coming from medical schools with M.D. degrees, although the largest number of professionals in this area come from graduate schools in the sciences with Ph.D. degrees. These are the professionals who are trained to take the leadership in the development and administration of programs of preventive medicine.

There are numerous career opportunities in preventive medicine. The range of opportunities stretches from medical careers in hospitals with direct preventive medicine responsibilities to teachers or professors in public schools and colleges with teaching assignments in the health education field. There are many such career opportunities in community-based health agencies dealing with sanitation, ecology, disease control, and other fields that deal directly with society in securing public health and living conditions conducive to promotion of high health standards.

Preventive medicine has a different emphasis from specialities in the rest of medicine. Preparation in preventive medicine needs to include sciences that take into account the complete individual and all his functions. In this respect such disciplines as sociology and psychology are important; the biological and physical sciences are particularly important. The professional roles of workers or professional leaders in preventive medicine include (1) the direct teaching of various facets of preventive medicine and (2) introduction of preventive medicine content into all the health disciplines in order to approach all health problems with an emphasis on prevention.

Professional Domain: The Conceptual Structure of Physical Activity in Preventive Medicine

The advancement of the role of physical activity as an integral component of preventive medicine has been most rapid in the past few years. The first emphasis on physical fitness came during World War II, when it was found that it aided rehabilitation following injury and helped maintain health at all times. Preventive medicine has gained momentum and stature from the contributions made by physical activity. These contributions can include sports, athletics, physical recreation, therapy, rehabilitation, conditioning, physical fitness activities, formal exercise, and other unique activities that have specific effects on the organism. These serve to contribute to improved health and prevention of illness.

The foundation for physical activity as an integral phase of preventive medicine is supported by sufficient evidence to emphasize physical activity programs directly designed as preventive medicine programs. Studies have discussed the preventive effects of exercise in providing direction and emphasis for physical activity. These reports indicate that exercise will prevent obesity and, thereby, the degenerative disease that results from it. Physical activity will act to inhibit the vascular degeneration characteristic of coronary heart disease. It has a delaying effect on aging and appears to have a favorable effect on longevity. Physical activity will also condition the organism, thereby aiding in meeting disease and injury emergencies more effectively and with less damage to the individual.

The search of the relevant literature in the preparation of this chapter had two objectives: (1) to identify and classify the concepts within the context of physical activity that could be identified with preventive medicine (List 11) and (2) to search for information and data on the established concepts and conceptual structure of preventive medicine in order to establish the contribution of physical activity to the discipline of preventive medicine.

Health Maintenance. Developing health and maintaining it constitute one of the essential components of preventive medicine. Physical health is a fundamental requirement for an active life; it is the basic prerequisite for all human activity.

One's environment is important in personal health. It can have either favorable or unfavorable effects on the individual. Temperature, humidity, and pollution are some of the elements of one's environment. Pollution alone is causing many respiratory health problems, yet elimination of the easily diagnosed cause is not easy.

Stress, fatigue, and insecurity in work and interpersonal associations

List 11. Conceptual structure: The professional domain of physical activity in preventive medicine

1. Health maintenance.
   a. Aging factors.
   b. Automation effects.
   c. Environmental factors.
   d. Fatigue reduction.
   e. Nutritional balance (weight control).
   f. Personal health considerations.
   g. Physical fitness.
   h. Physical security.
   i. Psychological factors.
   j. Recreational and leisure activity.
   k. Sociological factors.
   l. Tension and stress reductions.

2. Disease prevention and control.
   a. Alleviation of pulmonary disease.
   b. Community influences.
   c. Environments.
   d. Food-intake restrictions.
   e. Functional capacity improvement.
   f. Health education.
   g. Health practices.
   h. Immunization.
   i. Management of diabetics.
   j. Minimization of degenerative diseases.
   k. Physical activity and exercise.
   l. Reduction of blood cholesterol levels.
   m. Skill development.
   n. Sociological and psychological factors.

3. Injury and accident prevention.
   a. Acclimatization and condition.
   b. Clothing and protective devices.
   c. Environmental factors.
   d. Equipment improvement.
   e. Health practices.
   f. Interest in participation.
   g. Knowledge.
   h. Personality characteristics.
   i. Psychological factors.
   j. Regular exercise habits.
   k. Relaxation.
   l. Security influences.
   m. Tensions and stresses.

4. Rehabilitation and therapeutics.
   a. Disability limitation.
   b. Educational aspects.
   c. Facilitating social conditions.
   d. Health knowledge and practices.
   e. Nutrition.
   f. Personal factors.
   g. Physical factors and devices.
   h. Postoperative exercise.
   i. Psychological conditions.
   j. Psychological elements.
   k. Relaxation techniques.
   l. Treatment therapies.
   m. Vitamin medication.

5. Mental health.
   a. Adjustment.
   b. Anxiety.
   c. Bias and prejudices.
   d. Emotional expression.
   e. EMR activity programs.
   f. Fitness.
   g. Negative attitudes.
   h. Play relationships.
   i. Psychiatric methods.
   j. Psychosomatic influences.
   k. Recreational therapy.
   l. Stress adaptation.
   m. Stresses and tensions.
   n. Tolerance.

are elements of one's social environment that generally have destructive effects on individual health. If these conditions are not reduced or compensated for, their results on health will be evident in just a few years. This is particularly true for individuals in the middle age or older age brackets. These ages also coincide with the time when these stress factors are most common on the job and in individual personal associations.

Dietary practices and use of alcohol and drugs all have an influence on health. Overindulgence or lack of discretion in the consumption of food, alcohol, or drugs will have most negative effects.

Exercise is essential for developing and maintaining optimal health levels. Physical activity is a major health requirement and cannot be on a part-time basis; it must be scheduled daily. Losses in health resulting from physical deconditioning are rapid. Developing a high level of fitness is difficult, but if exercise is continued on a daily basis it becomes less drudgery and more a part of one's routine.

Social factors are also important. Sociological and psychological factors can have negative effects on individual health.

The periods of middle age and beyond, into the beginning of old age, are extremely important from the personal health standpoint and must be recognized and managed accordingly. Aging effects can be reduced by maintenance of health levels of early middle age.

Disease Prevention and Control. Prevention and control of disease are major factors in health and preventive medicine (List 11). The concepts and composition of this category include several important elements that will guide one toward achieving this goal.

Education in disease prevention and control is needed by all. One must understand these preventive requirements and put them into practice in his daily life. Immunization, for example, at the proper intervals is needed by all in order to avoid communicable diseases. Health instruction includes providing this information to children in schools from the primary grades on. Adult instruction comes largely from mass media.

It is important to minimize the effects of any disease with which one must live (e.g., diabetes). Diseases can often be controlled by individual health practices. Cardiac deficiencies, if properly diagnosed, can also be controlled by individual practices, so that it is possible to live a nearly normal life.

An individual's personal life practices are perhaps his single most important responsibility. Protection against environmental influences, desirable daily health practices, and maintenance of normal body weight are factors that will aid in disease prevention and control.

Injury and Accident Prevention. Injury is the most common cause for reduction in human abilities among most individuals. In some instances, injury is so severe that death results. The number of automobile accidents runs into the thousands in the United States over a normal holiday week end. Preventive medicine, which in this case would be largely accident prevention, needs to be practiced by everyone (List 11).

One of the most common causes of accidents is the psychological state of the individual. An individual who is in a state of frustration, emotionally upset, or under a great deal of tension is accident prone. One cannot respond efficiently in such an unsettled state.

Maintenance of physical fitness that will reduce the effects of fatigue and ensure normal physiological functioning of the organism is important in avoiding accidents and resulting injury.

Protective clothing and equipment in sports help in avoiding accidents and injury. It is possible to apply this concept to areas outside of sports. One should be aware of areas where accidents could strike and then protect oneself accordingly.

It has been firmly established that one of the most significant deterrents to accidents is adequate knowledge of safety procedures. If an individual is aware of the possible consequences of some act, the concern for protection becomes very meaningful.

Physical activity during leisure hours will add to the general state of relaxation of the individual. An individual who is relaxed both mentally and physically has an added measure of protection from most accidents.

Rehabilitation and Therapeutics. Based on the principles of organic strengthening or compensation many of the injuries that affect normal human movement and skills needed for daily activities are correctable to nearly normal levels. Psychological factors must be considered essential to positive rehabilitation. Interests, motivation, relaxation, tension, security, and confidence are some of the personal psychological conditions that aid in successful rehabilitation. Successful rehabilitation from any abnormal condition takes personal determination.

Nutrition is an important element in the process of rehabilitation and therapy. This applies to individual handicaps that are both physical and emotional.

Knowledge, treatment procedure, physical condition, therapy equipment, and special prosthetic devices are important in rehabilitation. Cold, heat, electro, hydro, sauna, light, and X-ray therapies all have significant places in the rehabilitation process. If available to the individual and used properly, these various therapies provide an essential resource to the rehabilitation of the individual.

Physical activity through sports and athletics is now recognized as significantly contributing to the rehabilitation of the individual in physical, mental, and emotional difficulties. Preventive medical practices in hospitals and other social or rehabilitative agencies now apply sports and exercise procedures as part of their total preventive medicine program.

Mental Health. The role of physical activity in mental health has increased dramatically in recent years. This is chiefly due to the recognition of the physiological base for the mental health status of the individual. Maintenance of the physical status of the organism at an average or preferably above-average level will add considerably to the mental health status of the individual. The possibility of mental deviation or maladjustment will be sharply reduced under these conditions. Barring inheritable disease of structural malfunctions, mental health can be achieved and maintained through the broad scope of physical and mental activities.

The physical fitness of the organism, play relationships and associations, and positive physical recreation during leisure are important positive factors in securing and maintaining mental health. A positive self-image within the setting of sports is in itself desirable for mental health and adds to security in meeting associates in both social and business activities.

The adjustment of an individual to others and the neutralization of the effects of stress and anxiety are elements of physical activity that strongly aid in the maintenance of positive mental health. It is more difficult to be negative in sports than positive. The team, even in recreation activities, has a strong motivation to win. This provides a strong positive base and adds to the positive thinking of the individual, which is a contributing factor in both mental health and preventive medicine.

Mental and physical tolerance and emotional and intellectual bias and prejudice are also factors basic to mental health (List 11). Again, physical activity through sports can reduce these negative influences and often almost totally eliminate them. There are any number of sportsmen that have no bias or prejudices about their teammates. Personal differences are at a minimum under the heat of sports competition. Under strong leadership, these positive social benefits can be maintained.

Professional Domain: The Physical Activity Content Structure in Preventive Medicine

The previous section presents the concepts that can be supported as elements of physical activity that contribute to preventive medicine. They are the elements that add to health and, thereby, serve to arm the individual against disease and illness. Although in the presentation of the conceptual structure some content statements are included, this section will deal with that content per se and an attempt will be made to avoid overlap or duplication. In order to understand the structure of physical activity fully in preventive medicine, it is important to understand both sections.

Health Maintenance Content. Regular exercise and physical conditioning help prevent overweight. They also add to the status of the physiological functions of the body and are therefore most desirable in health and preventive medicine. Physical activity is an essential ingredient for proper weight control by most persons.

The effects of physical aging, senility, and emotional depression can be reduced through involvement in physical activity and sports. Daily physical activity of sufficient intensity must, however, be a part of one's life from childhood up until the time of death.

Preventive medicine and the role of sports and physical activity in health have been emphasized in recent years because of the nearly complete absence of physical work in many of today's occupations. Recreational sports are now sponsored by nearly every community institution to maintain the fitness levels of its adults.

Active participation in sports is, of course, considerably more desirable than a spectator role. The spectator is deprived of the desirable effects of physical activity and may worsen his overall health status through emotional tension and excessive emotional involvement. An individual should be a spectator and participant. Physical participation is not possible at all times during the day and being a spectator during some of this time is to be encouraged.

As an individual grows older, more time should be spent in physical activity but with less intensity than when one is young.

The psychological and sociological effects of participation in physical activity and sports benefit both health maintenance and preventive medicine. One's self-regard and regard for others are elements that can also add significantly to mental health, if properly applied. A positive approach to physical activity will reduce tension and anxiety, which put a physical drain on the body.

Disease Prevention and Control Content. Physical activity has many positive contributions to make toward disease prevention and control. Some are direct contributions (e.g., combating cardiovascular difficulties) and others are indirect (e.g., sustaining desirable levels of physical fitness). The maintenance of normal weight levels is a major concern in a number of diseases, such as atherosclerosis and diabetes. Exercise will retard the vascular degeneration characteristic of coronary heart disease.

Working toward the goal of longer life should begin in childhood. This will help prepare the individual for an active life in which physical activity plays a prominent role and in which it will be continued throughout life. Exercise cannot reverse the aging process, and it will be much more difficult to lift an individual's fitness level after the deterioration associated with old age has set in. The physical laxity of the past will be most difficult to erase.

The physical fitness level and condition of the organism are important in the avoidance of accidents, injuries, or diseases that will reduce the functioning capacity of the body. A physically alert organism that is not easily fatigued has a measure of added protection. The unfit, emotionally unstable individual is most susceptible to injury and disease. Although an excellent physical status does not guarantee an individual freedom from all maladies, it does help avoid many diseases; and if disease does strike, the good physical condition of the body will aid in the fight against disease and speed up the recovery process. The content of physical activity in these respects is an important element in the work of preventive medicine.

The modern problems of pollution and the social environmental stresses of urban life affect the health of the average individual in a negative way. Some respiratory difficulties are directly related to air pollution. Automobile exhaust alone causes significant respiratory difficulties in most large urban centers.

Injury and Accident Prevention Content. Physical activity is important in avoiding injury and preventing accidents. Physical fitness will make the individual alert, remove dangerous fatigue levels, and serve as a positive factor in avoidance of accidents and injury.

Safe participation in physical activity toward positive ends is a planned, designed procedure. Knowledge of correct procedures for the protection of the body is a virtual science; necessary skills for the protection of the body must be learned through well-planned programs. To afford protection to the body, knowledge is needed about the mechanics of the skills used by the organism in physical activity; this includes knowledge of physiology and anatomy.

In educational institutions an individual must be prepared to protect his body during sports and physical activity. Trained instructors in sports and physical education safety are needed to teach students self-protection. Leadership by teachers and coaches is also needed in schools, colleges, and other social agencies in order to provide adequate protection during participation. Rules and their enforcement are essential to strong leadership. The supervision process prepares the participant for the safe enjoyment of physical recreation.

For the athlete, superior physical conditioning is necessary. The *overload* principle is applied in best utilizing the conditioning process. The physical condition of the individual then exceeds the level needed for participation in a sport or athletics. Fatigue levels will never reach a dangerous point and physical resources will be maintained at a higher than normal level, thus providing protection to the organism.

Both social and physical environments are important factors in injury and accidents during physical activity. The playing fields, facilities, equipment, and participant's attitudes are all environmental factors. Such environmental factors can cause injuries and accidents that could have been avoided. Available safety guides must be applied by those who direct sports and athletics in an institution or community.

The emotional status of an individual corresponds directly to the likelihood of an accident occurring to that person. It has been demonstrated that individuals who are unstable and who are easily frustrated have the most major accidents.

Knowledge about the body and skills for its protection are necessary to avoid injury and protect against accidents. It has been found extremely important for schools, colleges, and social agencies to include safety content in educational programs.

Sports, athletics, and physical activity have positive physical effects only when participation is planned for such results. Unwise physical participation or the lack of adequate protection can cause serious injuries in sports. Each year many young athletes die because of ignorance or lack of supervision in football. The inability of the body to release excess heat through sweat on very hot days is a common cause of many deaths each football season. These conditions must be controlled.

Rehabilitation and Therapeutics Content. Research and clinical experiences have advanced the applications of physical activity, sports, and physical recreation in rehabilitation and therapy most significantly in recent years. Physical activity as a means of rehabilitation from disease, injury, or surgery is considered a vital part in returning the individual to normal life. It has been found that appropriate physical activity will hasten the return of normal physiological functions.

Rest and physical activity are major components in the process of returning the individual to a normal physical condition. The individual or physician who overstresses rest during the healing process will hasten the rate of atrophy to a level that makes normal rehabilitation most difficult. For older individuals normal bodily functioning may then be impossible to attain. There are a large number of physicians who do not utilize physical activity to its maximum in the rehabilitation process because they are overcautious. The patient often agrees, because of his fear of the unknown, but physical losses are rapid during such a period.

Nutrition plays a part in rehabilitation and therapy. Of course, the specific practices are all related to the injury, disease, or malfunction of body organs. Each individual will need a specific rehabilitative program unique to him, but the positive benefit provided by good nutrition will aid in the rehabilitation process. Good diet promotes efficient functioning of organic systems and is of major consequence when illness has resulted in considerable muscular atrophy.

The psychological status of the individual—his personality, attitude, sense of well-being—is a factor in both physical and mental-emotional rehabilitation. It has been found that leisure recreational activities and sports can add considerably to the rehabilitation of the individual. Sports and physical activities of various kinds are now common among rehabilitation agencies, and gymnasiums, play fields, and swimming pools have become integral parts of modern rehabilitation facilities.

There are many forms of therapy, including specifically designed physical activity. In many instances prevention of further degeneration is planned by the scientific therapist in order to speed recovery as much as possible. These preventive medicine practices can save the individual from possible permanent loss.

The *individual* is a major part of the process of rehabilitation and therapy. In this instance, knowledge of the disease, injury, bodily malfunction, and physiology of the rehabilitative process is essential for achievement of desired results. The patient must be thoroughly informed in major surgery of the length of time and type of rehabilitation necessary for normal recovery. In some cases recovery is not influenced by therapy or requires complete inactivity. These are unfortunate conditions because inactivity adds to the functional reduction caused by disease, but in some cases physical activity must wait until the body has regained enough strength to respond favorably.

For successful personal rehabilitation the individual must be more than a knowledgeable layman. One's attitude is fundamental in the will to regain normal functioning and become fully rehabilitated. The alcoholic, for example, must want to change. He must have goals that are stronger than the need for alcohol. Without this desire on the part of the patient, little progress can be made, for rehabilitation is long and arduous. In some cases, the process of rehabilitation may continue throughout an individual's lifetime, simply to maintain his current status.

Mental Health Content. Mental-emotional maladjustments and mental illness have increased considerably during recent years, and this increase appears to be continuing. The reasons for this include our fast-paced modern life, intense professional and social involvements, crowded urban centers, transportation difficulties, and other forms increased stress put on individuals by a competitive modern society. These conditions must be countered with leisure and occupational activities that have positive results.

Physical recreation, maintenance of acceptable levels of physical fitness, and sports for everyone in the community are beneficial conditions for mental and emotional health and personal adjustment. These processes have physical requirements, and if fitness status is low, the individual is hardly able to function. Those who do so while in poor health are definitely the exceptions.

Physical activity as sports and recreation has a prophylactic effect, for it helps to neutralize the effects of stress in daily living. Continued stress can only be expected to have a lasting, irreversible effect on the individual over a long period of time. For the physically weak individual the period before damage results is considerably shorter than that for the strong individual. Physical activity, rest, and enjoyable intellectual and social interests are all conditions that compensate, both physically and mentally, for the negative aspects in life.

The social tension, prejudice, and anxiety typical of modern life take a heavy toll on the individual. These conditions result from modern transportation and the automated machinery, which increase the daily pace, and from racial, religious, and national prejudice, which have existed, unfortunately, in all times but continue to add to the unhappiness of life.

Physical Activity: A Preventive Medicine Profession

The effects of ill health and the high costs of medical services influence many of the ills afflicting modern society; reducing the amount of poor health and medical costs can also reduce other societal ills. In most countries considerable emphasis in medicine and education is placed on diagnosis and cure of disease. Although efforts have been made by health agencies and the government for disease prevention in recent years, this effort is considerably behind the demand for such programs by society.

Research on the value of sports, athletics, and physical activities to the health and well-being of the individual is essentially limited to student research on the university level. These studies deal largely with the understanding of physical performance, and there are few long-range studies of the preventive value of physical activity.

It is a commonly accepted truism that prevention is better than cure, but it appears that governments and agencies do not have the confidence to invest sufficient funds to investigate the various factors that appear to have disease-preventing potential. In this chapter we deal only with disease-preventing potential of physical activity. In the full context of preventive medicine, physical activity is only one of a number of components. The effects of physical activity on health have been emphasized less than the effects of the environmental conditions. Of course, immediate disease-producing environments must have first attention, but it is also important to consider the long-range effects of disease and the effects of man's life practices on his health. Unfortunately, scant attention has been given to these conditions.

In this text and chapter we consider physical activity in all its possible professional roles so that one can objectively judge whether these practices are worthy of professional classification. We ask the question, "Is it possible to identify physical activity as a professional component of preventive medicine, so that physical activity is accorded a professional status unrelated to disease prevention?" It is possible to view through the literature in this field the powers of physical activity in its application to preventive medicine.

Physical activity as it contributes to the goals of preventive medicine is set into a conceptual structure that identifies its various elements; these elements consist of human qualities that are influenced by physical activity. This structure served as a basis for a search of the literature and research studies that would provide information about the concepts and the conceptual categories of physical activity as a whole, thereby providing a presentation of the professional nature of physical activity in its role in preventive medicine. This role is identified as contributing to health maintenance, aiding in the process of disease prevention and control, preparing for injury and accident prevention, serving as a medium for rehabilitation and therapy, and providing a setting in sports and physical recreation for mental and emotional adjustment with the idea of helping the maladjusted individual toward a normal level of mental and emotional functioning. These roles of physical activity are reviewed in this chapter with supporting statements on the nature of the contributions that can be made by physical activity. The value of physical activity is reviewed largely within the scope of preventive medicine and as a part of the larger field of general medicine. The role of physical activity is of major significance within the profession of preventive medicine.

Without question considerably more emphasis must be placed on preventive medicine than has been the case until now. The need for preventive medicine does not imply that less time and money should be spent on curing individuals once illness strikes, but it is known that many injuries, diseases, and cases of poor fitness and lack of energy can be managed by the individual himself, largely without professional help. It is generally possible to prevent disease and injury. Society must be informed about disease and its symptoms, but of more importance is motivating people to work at constant good health. Many know what to do but still do not do it.

In addition to the content in this chapter, the reader should refer to the *Encyclopedia of Sport Sciences and Medicine* (Macmillan Publishing Co., Inc., 1971), Area VII on "Prevention of Disease and Injury." This encyclopedia is designed as a review of knowledge now available in order to provide an understanding of sports and physical activity and its worth for human development and the personal welfare of the individual. The section on prevention contains five categories of content: prevention through behavior, prevention through sociopsychological development, prevention through physical and physiological development, prevention through social and physical environmental controls, and prevention of sociopsychological disorders. The content of this section is directly applicable to this chapter and to the understanding of the contribution of physical activity to preventive medicine.

It can be safely concluded that physical activity in its application to sports, athletics, recreation, rehabilitation, and so on, has significant professional content for the preventive medicine field. The prevention of many possible negative results from daily activity; the maintenance of a satisfactory level of physical fitness; the interest in sports as an observer and follower through the medium of newspapers, radio, television; and the participation in outdoor life of camping, hiking, and hunting are all applications of physical activity designed to maintain and advance the health of the individual. All of these activities help promote normality and contribute directly to the profession of preventive medicine. It is anticipated that the sports activities begun within the past two or three decades in the preventive medicine field will be significantly increased within the next few years. The costs of disease and illness alone will provide a strong motivating force, as well as the primary reason for preventive medicine, namely, to avoid risking the health of the individual whenever possible.

Chapter 15

Recreation

Recreation is more than physical activity. Regardless of the form it takes, whether sports, athletics, hiking, camping, or any one of a number of possible activities, recreation has more than purely physical benefits. The form recreation takes depends upon the attitude of the individual toward the activity selected and the amount of enjoyment he gains from participation. It encompasses a multitude of personal choices and preferences, and recreation is as broad a field as the choices it offers to society for leisure utilization. To some individuals recreation is social involvement and activities entirely free from physical work or activity; for others recreation means spending their free moments in activities that require strenuous physical effort. Satisfaction to those who enjoy strenuous physical effort comes through the strain placed on large muscle groups. To individuals unconcerned with the physical component of recreation, social activities usually fulfill all recreation needs.

There are as many types of recreation as there are individual human interests and desires. Recreation involves all ages, from children at home to retired, aged, or handicapped individuals, to whom recreation is especially important. Recreation ranges from vigorous sport activities to quiet study, from watching an activity to participating in it, from solitary enjoyment to group activity, from spontaneous participation to highly organized teams, and from activities requiring no leadership to those requiring highly skilled professional specialists.

Recreation usually involves a change of pace that refreshes the individual and allows him to maintain physical, mental, and emotional well-being and equilibrium. It may also involve the same activity as that with which the individual is vocationally linked, but merely a change of focus from work to pleasure. For example, a swimming coach may play the piano for recreation or he may prefer to go swimming with friends. In the first instance, the coach has changed his activity as well as his pace; in the second, he has changed his mental focus while still participating in the same activity.

An individual's recreational choices may contribute to health and fitness or may undermine them, may bring joy and excitement or may become boring and frustrating. Whatever the situation, recreational choice is completely free and personal. An individual can do as he chooses within the boundaries of the law and his physical and financial resources. Realizing the importance of personal recreational choice to the welfare of the individual, professional and community leaders are now more concerned with the recreational resources and interests of society than at any time in history. The main reason for this increased interest in recreation is that man has more free time than at any period in history, and this free time is increasing rapidly. It has been said, mostly without conviction, that in the future the work needed to maintain society could be accomplished largely by machines, with a miniscule portion of society actually needing to work. No longer can work be thought of in the food-shelter terms of earlier societies. Modern resources and commodity advantages come largely without individual physical work. If modern technology continues its rapid advance, the work week may be reduced to less than the twenty hours now spent by some individuals. Certainly there is a need to prepare each individual for constructive leisure activities. Future preparation for professions or occupations will be less demanding. On top of all these advances, discussion is now under way about lowering retirement to fifty or fifty-five years of age. The tragedy of this is that this period, from fifty to sixty-five years of age, is often man's most productive time.

It is the hope of most experts that the increased opportunities for recreation will develop wholesome, constructive, and socially acceptable activities as a means to improve personal life and to elevate the cultural levels of the community. Worthwhile activities can bring with them personal challenges and social approval in home, community, and national life that are the basis for all other professional activities and work necessary to that society. An individual's leisure activities are closely related to other cultural programs in a society. Recreation is related to work, social welfare, education, religion, and health, yet does not fall into any of these categories.

An individual's occupation is not recreation even though it may be pleasurable and the individual may spend most of his time at it. Generally, individuals are motivated to work by the financial returns, prestige, and satisfaction the job provides. For some individuals the job might meet all their needs for an entire lifetime, but most require escape from jobs that are only partly satisfying or fulfilling.

People have always had time for recreation. During preautomation days in the United States, the individual typically worked six days a week, ten hours per day. The work was physically demanding and after-work hours were necessarily devoted to rest. Recreational interests were held to a minimum because of the lack of free time. Today recreation is recognized as important not only because it fills the activity void created by increased free time but because it is a vital part of society and its cultural structure. Recreation now stands along with education, vocational professions, and religion as a necessary ingredient for a well-balanced life. Recreation, like any other activity in which an individual takes part, is based upon satisfaction of certain basic needs or desires. For many people, particularly those in intense, demanding professional work with a great deal of accompanying stress, recreation provides balance to life.

Professional Status of Recreation

A profession has its roots in the need of people for professional services. Recreation, like other social services, grew out of society's need for community programs geared to leisure activities of interest to individuals during periods when they were not at work. Leisure planning began in the schools. From its beginning in the school systems, social agencies grew in number until today there are thousands in communities of only moderate size. These agencies developed around sports, the church, social clubs, and fraternal organizations. This provided the beginning of a recreation profession, of which physical activity constitutes a subprofession.

This section will review recreation and present its status as a profession. This will serve as the basis for the next section of this chapter, which deals with the physical activity domain of recreation and its role in the total field of recreation as a profession. This section will show the role of physical activity as recreation and provide a basis by which to judge its professional potentials.

Carlson et al.[1] report that for recreation to be judged a profession, it should meet several requirements. To be recognized as a profession, recreation would require the general acceptance of the public, must have a specific body of knowledge, must have and support basic research, must operate professional education programs for leadership in all phases of work, must develop and continue to revise certification standards consistent with advancing profession and social changes, must develop standards for personnel and recruitment practices, and, of considerable importance, must plan a professional organization that manages the activities of the profession in order to render to society services of high quality.

Planning for recreation programs requires a considerable body of knowledge. The professional worker must have a philosophy about

[1] R. E. Carlson et al., *Recreation in American Life* (Belmont, Calif.: Wadsworth, 1963), pp. 349–370.

people, their needs, and programs to fill those needs, while also serving the best interests of society. He must also recognize society's many differing opinions in philosophy and ways of life. The professional must understand the people and the community and have the knowledge and skills to work with each individual, not only to meet their needs but also to direct them into desirable areas of interests and activities. The leader must lead, not follow traditional interests. The requirements for recreational leadership are as broad as the social life of the people.

A vital and progressive profession has both basic and applied research programs. Quality recreational services come only from programs that are researched to establish the procedures by which the needs of society can best be met. The research requirements for recreation are more difficult than those in the biological sciences, because the social sciences include all conditions that influence people's choices, and these variables are more difficult to control in research.

Preparation for leadership roles in recreation is recent in the United States. Universities now offer degrees in recreational leadership through the doctoral level. There are now many recreational graduates throughout the country who have significant professional positions in recreation as trained recreational leaders. There are some 100 or more educational institutions in the United States alone that now have degree programs in recreation. This number would be significantly increased if one counted those individuals with training in that phase of physical education that deals directly with recreation. (Over 1,000 institutions in this country offer degree programs in physical education.) In addition to university programs, the number of institutions, clinics, workshops, and special recreational leadership programs in each state is so large that an estimate cannot even be made.

The curriculum for preparation in recreation leadership includes studies in the humanities, natural and biological sciences, communications, education, business administration, public administration, public relations, health and safety, group processes, and philosophy as well as field experiences for the undergraduate that make up a significant part of his curriculum. Professional recreation preparation is now established as a profession. However, unfortunately leaders are often selected in the recreation field for areas in which they have little preparation or competence. Employers should be more aware of job specialization.

There are additional aspects of a profession that indicate its status. For recreation these include recruitment practices, certification, standards for personnel, a code of ethics, and professional organizations.

Recruitment practices in the past resulted in a gap between supply and demand in the recreational field. In recent years, this has been corrected. During the past two decades, a significant number of qualified personnel have been prepared for recreational leadership positions. This is particularly true in the areas of supervision and administration. Many recreation positions are available in local communities, particularly on the program level. The development of recreational programs by commercial agencies for their personnel has also increased the number of leadership opportunities.

Certification of personnel, personal standards, and employment practices in the field of recreation appear to be in the early stages of professional development. State and national recreational organizations, however, have accomplished a great deal toward upgrading standards for professional practices. The difficulty of this endeavor is in the implementation of these standards by local, state, and national agencies employing recreational personnel. Many of the agencies still appear to believe that formal preparation is not needed for this work or that the preparation in other fields (e.g., physical education) is of equal value.

Workers in recreation have organized into professional associations. These organizations are numerous and include park authorities with jurisdiction over recreation; education for recreation personnel heading school and school-community recreation programs; private agencies, such as the YMCA and YWCA, with major portions of their programs recreational; and finally many special groups, such as camping organizations, recreational therapy groups, sports and hobby clubs, and so on. These workers are all concerned with their status and are, indeed, aware of the professional requirements of their vocation. They are making progress in upgrading each application of recreation as it meets recreational objectives.

This chapter is concerned with the professional status of recreation. What is the current professional status of recreation? If recreation is compared to the more-established professions, such as law and medicine, its present status would certainly fall short of those professions. In the final judgment, controls by the members of the profession themselves should be established that explicitly detail the standards for all facets of work that must be met before the individual is certified to practice the profession. This has not been done in recreation. This is, in part, because of the uneducated views of the public on the need for recreation and the degree of leadership specialization necessary to render such services. For many communities, special requirements are not necessary. Professional workers in the recreation field who know the value of specialization, however, have a much more sophisticated view of the value of recreation. Advancement of the professional status of recreation must come from the resolution of these two differing viewpoints.

This section is designed to provide a setting for the study of the role of physical activity as recreation, the role of physical activity in the recreation profession, and the role of physical activity as a profession itself or as a part of a larger recreational profession.

Professional Domain: The Conceptual Structure of Physical Activity in Recreation

In meeting the objectives of this chapter, two requirements were set for study and for securing supporting literature: (1) to analyze physical activity in its various forms in order to identify those segments that could be classified within the recreation context and (2) to identify the appropriate physical recreation literature for evidence supporting physical activity's fulfillment of the recreational needs of society. Achieving the first objective calls for the preparation of a conceptual structure that establishes a definite framework into which it places the concepts, human values, and elements of physical activity that meet these recreational goals and, in addition, classification of these concepts into categories that represent unique and independent concepts of physical recreation. This structure is presented within five major categories (List 12).

In meeting the second objective, the literature was reviewed for supporting evidence of the recreational content of each concept and category. These statements represent the content of physical activity in its professional recreational roles.

List 12. Conceptual structure: The professional domain of physical activity in recreation

1. Values (individual and societal).
   a. Aesthetic.
   b. Application and acquisition of skills.
   c. Community spirit.
   d. Creative experience.
   e. Cultural values.
   f. Democracy.
   g. Fitness and health.
   h. Integration.
   i. Intellectual values.
   j. Moral leadership.
   k. Personal satisfaction.
   l. Physical well-being.
   m. Provision for challenge.
   n. Psychological safety.
   o. Social adjustment.
   p. Social development.

2. Recreation programs.
   a. Arts and crafts.
   b. Camping and outdoor activities.
   c. Church.
   d. Commercial programs.
   e. Community relations.
   f. Deprivation.
   g. Family recreation.
   h. Fitness and health.
   i. Hobbies.
   j. Industrial.
   k. Leadership.
   l. Parks and playgrounds.
   m. Physical activities in leisure.
   n. Programs for the handicapped.
   o. Recreational games.
   p. Rehabilitative programs.
   q. Safety and protection.
   r. Social agencies.
   s. Sports and athletics.

3. Government.
   a. City redevelopment.
   b. Commercial activities.
   c. Community administration.
   d. Democratic government.
   e. Environmental protection.
   f. Equality and opportunity.
   g. Facilities.
   h. Leadership.

List 12. Conceptual structure: The professional domain of physical activity in recreation—Cont.

i. Long-range plans.
j. Policy structure.
k. Programs and service.
l. Recreation and parks.
4. Leadership.
    a. Administration.
    b. Coaches, players, and students.
    c. Environmental understandings.
    d. Guidance and supervision.
    e. Human development and understanding.
    f. Interdisciplinary understandings.
5. Philosophical determinants.
    a. Attitudes.
    b. Automation.
    c. Education.
    d. Ethics.
    e. Experiences.
    f. Facilities.
    g. Health.
    h. Human understandings.
    i. Human values.

m. Social integration.
n. Social organizations.
o. Societal responsibilities.
p. Urbanization effects.

g. Interpretation of aims and objectives.
h. Knowledge.
i. Press, radio, and TV.
j. Professional leaders.
k. Public relations.
l. Skill teaching.
m. Special qualities.
n. Teaching techniques.
o. Volunteers.

j. Motivational goals.
k. Opportunities.
l. Outdoor life.
m. Safety and protection.
n. Security.
o. Skills.
p. Spectatorship and participation.

Values (Individual and Societal). The purpose of recreation is to develop human values and qualities that are important to the individual and to society. If physical activity is applied as recreation under proper supervision and in an appropriate setting, human values will be affected by participation.

Social adjustment is one of the major reasons for participation in sports. This, of course is not the only purpose, but social association in sports is high in importance among the desirable values of sports.

Cultural, aesthetic, social, and moral values are also part of the informal value system of physical activity in recreation. Physical activity is cultural itself, largely because of the role it plays in an individual's social life. When sports are sponsored by educational-recreational institutions, these values are especially stressed in individual and group programs.

Every individual has an inherent need to be *challenged*, to have opportunities to be creative and become involved in situations that stimulate the psychological being. These qualities are found in the competitive context of sports and athletics. The nature of the result, however, will be determined by the social environment of the participation. This is an integral part of the conceptual domain of physical activity in recreation.

Physical activity through its recreational context can help the individual toward greater personal skill, fitness and health levels, awareness of safety skills and ability to employ them. This quality of physical activity certainly is a part of the conceptual structure of physical recreation.

Leisure experiences are both emotionally and intellectually oriented. Individuals must understand the benefits of physical activity yet maintain the emotional enjoyment of them over a long period of time. Leisure experiences should be democratically planned and programmed in order to integrate each individual's attitudes and aptitudes into an enjoyable leisure program. These benefits of physical activity as recreation are inherent in the process of participation. They do not happen by chance or through unsupervised play, but require planning and hard work by recreation leaders. The absence of adequate leadership could result in disorganized activities with few personal benefits. This permissive atmosphere can lead to participation in riots, fights, and property damage. Social organization is most difficult to achieve; supervision is essential.

Finally, physical recreation promotes pleasure, personal satisfaction, and meaningful social adjustment. This is one of the principal reasons an individual desires to participate in such sports as golf, tennis, and swimming. The ability of leisure sports to meet the need for companionship is one of their most attractive aspects.

Recreation Programs. Physical activity constitutes a large part of recreation. Physical activity as a segment of recreation has grown significantly in recent years because of the need for it and because of the extremely rapid development of school and community facilities. Some social agencies (e.g., YMCA) plan most program activities around physical activity (about 60 per cent) and therefore must employ recreation and physical education leaders.

The most common physical activity programs in recreation are run in conjunction with parks, playgrounds, camping sites, community swimming pools, gymnasiums, and other community facilities. These programs are particularly valuable for youth, who often have a considerable amount of free time.

Sports and athletics are major portions of the recreational programs in every community, both for participants and spectators. The growth of sports and athletics in the schools, colleges, and universities reflects their value to the community at large, as well as the rapid growth of commercial sporting enterprises in nearly every sport and on every level.

Recreational games, informal family activities, and family play on a holiday fall within the physical activity context of recreation, although they may not involve vigorous physical activity. This area of low-key physical activity is growing rapidly.

There is also a recreational aspect of physical activity in rehabilitation programs for the injured, physically handicapped, or socially deprived. Here the aim is to contribute to the process of normal self-actualization as well as to provide enjoyable experiences to the participant. Recreational therapy utilizing physical activity is now a common practice in hospitals and rehabilitation centers and has proved to be a positive aid in rehabilitation. The continued high level of positive results gives continued support to these programs.

Industrial agencies, churches, social agencies, and commercial organizations have physical activity programs that they utilize as recreation for their employees. These programs are important for upgrading employee morale and physical well-being. Their importance has been demonstrated by substantial production gains and improved human relations between labor and management.

Clubs and social groups program physical activity for their organizations in many varying forms, including arts and crafts, hobbies, hiking clubs, woodworking, gardening, and so on, which bring people together in close informal association. This is a designed attempt by the community to improve its culture, social interaction, and human understanding of its citizenry. These social-recreational experiences are found to be extremely valuable. They represent a continuing program for everyone in the community in which they can find self-expression and enjoyment through some form of physical activity.

Government. Governments on all political levels have supported sports and athletics. Public recreational facilities have been provided by the federal and state governments, which have also supervised and operated recreational programs. Local governments have also provided and supervised community sports and recreation programs. It is now common practice to open schools and public facilities for adult leisure sport and recreation activities. The governmental domain in the United States is today a major force in sports and recreation. In some countries, the role of government is considerably more tangible than it is in this country.

Government is the science of human management in the pursuit of desirable social goals. Perpetuation of the social standards of the culture is one of the foremost goals for any government, regardless of political philosophy. The government is responsible for all community activities that aid in the achievement of more democratic and efficient government.

Federal, state, and local governments provide sports and recreational facilities for the public, which provides the major support for physical activity as recreation. In many instances, governmental facilities are willingly provided without the necessity of associated programs or leadership, but simply as a convenience for the recreational use of its people.

Democratic government, community responsibility, public administration and political leadership are important goals of government. An ideal relationship is based on local autonomy. This goal, however, is most difficult on the community economically, desirable as it may be socially, culturally, and politically. If local government fails, it will be most difficult to manage adequate community programs on the state or federal levels. Most communities generally succeed in being autonomous. Community life is essential for this goal. Sports, athletics, and recreation aid the development of desirable community life and contribute toward the maintenance of a satisfying personal life as well.

The protection of society in its various social and physical environments and the neutralization of urban effects on community life are governmental responsibilities. Generally it is possible to achieve this lofty goal on a private, communal basis. These private developments are available to the public. Based upon the principles of commercial enterprise, they contribute to personal welfare and gains in community socialization and help to strengthen government by strengthening the individual.

Social integration, ethical behavior, equality of the individual, citizenship in leadership roles, and communal activities directed toward social needs are all important political activities within the community and the nation. When sports are programmed for the citizens, government is significantly aided. Political goals, in part, can also be achieved through sports by community leadership through the development of sports and recreation programs. Most of these programs are developed by civic-minded volunteers who are deeply interested in citizenship and individual participation.

Leadership. Physical activity programs designed for recreational purposes must be organized under qualified leadership in order to yield positive results. For physical recreation programs, leadership for the large number of organized activities is generally supplied by citizen volunteers. It would be impossible and probably undesirable to put the responsibility for all leadership on the paid professional. It is extremely valuable for a community to involve as many of its citizens as possible in the leadership as well as participation phases of physical recreation and sports programs. The lack of professional knowledge and skill is outweighed by the personal associations of the citizen leader, which provide him with close knowledge of the people of that individual community. Leadership is probably more extensive in physical recreation programs than in any other community program. Recreational leadership can be provided by both volunteer and professionally prepared individuals. Both are definitely needed.

Professionally prepared leaders serve in numerous capacities, including administrators of community recreation programs, teachers and coaches in school and community sport programs, school administrators and supervisors, social agency directors, and sport specialists. Each of these individuals is a professional charged with the responsibility for school, agency, and community programs in sports and recreation.

Citizen volunteers are essential in school, community, and social agency sports and recreation programs. Most social agencies have a minimum number of paid workers; most of the actual supervision is handled by the large number of volunteers who serve as program leaders.

Knowledge of leadership in sports and recreation requires knowledge of people, community needs, social problems, cultural differences, program values, human development, and society and the role of sports in the solution of many human problems. Narrow-minded views of sports as ends in themselves will do little to solve social problems.

Radio, TV, and newspapers can do a great deal to add quality to recreation programs. By placing sports in an acceptable social perspective, these media can make maximum contribution to community life and public standards. High-quality sports, athletics, and recreation programs add to the overall quality of life in the community.

Establishing the proper environmental setting for sports and recreation in a community is another domain of physical activity in recreation. Social and physical environments have a significant influence on sports and recreational activities. Dirty, unsafe, and unplanned physical environments for sports and recreation can hardly generate enthusiasm for participation. This is certainly also true for the social environment, because its influence is considerably more obvious than the physical setting. Social forces are so strong that an individual could hardly survive if he did not become a member of the group. Individual influences on the mores of a social group are most difficult to assess.

The leadership domain of physical activity as recreation, whether it be volunteer or professional, is of major consequence to society. The events that occur in the other components of this structure will be determined largely by leadership. It is unfortunate that sports and recreation are not viewed by many political professionals as a vital force in a community. The political structure and government of a community without constructive programs for the people will run into difficulties, for its community life will lack vitality and fail to satisfy the deep desire of its citizens for human association. Providing this association is the basis of constructive community programs. For this, leadership is necessary.

Philosophical Determinants. Philosophy exerts a direct force on all human activity. Certainly in programs that have close community and societal relations the program must be planned and designed within the context of those human values. Philosophy is the discipline incorporating knowledge and history of events in order to provide guidance to thought in the establishment of programs for the achievement of societal goals. This is certainly true for educational programs and the possible roles of sports and physical activity in recreation.

The essential domain of philosophy in physical activity as recreation is in the establishment of *human values* directed toward intrinsic needs and desired goals. Sports and physical activity are programmed, and their leadership is directed by philosophy. For example, pragmatism is a philosophy that guides most coaches in sports and athletics. Success to them is foremost, and winning is the criterion for success. Human values in this philosophy assume a secondary role. Human values in sports deal with man's feelings, attitudes, behavior, social or antisocial acts, emotions, integrity, and so on.

Philosophy guides educational programs in the community, the preparation of the individual for ethical life and behavior, the formation of attitudes in human associations, the development of personal security, and other qualities that provide meaning to life. The role of sports and recreation within these contexts of philosophy is a major one, because human associations in informal sports provide experiences that, if directed by the proper philosophical application, can lead to meaningful personal accomplishments.

Philosophy provides the basis for judging personal matters of health, safety, understanding of oneself and others, daily habits and leisure practices, and any other personal guidelines. This influence of philosophy provides the individual direction for the advancement of health and fitness or their deterioration and destruction. Choices each day will determine the direction and end result.

Philosophy also directs views on sports and physical activity. Social philosophies encourage sports, athletics, and recreation for personal well-being, participation enjoyment, enjoyment in the role of spectator, development of motivation, and development of interest in desirable leisure programs. The basic philosophies of pragmatism, realism, and, to some degree, idealism provide direction to the individual interested in sports for personal development that helps to prepare him for his responsibilities as a citizen.

Each individual's concept of balance and fullness of life reflects his own philosophic views. Those individuals who took to leisure for relaxation and enjoyment and those who seek leisure activities to provide satisfaction and personal development will gain most from recreation. Sports have numerous contributions to make to an individual's life, and because they provide variety to living, they should be a part of each person's daily life.

Professional Domain: The Physical Activity
Content in Recreation

In the preceding section, the conceptual domain of physical activity in recreation has been presented. The conceptual domain is that part of recreation that utilizes physical activity in all its forms for recreational purposes. This section deals with the potentialities of physical activity for meeting the requirements of recreation. One must know the value of the current recreation program and its potential for the future before one can modify a recreation program.

Values (Individual and Societal) Content. The loss of physical work that has resulted for many people from automation has made physical recreation a modern health necessity. Recognition of this fact has led to major advances in physical recreation of all forms from lawn games to professional sports. Camping, as only one example, enjoyed a virtual metamorphosis and is today America's favorite recreational pastime.

The value of physical recreation as a *socializing force* or *medium* is now well recognized by workers in sociology and psychology. The qualities of the human personality that can be most greatly influenced by physical recreation include social adjustment within sports and social recreation and elevation of cultural interests through properly organized and administered community sports and recreation programs. The sports program itself, under proper regulations and leadership, constitutes a major contribution to a society, and this does not happen by accident. It requires careful planning and leadership on the part of community leaders.

Physical recreation provides a setting for creative experiences. Sports hobbies, such as gardening, represent activities that are different and distinctive, but they are also physical in nature as well as recreational. With the freedom of choice and thought enjoyed in this country, creativity in an infinite number of recreational activities is certainly possible. An individual's aptitude will be best reflected by the experiences one gains from simple trial-and-error experiences.

Democratic human values, social standards, and moral judgments are all fundamental elements of participation in sports and physical recreation. Sports participation requires close interpersonal relationships. Democratic human values can be the spin-off product of relationships with teammates striving for the same common goal in sports participation. Positive social standards and moral judgments in the context of sports participation are essential for group cohesiveness and interaction as well as for promotion of individual satisfaction from the group experience. Antisocial group associations cannot be deeply satisfying or productive.

Physical recreation and sports have been shown to have cathartic effects on the individual. These effects essentially reduce the individual's tension levels, which have negative physiological effects. The relaxed individual also reduces his caloric need in all activities, both mental and physical. Psychologically, the individual will enjoy improved command of his own personal attitudes and social behavior within the bounds of individual ability and prior learning.

Fitness, health, and personal well-being are important to every individual. Their value today has increased because of our sedentary ways and the increased stress to which we are subjected. It is impossible to reach high levels of health and fitness in any way except through careful planning of one's time so as to allow a period for daily physical activity. Because physical activities have highly specific results, one must decide the general level of health and fitness desired for his daily living and plan his physical recreation program accordingly.

Sports and physical recreation have the potential for identifying psychiatric disorders as well as for serving as a medium for the prevention of these disorders if their causes are recognized soon enough. The social and psychological value of sports can strengthen the individual and provide emotional stability through the positive social setting of physical recreation. This will help to maintain the individual psychologically against the stresses of daily living. Sports and physical activity programs can help those with mental disorders as well as those with physiological disorders.

Sports and recreation form major segments of community social programs. They represent the culture and mores of society as well as the potentials for advancement of its social values. Bias and prejudice in most societies are strong influences that can render great psychological damage to individuals and groups in a community. Riots are caused by such feelings. Sports and physical recreation planned in conjunction with groups who provide inviting facilities and professional leadership can add considerably to the elimination of such antisocial behavior.

The value of sports and physical recreation as an integrating force in society is recognized by professional workers in many fields. The informal nature of sports and the physical recognition of performance are conditions that contribute to human understanding. In the United States, sports have made major public contributions toward the elimination of a major share of social bias. With few exceptions, an individual in sports is accepted on the basis of his ability and not his social persuasion.

Content in Recreation Programs. A large segment of community recreation is now planned as physical activity covering the full range of possible movement activities. These programs also contribute to the physical welfare of the individual. They range from the most basic individual activity to highly organized athletic programs directed by professional coaches. Each of these activity programs has considerable value to society.

Programs in sports and physical activity also provide valuable leisure activities. Sports can be fun and a great source of enjoyment. Community recreation programs provide physical activities that incorporate nearly every interest and skill of its people. These programs are heavily supported by the community.

Physical recreation has therapeutic value, both for those with physical handicaps and for those who are mentally or emotionally maladjusted. These programs are geared to the physical and mental condition of the individual and are designed to allow normal participation and behavior consistent with individual capacities and societal goals. The demonstrated value of physical recreation programs has resulted in increasing support from the community.

Sports, athletics, and recreation programs complement each other and provide a balanced community program. These programs are implemented to include abilities ranging from the highly skilled individual with strong athletic aptitudes to those individuals desiring participation in physical activity that requires little skill or athletic aptitude. Athletic programs do not even totally meet the needs of the athlete. He, too, needs a variety of leisure or recreational activities in addition to athletic participation.

Recreation and sports programs are planned to promote social integration. Race, religion, nationality, cultural background, and occupational differences all can divide the community into different groups or factions. Programs must be provided to include the entire community. Success has been noted in many communities as a result of these efforts. Greater emphasis is being placed today on the use of public facilities for these programs on week nights, week ends, and holidays.

Outdoor recreation and lifetime sports programs are part of school physical education and recreation programs aimed at preparing the individual for future leisure opportunities. There is no excuse today to graduate from high school and not have the physical recreation skills necessary to fill the leisure role afforded to nearly everyone.

Transportation and facilities have played a significant part in helping to stimulate program growth and developments in physical activity. There is scarcely a community today that does not provide its citizens with playgrounds, gymnasiums, swimming pools, and camping grounds for full use of all its citizens. Some of these facilities were built as a part of the school system, but they are readily made available to the people of the community. Transportation has advanced recreation throughout all parts of the country and around the world. Most people now have automobiles and most travel during holidays and on vacations. Mobility throughout this country and around the world has become a fact of life. The old concept of the self-contained community now encompasses the country as a whole. Planning sports and recreation programs now involves planning on the state and national level as well as in the local community.

Communal sports include all spectator sports at an economic level that influence the economic planning of a community and to some extent a nation. Huge investments are made in facilities, and this has a definite impact on the economy of a community and of the nation.

Industry has invested in sports and physical recreation programs for its employees. It has found that this is an aid in improving employee morale and general fitness for work. Recreation pays off in increased production and, of course, provides personal benefits to each employee in the form of improved enjoyment, fitness, and personal well-being. The church and social agencies of the community are also involved in establishing sports programs. They have found that these programs contribute to the achievement of the goals of their institution.

The number of program activities available in sports and physical activities for community planning is very large. The possibilities for physical activity provide numerous choices for each individual, regardless of skills or aptitudes. They cover all possible interests of that segment of society that wants some physical activity. Although the results of physical activity will differ with each activity, each does provide the singular general result of personal refreshment and well-being. One must, however, be interested in participation with sufficient intensity if he expects to receive maximum results from his activity.

Government Content. Governments on all levels are organized to represent in some manner the people and their welfare. This includes political management for providing law and order for the protection of society. Simply protecting society is not enough; government must be concerned about the total quality of life enjoyed by that society. These responsibilities exist at the local, state, and federal levels.

Recreation and sports require space and facilities beyond the resources of individuals, local communities, or states. The federal government provides in many instances land and facilities for the recreational use of society on a national scale. In some instances, leadership is also provided by the federal government.

Parks, recreation facilities, and recreational leadership are generally highly developed in each community with sufficient size and resources to afford such leisure resources. Local governments provide the funds and leadership for these programs as well as supervision. *Governments purchase* land in urban areas in order to provide the people with adequate park space. The parks of London and Central Park in New York City are fine examples of this concept. These facilities are enjoyed by nearly everyone in those large urban areas.

Governments also cooperate with commercial sports enterprises in providing recreational parks and facilities. Nearly every large urban center today has a sports stadium. These facilities seat 50,000 spectators or more and provide an ideal showcase for amateur or professional teams. Efforts are made by local governments to provide protection for these facilities and tax relief or exemptions to help make it possible for sports promoters to provide programs at minimal cost to the public.

The natural recreational resources of a country must be protected and maintained through governmental control. These facilities (e.g., national parks) provide a natural, open landscape that gives relief from the congestion of urban life. Days spent by individuals hiking and camping in these parks would be impossible without governmental support and supervision.

Governments, through the programs of social and educational institutions, provide support for leadership preparation and research. These programs include single-day clinics, week-long workshops, or lengthy graduate education programs leading to a doctorate degree. In the United States, leadership provisions have been made by federal and state governments in order to ensure a continuing supply of qualified personnel for sports and recreation programs.

Sports and recreation programs have had special emphasis internationally during recent years. International sports are now quite common and many new countries are emerging as sports powers. This is only the beginning of an athletic renaissance and should produce major gains in sports achievements in the next few years. International sports programs have grown principally because of the availability of rapid transportation and mass communication.

Governments have been very direct in providing leadership to sports-recreation programs. The emphasis on physical fitness during the Eisenhower and Kennedy administrations is an excellent example. The United States government has readily provided funds for leadership on the federal level to aid state and local governments in the development of sports programs. The objective of governments is to help individuals recognize what constitutes poor levels of fitness and to provide knowledge and leadership for fitness improvement.

Without government and political interests in sports and recreation, one can easily visualize the self-centered individualism that would characterize a community. This would be especially disastrous today, with the abundance of free time available. The results of crime, vandalism, and antisocial practices would require government expenditures that would go considerably beyond the costs of these programs or other preventive programs designed to upgrade community life. In this respect, it is well known that a highly educated individual well schooled in the principles of citizenship has considerably less need for governmental resources than his less-educated neighbor.

Leadership Content. As in all successful enterprises, the leadership in each phase of work will determine the degree of success of a project. There are infinite numbers of institutions that have failed, not because of their program or business practices, but because of the people they employed. An institution cannot survive by its structure alone; its employees must believe in the institution and be anxious to make it work. In fact, some programs with little appeal can be highly successful when performed by highly motivated employees.

The quality of sports and recreation depends primarily on quality of leadership. Some believe that the activities in which one participates during his leisure hours should be based upon complete freedom of choice. In truth, however, the range of opportunities available to an individual and the effects of his recreational choice are so important to his health and welfare that the highest order of prepared leadership is needed both in selection of and participation in leisure pursuits.

Directing the recreation, sports, and play life of the individual, particularly during youth, provides an infinite number of opportunities for the physical and social development of the individual. In families in which both parents express concern for the health of their family and have some preparation in positive health and fitness procedures, there is often little delinquency, social deviation, or maladjustment problems among the children. In broken and unhappy families the opposite generally occurs unless the children are strongly influenced by leadership in schools, churches, or other social agencies.

Adequate preparation for leadership in sports and recreation requires an individual to be broadly prepared in the human service philosophy and the potentials of sports in the development of the individual. At the present time, sports and recreation professional leaders need a college or university preparation equal to that required of any profession that deals with societal development. For sports, the scope is larger than that for most professional endeavors, because the individual must have an understanding of the community, its people, and community agencies as well as a physical and biological science base; in addition, a social sciences background is desirable. Preparation must also include philosophic understanding of the individual and the people.

Sports and recreation programs in a community could not survive without voluntary leadership from its citizens. Volunteer leaders, however, must be prepared by professionals in the field in order to provide the best setting and instruction for learning and development in the recreation area. In social agencies, a considerable amount of programming is planned by volunteer leadership.

The mass media have a potent influence on sports. The role of sports in a school or in a community is undoubtedly influenced by the media. In commercial sports, at this time, it is a disgrace to lose. The goal usually is to win at all costs, and if the team does not win often enough, it may not survive. Unfortunately, this attitude is also becoming prominent in high schools, colleges, and universities, where sports should be played well for the learning and developmental experiences they afford rather than as a self-sustaining subcommercial enterprise within the confines of an educational institution. The influence of the mass media on recreational sports is, of course, much less than that on commercial sports, but through favorable publicity the media can aid in providing the facilities and leadership needed for these programs.

All social institutions are responsible for the status of society within a community. Sports and recreation teachers and coaches are particularly responsible because of their considerable influence over their pupils. One can characterize a team simply by knowing the attitude and preparation of the coach. Well-disciplined pupils behave in the way they are taught. This is particularly true with a successful coach, who is generally concerned about the player as a responsible individual or citizen.

For positive results from sports and recreational programs, there is no substitute for qualified leadership. Any compromise of this requirement is foolish economy. Moreover, such a compromise may involve the social loss of individuals that could have been useful and successful citizens. Leadership in voluntary sports or recreation is particularly needed in order to influence people to cooperate and establish desirable and satisfying goals.

Philosophical Content. One must have opinions, a definite philosophy about life and his own personal goals. This is the basis for all choices an individual makes in life, including selection of profession and direction his adult life takes as a result of his recreational interests. The manner in which an individual uses leisure is directed by his own personal philosophy, but the results of leisure are judged by personal results and rationalized through various interdisciplinary scientific experiments.

Because man has complete freedom of choice in leisure and recreation, he must be guided by a definite and desirable philosophy in life to achieve the greatest positive results through constructive physical or social experiences. It is important to understand the value of leisure activities in personal development.

Leisure, recreation, and sports should be regarded as complementing work. Each person should understand why both work and leisure are essential to a balanced life and optimal human development.

Industry and commercial enterprises are changing their philosophy and now evidence a concern for employees beyond the boundaries of the normal workday. Sports and recreation programs are planned to boost morale as well as to maintain the fitness of the worker, which benefits the person and the institution.

Most educational institutions in the United States are guided by a social philosophy that takes into account the whole individual. This philosophy is concerned not only with the mind but with the behavior and fitness of the individual. It aims at involving the young in the democratic process. Sports and recreation occupy important places in educational institutions because of this philosophy. Educational philosophies state that sports represent activities that contribute to the improvement of the quality of human life as well as to the maintenance of the physical body for a longer and more efficient life.

It is recognized by recreation leaders that there are many recreational choices and not all of these are physically oriented. Recreation is more than physical activity, and this is as it should be. A balance in recreational activities is also needed. The individual with many interests and skills is best equipped for a constructive and purposeful leisure life.

All leisure activities, with the exception of purely sedentary ones, require physical effort or work. One cannot enjoy leisure if he does not have good health and the necessary physical fitness level to be active.

The philosophy of many Americans delves very deeply into the realm of realism and pragmatism, or those philosophies that recognize facts about their field that stem from the sciences and medicine. People are aware of the conditions that will help them to improve, although some may not practice them.

Physical Activity: A Recreation Profession

Freedom of choice in recreational activities is as important as the activity selected, and the activity or activities selected certainly should be those forms of recreation that provide satisfaction and enjoyment to the individual. These basic facts have spawned the growth of recreation as an institution on a par with other strong professions. Recreation is, indeed, a profession, as demonstrated by the recent formation of professional associations. Whether recreation is a profession equal to medicine, law, social work, and others has yet to be fully judged. The application of the criteria by which professions must be judged will aid in analyzing the quality of these various professions in order that differences between them can be distinguished. This analysis is not the purpose of this chapter. This review of recreation is simply to note the role of physical activity and to determine whether that role is sufficient to infer professional status for physical recreation in itself, or as a phase of recreation as a whole, or both. Some impressions will be briefly reviewed.

The knowledge that must be known by workers in this field and needed by those individuals who participate in physical activity is probably the most essential ingredient of recreation as a profession. To plan, administer, and operate recreational programs properly, basic knowledge is definitely needed in the fields of sociology, psychology, biological sciences, philosophy, government, history, literature, and speech, in addition to other subjects intrinsic to a basic liberal education. In addition, the individual must be specialized in the professional education and recreation career fields, which provide the knowledge and skills necessary to understand society and plan programs that contribute to individual welfare. The requirements are essentially the same for physical activity. The only major difference is that the individual becomes a recreational specialist in sports, athletics, and physical activity in all its forms.

To be classified a profession, it must be judged according to society's requirements for specialized services. Regardless of the influence of the professional worker, if the services rendered are not considered essential, they will not be recognized as of professional caliber by the public. Sports, athletics, rehabilitation, and preventive medicine as applications of physical activity have been professionally organized in order to provide guidance for professional services. Similarly, physical activity is organized as a recreational profession, which has been demonstrated by the employment of coaches, teachers, and specialists in nearly all social functions or interactions that serve society.

The requirements for certification, registration, accreditation, and licensing of institutions and personnel are also indications of the quality of a profession. In law and medicine these requirements have been reasonably established; in recreation and physical recreation they are less established. Requirements are recognized, nevertheless, and it is now a matter of time and perhaps motivation on the part of the recreation community until professional quality is assured from the members of this body. Professional ethics hold that practices cannot be accepted unless they fall within the standards set by the profession. If recreation is willing to set high standards and it enforces these requirements, it will be accepted as a profession and will grow rapidly.

The heart of any profession is the organization of workers in that field along definite standards. Unfortunately for physical activity, no "overall" regulating association has yet been established. There are many groups organized around a sport as a result of common interests, but they are planned for the promotion of the sport itself rather than for the promotion of the organization as a professional regulating body.

The motivation behind the development of a profession is not to instigate a "control" force for autocratic rule, but to establish regulations that must be met before institutions can prepare recreation leaders or individuals can practice the profession in service to society. These requirements call for internal self-regulation by the associations of recreation members if recreation is to be considered as a profession. These requirements, of course, will improve the status of the member and certainly the quality of services to society. The professional status of recreation should grow as improvements and satisfying results follow in the wake of this upgrading process.

Chapter 16

Rehabilitation

Rehabilitation is the restoration of the handicapped individual to the fullest physical, mental, social, and economic usefulness that organic functions allow. Self-respect and usefulness are within the grasp of every man, no matter what his handicap; it is imperative that rehabilitation aid every handicapped individual to find his niche in life. The restoration process can help that individual reach the highest possible level of adaptation to work, home, and family life, as well as a happy leisure life. In this chapter we shall examine the role of physical activity in restoring the handicapped individual to a normal life. Physical activity definitely contributes to this goal; this review is simply to identify its roles and to judge the value of physical activity in rehabilitation. Physical activity in rehabilitation is an accepted and established profession, which opens its resources to many.

There are many conditions in the world today that may lead to disabling injuries. The four wars during the twentieth century that directly involved the United States alone have resulted in injuries and disabilities that number in the millions. In addition to this, during the four-year American involvement in World War II over 1 million civilians were permanently disabled by accidents in the home, in the community, or on the highway. Tension, drugs, alcohol, and poor health practices cause disabling injuries of staggering proportions in this country each day. Cardiac arrest has become the major cause of death in the United States today. In the case of a heart attack, medical attention is desperately needed to save the life of the individual, but after these services have been rendered, the individual faces the even greater challenge of restoring his heart and circulatory system to a normal capacity. If rehabilitation is limited to rest alone, the individual will progressively lose power in the remainder of the body, until the slightest illness will place additional stress on the heart and make death more imminent. The individual with a weak or ailing heart already has disadvantages in the fight against any other disease or injury.

The concept of physical disability has undergone radical change as the result of advances in science and medicine. These changes place an obligation on science and medicine not only to heal disease and injury but actually to return the individual to a relatively normal life. The rehabilitation process often takes considerably more time than either the onset of disease or the healing process. Postoperative rehabilitation also goes beyond the strict bounds of the medical profession. It combines the efforts of the biological sciences and the potentials of physical activity in restoring normal bodily functioning within the limit of the individual's capabilities, which, of course, may have been considerably reduced as a result of disease or injury.

It is estimated that there are more than 30 million persons in the United States who have movement problems. They either have difficulty in physical movement or cannot move without assistance. Although it is difficult to estimate, a conservative figure is that 25 per cent of these individuals could be returned to useful life.

The increasing life-span of today's citizen adds to the rehabilitation problems. Experts estimate that by 1980, 25 million people in the United States will be sixty-five years of age or older. Physical problems requiring rehabilitation increase drastically in this age bracket, as do the social and emotional conditions that require services.

Cardiovascular disease is most prevalent among the aged. A large percentage of those in this age bracket are disabled. Each of these individuals could benefit from rehabilitative services, but many cannot afford these services. Moreover, rehabilitative personnel often are not available. Some of our elder citizens philosophically accept these disabilities and strive to meet only their immediate requirements for life itself. Estimates state that chronic disease, a major cause of physical handicaps, accounts for nearly 90 per cent of all cases that could possibly benefit from rehabilitative therapy and training.

Rehabilitation is more than individual or personal; it also has a strong economic base. If the number of handicapped continues to increase, it will not be long before society is overwhelmed by the physical and economic dependency of a large segment of the population, including the poor and the aged as well as the physically disabled.

Rehabilitation is also extremely important mentally and emotionally. The whole individual requires rehabilitation, and this must be accomplished by specialists that deal directly with all traits and functions of the human being and his personality. In many instances the psychological problems of rehabilitation are more difficult than the physical ones.

Science, especially the biological sciences, and medicine are directly associated with the process of rehabilitation.[1] In the past few decades the

---

[1] See *Physical Medicine and Rehabilitation*.

use of physical exercise and sports in rehabilitation of physical, mental, and emotional conditions has significantly increased. Exercise and physical activity as sports in the rehabilitative process were found to be especially useful during the years of World War II and after. Activities range from a precise group of exercises to rehabilitate a specific movement to sports used in hospitals as aids in the process of rehabilitating the mentally and emotionally disturbed patient toward normal associations and a satisfying life.

Professional Status of Rehabilitation

Institutional rehabilitation is a multidisciplinary effort; specializations include internal medicine, pediatrics, orthopedic surgery, neurology, neurosurgery, plastic surgery, cardiology, and preventive medicine. The rehabilitation team also consists of specialists from the sciences in physical therapy, occupational therapy, rehabilitation nurses, social workers, clinical psychologists, vocational therapists, speech therapists, and exercise specialists. In rehabilitation, success results from the knowledge and skill furnished by this team. The rehabilitation program is designed by a group of specialists, and no single person or discipline is dominant in the overall process. Medical services are generally applied for corrective purposes, and then the rehabilitation process starts for functional improvements of the organism. In a fracture, for example, the orthopedic surgeon sets the fracture, and when healing is complete, the process of restoring functional movements to the limb begins.

Because rehabilitation is multidisciplinary, professional status must be judged by not only each discipline but also the combinations of disciplines in meeting the various rehabilitative requirements. The basic status of a profession is essentially established by the needs of society and the skill of professionals in rendering services. These two requirements will be reviewed to provide insight into the current status of rehabilitation as a profession.

Professional Services. It is obvious that total rehabilitation of the handicapped individual must be an interdisciplinary effort. Any handicap, no matter what it is, goes beyond its own immediate impact, important as it is that this be corrected. To restore the individual to his fullest physical, mental, social, and economic usefulness and capability the disciplines must plan together to meet individual needs. The process of becoming a completely useful citizen is a basic goal for everyone, and this process is as much psychological as physical.

Teamwork in providing rehabilitative services is an essential requirement. Specialists use their knowledge in medicine, surgery, therapy, psychology, and psychiatry as well as their personal patience and kindness in their efforts to help the physically handicapped person in the process of re-education and vocational preparation.

The professional status of rehabilitation is the product of coordination, communication, and interaction among these various disciplines. The coordinated services must be specifically directed toward the ill or the physically disabled person on an individual basis. The professional goal of coordinated services is the establishment of a well-directed program for all established rehabilitation institutions. This is a goal for all those individuals who are professionally prepared to work in the rehabilitation field. For physical activity applied in rehabilitation, it is recognized that these services fall within the complete context of all functions and abilities of the individual. Successes in physical restoration alone are not enough.

Professional Preparation. Personnel for rehabilitative services include all individuals in the institution who have contact with the handicapped individual. These range from the custodian to specialists in each of the various disciplines of science and medicine. Everyone must understand the possible frustrations suffered by the handicapped individual in his drive for normalcy. An institutional environment with friendly and always helpful personnel is the type of climate suitable for the handicapped individual. Changes in the handicapped are not easily accomplished, but require long, hard work that can become boring and extremely difficult to continue over an extended period of time. Progress is extremely slow and not easily recognized.

The preparation requirements for a rehabilitation specialist are lengthy and difficult. For the M.D. or Ph.D. in this discipline, a professional license requires eight years of university preparation and, in addition, resident clinical practice that further adds to the requirements.

Personnel on rehabilitation teams focus their efforts on using their professional understandings and skills to bring about constructive changes. In each instance, a thorough knowledge of the human organism is essential. The specialist must be fully acquainted with the individual and know the full nature of his handicap. The skillful application of rehabilitation programs based upon this background will then most likely result in substantial progress. Of course, the handicapped individual must understand the program and its requirements and cooperate to make the results as successful as possible.

One of the strongest components in determining the professional status of rehabilitation is the personnel in institutional rehabilitation programs. Rehabilitation is a profession with many disciplines, but its status is directly determined by the quality of the results of the professional services rendered to the handicapped individual. This is, indeed, a pragmatic requirement for professional status. The advances in these programs provide evidence that specialists have given a high-level status to this profession.

Professional preparation of rehabilitative personnel for handicapped services is an established professional requirement. The only difference between rehabilitation and other professions is that the specialists come from several different disciplines, but in each case special preparation is made in applying the discipline to the handicapped individual. Physical activity as physical education and recreation are both used extensively to aid handicapped individuals to adapt to society and meet daily personal requirements and needs.

Institutional Resources. There are numerous public and private agencies devoted to providing services for the handicapped. These agencies cover the complete range of requirements for the handicapped individual, from personnel and health needs to economic requirements for daily living.

Involved agencies include rehabilitation centers and rehabilitation agencies. These rehabilitation centers coordinate the activities of various specialists, including the psychiatrist, orthopedist, internist, pediatrician, psychologist, physical therapist, occupational therapist, speech therapist, rehabilitation nurse, vocational counselor, and social worker. The group also includes the physical recreation therapist and the exercise specialist. These specialists working as a coordinated team are able to provide a program for each handicapped person that is individually planned and directly involves the specializations necessary for that individual's rehabilitation. A specialist from a single discipline, in most instances, cannot render all the services necessary for successful rehabilitation without the aid of other disciplines.

Teamwork in rehabilitation is equally essential for governmental and voluntary agencies, professional groups, and other societal agencies that serve the disabled. At the interagency level, where handicapped individuals are separated physically according to functional disorders, however, coordinated teamwork is more difficult than on the institutional or community center levels.

Interagency difficulties are not surprising when one considers the size of this team. The number of cooperating members on all levels runs into the thousands. In each discipline alone, this number may easily run into the hundreds. Liaison relationships are now used to tie institutional services to individual needs and, of equal importance, to reduce duplication of effort and fill gaps where services are needed. With so many disciplines and public, private, and voluntary agencies, the boundaries and clienteles of each agency become a matter of jurisdictional concern, and many times, because of this fact, conflicts arise. It is indeed unfortunate that in numerous instances an agency renders a service without attempting to identify similar services, which might prevent duplication of effort. Competition begins in an area that should be cooperative. Such differences, however, are gradually being resolved, and the proper role for each discipline and agency is being established.

Research. Although considerable research is now under way at various institutions and rehabilitation centers, there is a great need for both broader and more-intensive research programs. This need encompasses the many classes of handicaps and disabilities. Research in rehabilitation is generally devoted to a synthesis of the knowledge of a number of sciences and medicine about a solitary organic system. The purpose of this research is to solve the problems surrounding the concept of the individual's functional adequacy in relation to environmental demands. Analysis of the causes for disabling diseases are de-emphasized in order to concentrate on the pressing problem of returning the individual to a useful life in which he finds a measure of personal adequacy and fulfillment. Funds available for research in rehabilitative medicine have been considerably below those found in other phases of medicine. The role of physical activity in rehabilitation is now gaining support in competition for research funds, but the actual amount of money available for research in this area is insufficient to make a significant impact on the understanding of physical activity in rehabilitation.

Krusen [2] has classified the research needs as they apply to rehabilitation. This classification considers the full needs of the individual. The rehabilitation process, including the role of physical activity, is related to individual needs.

1. The physiological adaptability of the individual.
   a. Effects of age on abilities.
   b. Mechanisms of compensation for disabilities.
2. The physiological demands of our society.
   a. Self-care.
   b. Ambulation.
   c. Vocational demands.
3. Psychological aspects of rehabilitation.
4. Adaptation of vocational activities to limited physical abilities.
5. Mechancal substitutes for functions lost through disability.

Krusen states that "there is also need for research and development in the area of intensive scientific evaluation of our aging citizens. Greater accuracy in identifying and classifying needs could help us better determine the type of care required." This report is now about ten years old; and although the support for rehabilitation research has increased considerably, the problems listed and the report itself remain today essentially unchanged. This, however, does not mean that insight into the problem has not been gained or that no progress has been achieved. A

2 Frank H. Krusen, *Concepts in Rehabilitation of the Handicapped* (Philadelphia: Saunders, 1964), pp. 46–47.

good deal has been accomplished through the insights of the teams of specialists dealing with these problems and by trial and error in daily work and clinical experiences.

It is important to note that the emphasis in research must be placed on human abilities and their potentials within the limitations of individual disability. The role of physical activity then becomes paramount in the rehabilitation process, for it is basic to advancing the ability of the disabled individual to perform the movements required in normal life activities. The need for rehabilitation services comes only when surgery and the other required medical disciplines have removed the individual from danger and stabilized his condition. Physical activity assumes a place within other life essentials, such as diet, health practices, and so on, in contributing to optimal readjustment.

Research into attitude changes in the rehabilitation setting is needed for the benefit of both the general public and the disabled. This is true for every handicapped individual, but it is particularly important for the aged, convalescents, or the permanently handicapped. The effects of attitude upon rehabilitation and adjustment are unanswered problems that require careful study.

The professional status of rehabilitation research is on a par with that of other recognized social professions. Although research is not as extensive or thorough as one would like, there can be little question about the value of programs projected and implemented by trained rehabilitation specialists.

Professional Associations. In order to gain professional recognition, members must be professionally organized. The organization of members of a discipline into a working profession is one of the most important goals to be accomplished by any fledgling profession. Growth and advancement of any discipline cannot be accomplished by public interest and resulting activities; instead, it must come from its members, who are thoroughly familiar with the discipline and regard it as their life's work. A strong profession regulates all activities of that body's membership from professional preparation to licensing of graduates for commercial practices. There are, for example, few laws publicly regulating a profession that were adopted without the support of its membership. This fact has its basis in the lack of public knowledge about the discipline, as well as the fact that laws made without the support of professional members have little chance of being successfully implemented.

Rehabilitation is more a combination of professions than a profession itself. For those individuals who work as rehabilitation specialists, it very definitely takes on all the connotations of a profession, and these specialists may view rehabilitation as their primary profession. Each member actually comes from an individual discipline related to rehabilitation, however, and is probably also organized within his individual field of specialty. Athletic trainers, for example, are members of a professional association that deals specifically with problems encountered by the athlete and sports, but athletic trainers are also a part of the rehabilitation profession. Organization of subgroups such as athletic trainers into a profession should be encouraged. Athletic trainers must also participate with all other subprofessions in order to apply the best possible overall procedures in rehabilitation. The rehabilitation profession can have considerable influence on all practices of its subprofessions and in this way gain the support of the public, which is needed for the success of any profession.

There is a great need for utilization of the full professional resources of rehabilitation. Unless help is made available to the chronically ill and the handicapped, communities will be overwhelmed by these economically and physically dependent individuals. The vast increase in the aged population of this country also creates a serious strain. The need for rehabilitative services is rapidly increasing in all phases of physical maladies, whether precipitated by age, genetic deformity, or injury. If we are to meet each of these needs, the understanding and support of the public are necessary. Support is achieved through the efforts of the profession in bringing these problems to public attention. Acceptance of the responsibility for funding of rehabilitation must come from citizens through the voluntary efforts of each person in the community.

Like other successful professions incorporating multiple specializations, rehabilitation must function as a whole and not as individual parts. This does not reduce the value of the individual contribution of each discipline; on the contrary, the scope of their contributions will be considerably enlarged. The total rehabilitation program must be available to society as an organized profession, and not as disputed subgroups.

Certification and Accreditation. A basic requirement for any profession is the certification of personnel for practice in the profession. In connection with this, accreditation of the schools, institutions, or agencies that prepare personnel is also required. Both these requirements have been achieved, in part, by the various subdisciplines within rehabilitation.

The certification of personnel is generally handled by the state. This gives the state the responsibility for legal enforcement of certification standards. The state ensures through the certification process that services are provided to the public by properly prepared personnel. The standards established by the state are, unfortunately, generally minimal. If standards were established at levels above those in current practice, the services of many workers would be eliminated. Programs that have current practice standards will always be inadequate because of the lack of qualified personnel, but it generally becomes a question of some lower level of expertise or no program at all. To avoid this complication, the profession must establish preparation standards at a high level. Professions, if they wish, can be considerably more powerful and effective than either state or federal law in advancing the preparation of personnel. The rehabilitation profession could enforce higher standards through influence on preparatory institutions and by informing the public of the standards necessary for best possible results in the rehabilitation field. Such practices are not common, but some rehabilitation disciplines do exert powerful influences on institutions preparing personnel.

Certification and accreditation go hand in hand. Institutions must be accredited in order to prepare personnel, but the range in program accreditation in rehabilitation is a broad one, ranging from practically no standards at all to programs that are rigid and time-consuming. No general accreditation standards exist except those established through accrediting agencies. Their recommendations have only persuasive powers to wield against poor programs, unless the agencies can influence states to enact laws regulating accreditation. It is unfortunate that laws are not enacted in states in which practices vary so greatly. Some professionals probably do not want this lack of accreditation standards changed, because at present it is possible to find work in the rehabilitation field with only a minimum of preparation. Rehabilitation as a united profession consisting of a wide range of specializations has the potential to have a major influence on institutional programs. Rehabilitation, with its large number of highly specialized disciplines, should favor the development of a professional organization that coordinates all specialized programs that cooperate in total rehabilitation of the individual. This would place each discipline in a definite relationship with all other rehabilitative disciplines and emphasize the need for establishment of appropriate preparation standards. This appears to be a major professional need for rehabilitation.

Ethics. For a profession to form a recognized and influential organization it must have a code of ethics for all its professional members. The emphasis is on *all* and not just some of the organization's membership, ranging from building maintenance personnel to the most highly skilled specialist in the program. All workers should serve the handicapped individual in a professional manner. Ethics should cover all services rendered from rehabilitation skills to overall concern for the person as a human being. The latter concern is particularly important in rehabilitation, for the handicapped individual may be highly sensitive.

Ethics are now strongly developed within the disciplines of rehabilitation, covering all phases of practice, including salary, fees charged, personal behavior, responsibilities for the patient, training and retraining, commitments to the profession and its development, and other requirements that will result in high-quality services as well as public confidence in the specialist and the profession.

Professional Domain: The Conceptual Structure
of Physical Activity in Rehabilitation

Rehabilitation has long been considered a continuum stretching from
the onset of disease and its effects to the healing process and the further
therapy or treatment that return the patient to a normal health status.
During the early years of medicine rest was thought to produce the best
results in the healing process. In recent years, however, emphasis has
been placed on physical activity and exercise as aids to the healing
process by encouraging normal physiological functions. The individual
is placed in an exercise program planned specifically to improve bodily
functions that have been impaired by disease or injury and to advance
functions needed for the individual to return to participation in pre-
disease activities or levels of physical independence. The exercise or
physical activity programs applied are generally classified as passive,
active-assistive, active, and resistive. The type of exercise is determined
by the nature of the handicap. The more active and intense the exercise,
the more functional capacity or ability will result. The individual pro-
gresses as rapidly as possible in exercise tolerance programs, with the
original injury determining the limits of the program. Physical activity
in rehabilitation is equated with the individual's functional capacity to
obtain as much independence as possible within the limitations of the
underlying pathology. Because movement in every daily activity is a
physical process, physical activity must be used as the basis factor for
returning the individual to a relatively normal life with typical activities.

The concern in this chapter is the domain of physical activity in rehabilitation. In the previous section, a review was presented of rehabilitation as a total phenomenon. Now we shall examine the setting for
physical activity in rehabilitation, dealing with its conceptual structure.
The following section will deal with the content of physical activity in
rehabilitation to provide some indication of what can be accomplished.

Physical Domain. The physical domain or conceptual structure of
physical activity in rehabilitation consists of those concepts or elements
that provide for human physical movements. These range from relatively
simple activities, such as walking, to the highest level of skilled movements. Meeting the daily needs of the body is also a physical process.
Life itself is comprised of the physical functions carried out by the cells,
organs, and systems of the body. Any change in one single organ will
soon have an effect on some human ability. The effect may be minor or
may place the individual in a state of complete immobility. From the
point of view of rehabilitation, the concepts that provide assistance to
the individual in his restoration process are reviewed (List 13).

List 13. Conceptual structure: The professional domain of physical activity in rehabilitation

1. Physical domain.
    a. Active exercise.
    b. Cold therapy.
    c. Electrotherapy.
    d. Endurance.
    e. Functional capacity.
    f. Hydrotherapy.
    g. Light therapy.
    h. Muscle re-education.
    i. Neuromuscular therapy.
    j. Nutrition.
    k. Passive exercise.
    l. Planned continuum.
    m. Progressive resistance.
    n. Prosthetic services.
    o. Rehabilitative aids.
    p. Safety and protection.
    q. Sauna.
    r. Skill development.
    s. Sports therapy.
    t. X-ray therapy.

2. Psychological domain.
    a. Acceptance of limitations.
    b. Adjustment.
    c. Attitude determination.
    d. Health practices.
    e. Hobby interests.
    f. Intelligence.
    g. Leisure practices.
    h. Maturity.
    i. Meaningfulness of acts.
    j. Motivation.
    k. Personality characteristics.
    l. Plans and hopes.
    m. Play (cooperation and competition).
    n. Psychic states.
    o. Relaxation and rest.
    p. Security.
    q. Self-esteem.
    r. Stress reduction.

3. Social domain.
    a. Attitudes.
    b. Cultural demands.
    c. Environment.
    d. Fulfillment.
    e. Independence and dependence.
    f. Institutional effects.
    g. Interests.
    h. Isolation.
    i. Knowledge and understanding.
    j. Motivation.
    k. "Normality."
    l. Philosophy.
    m. Responsibility.
    n. Security.
    o. Social contact.
    p. Social integration.

4. Medical domain.
    a. Balance.
    b. CNS control rearrangement.
    c. Diet and nutrition.
    d. Drugs.
    e. Efficiency.
    f. Exercise prescription.
    g. Food supplements.
    h. Pathology.
    i. Protective influence of exercise.
    j. Regulatory mechanisms.
    k. Relaxation.
    l. Rest.
    m. Re-establishment of motor patterns.
    n. Restoration of function.
    o. Surgery.
    p. Training.

5. Educational domain.
    a. Adaptation.
    b. Attitude.
    c. Educative worth.
    d. Evaluation.
    e. Health practices.
    f. Individual needs.
    g. Interests and motivation.
    h. Knowledge of performance.
    i. Leadership.
    j. Leisure.
    k. Meaningfulness of activity.
    l. Motor habits.
    m. Quality of instruction.
    n. Recreational programs.
    o. Understanding of physical activity.
    p. Vocational counseling.

Planned *exercise programs* for the handicapped in order to restore the ability to perform normal bodily functions lost for some medical reason are a large part of the rehabilitation process. Exercise may be *passive, active, resistive,* or applied to provide optimal stress on a certain function or body part to contribute to the development process and help return the individual's ability to move. For example, following knee surgery a formal exercise program is planned and implemented to help the patient to regain the functional range of movement of the knee prior to injury.

Rehabilitative aids are an important part of the program of physical rehabilitation. They provide support during rehabilitation while active physical activity is in process. An example is the use of crutches by the patient before he is able to put full weight on the knee. The slow process of healing and regaining functional powers is entirely individual in its time frame and results. The individual eliminates the aid as soon as possible to hasten recovery, and such aids should not be used unless there is a chance of further injury. Caution against reinjury sometimes results in too conservative a rehabilitative approach. Because experts agree that stress on damaged body parts or bodily functions will hasten rehabilitation, the individual should take as much stress on the body part undergoing rehabilitation as possible.

Therapies are commonly used in physical rehabilitation. These therapies (e.g., electrotherapy, light therapy, X-ray therapy, sauna, and thermotherapy) are designed to reduce soreness, swelling, and pain to speed up the healing process. They advance movement only through their contributions to improved healing. Exercise is required for physical rehabilitation designed to regain lost or impaired bodily functions.

Sports therapy is also a common practice in rehabilitation. Use of games, sports, and athletics is an integral part of most rehabilitation programs. In each instance the sport is adapted to fit the nature of the handicap. Sports therapy provides personal interest by utilizing the individual's competitive spirit to yield more complete rehabilitative results. The individual becomes lost in the joy and enthusiasm of play and becomes less sensitive to his own handicap. Sports therapy is employed in mental and emotional rehabilitation programs in most hospitals today.

Prosthetic devices are devices such as crutches, braces, wheelchairs, mechanical limbs, and so on, that provide support for human movement. When injury has resulted in permanent disability, the aid may become a necessary part of the equipment required for the pursuance of relatively normal life activities. Generally, these devices are temporary and should be eliminated as soon as possible.

Safety and physical protection are important elements of physical rehabilitation. The handicapped individual requires protection in conjunction with his physical restoration. This includes special equipment to aid in rehabilitation. Protection guides help the individual not to overdo during physical activity and possibly reinjure himself. Diet, nutrition programs, and health practices are part of this program. Exercise or sports without adequate safety or protective guidelines and equipment can result in further functional losses.

Probably one of the most important physical requirements for rehabilitation is the restoration of *neuromuscular skills*. This includes muscular strength, physical endurance, and other physical movement requirements. The loss of a leg requires the individual to undergo training in the use of an artificial limb. The skillful individual will be able to walk employing the artificial leg with few noticeable effects. The knee following surgery requires strenuous, regular exercise and neuromuscular retraining to return its strength and normal range of movement. Acquiring physical skill to meet daily needs is a major consideration in rehabilitation.

Psychological Domain. The psychological elements involved in rehabilitation are major components of the overall program. In some cases the individual's mental and emotional needs become more important than his physical needs and, as such, direct targets for rehabilitation. The time required for rehabilitation is a common psychological factor (List 13).

An individual's attitude about his handicap is perhaps the single most important factor in his rehabilitation. With a strong desire and positive attitude toward achievement, the individual cannot help but see his good psychological frame of mind reflected in physical results. For some handicaps such as an emotional disturbance, the individual's attitude is a major factor. Disturbances may be the direct result of negative attitudes and uncertainties that do not permit normal adjustment.

Maturity, security, and *intelligence* are psychological concepts that become important factors in programs of rehabilitation. They are particularly major elements in some rehabilitation programs (e.g., for the emotionally disturbed), but the effects are felt either favorably or unfavorably in all rehabilitation programs. The mature, secure, and intelligent individual can plan and continue a program of rehabilitation to his optimal capabilities. Rehabilitation is so individual that if the specialist is unable to gain the individual's cooperation in the program, there will be few positive results. In fact, the injury is best diagnosed by the individual. In this manner, he shares directly in his own movement rehabilitation program. Of course, the specialist is needed, but he must gauge his efforts by the reactions of the patient.

The personal factors of *self-esteem, determination, motivation,* and *acceptance of the handicap* are basic to all physical, social, or emotional rehabilitation programs. Extraordinary results can be accomplished by an individual who truly wants to succeed, and physical rehabilitation cannot progress very far without the individual's acceptance of his problem and his formulation of a strong, positive attitude toward rehabilitation.

The nature of the *social* and *environmental adjustment* desired by the handicapped individual is an important consideration for any program of rehabilitation. The individual and the specialist must together set realistic goals that can be accomplished through hard work and perseverance. The individual must adjust to the limitations dictated by his handicap. He will be functionally limited under conditions of permanent disability, and judgments should be made within this framework.

Leisure interests, activity and play motivations, and *hobby interests* are important concepts of physical activity that can be pleasurably incorporated into the rehabilitation program. Even the individual with severe handicaps can make a satisfactory adjustment to life. The outstanding example of Helen Keller shows the adjustment possible despite the presence of a major handicap. The individual with many leisure interests is certainly able to gain more from rehabilitation, because he has alternative positive purposes in life. *Personality* is an important constituent of the total organism and must be given significant consideration in physical rehabilitation.

The individual who has acceptable *health habits,* can relax easily, and lives a life that is largely free of stress is also able to gain more from rehabilitation. These are generally supportive factors but in certain cases (e.g., cardiac) may have a strong and positive relationship to the outcome.

Social Domain. Rehabilitation has social requirements that are also important factors in physical activity. In some cases social aspects of rehabilitation have a more direct relationship to the overall process than the physical activity, which is applied because of its vast social potential.

The socially maladjusted individual desperately needs to be integrated into a group and society. Physical activity as sports and games can make significant contributions toward these ends. The informal nature of sports makes interpersonal relationships a prominent part of the overall participation experience. Social contacts *within this setting* provide the potential for socialization. This fact is demonstrated daily by many physically normal individuals, but for the physically handicapped, these potentials are even more significant.

Social responsibility, social dependence, and *social fulfillment* are all elements of human adjustment and can be achieved within the context of sports. Most individuals require social dependence as well as social independence, both of which may be achieved through sports; both are necessary for participation. For the handicapped individual, rehabilitation provides satisfaction through social interaction with others (e.g., wheelchair basketball). Developing personal independence promotes further adjustment and greatly adds to the process of physical rehabilitation.

Social philosophy, positive attitudes about self and others, and personal fulfillment are desirable elements in most human relationships, and in rehabilitation, these concepts are essential. For social rehabilitation these social characteristics become direct achievement goals, but they are closely related to rehabilitation goals for the physically handicapped as well. Maladjusted individuals in society reflect negative social attitudes that lack personal satisfaction. Sports have vast social potential and provide a setting for the achievement of satisfaction and adjustment.

Individual *responsibility* and *security* within the group and society are social elements that are extremely important to the handicapped individual. They can be learned within the context of sports and physical activity as they contribute to the rehabilitation of physical disabilities. Responsibility for self and personal security are important for everyone, but particularly important for the handicapped.

Institutions, education, and *social development* have special significance for the physically handicapped. Rehabilitation institutions are available to prepare the individual for vocational and leisure life. Strong institutional programs and leadership are even more basic in the preparation of the handicapped individual than the normal individual. All institutional personnel must have the motivation to exert long and hard efforts in the hope of achieving a high level of individual rehabilitation. Patience and kindness along with professional skills are necessary for personnel in rehabilitation institutions. Rehabilitation institutions must deal not only with the physical or social rehabilitation of the individual, but also with shaping an institutional atmosphere that fosters society as it should be. Physical activity as sports will add considerably to this goal.

Medical Domain. Medicine and medical disciplines play major roles in the rehabilitation of handicapped individuals. Handicaps, whether caused by congenital defects, age, or injury, need help from the various medical disciplines. Generally, the medical sciences begin corrective action within their scope and capabilities. This endeavor can be in conjunction with other disciplines or can precede them. Social rehabilitation results only after optimal results have been achieved through corrective procedures.

Corrective surgery may be a major part of physical rehabilitation. Sports, accidents in the home, accidents on the highway, and untold other factors result in injuries to organs and organ systems of the body that require surgery. In some instances, structural destruction cannot be rectified. Following the healing process, or as soon thereafter as possible, rehabilitation programs are begun. Rehabilitation works to restore the system to full functional capacity with the necessary compensations to allow normal activity. Physical exercise is the process through which normal functional capacity is regained. Every surgical procedure carried out as a result of an injury, no matter how successful, is a second injury superimposed upon the original trauma. Carefully planned, prescribed, and supervised activity for the patient and his particular surgical problem is then the keystone of rehabilitation. The patient who is able to see continuous improvement as the result of his efforts, even though the daily and weekly increment is small, will be encouraged to achieve functional, economic, and mental self-sufficiency, whatever his residual disability. Without qualified rehabilitation personnel, the lack of benefit from therapy generally leads to discouragement.

Proper nutrition is another aspect of rehabilitation. For successful physical activity following surgery, resistance against specific deleterious effects is essential. Special attention must be given to the stability or improvement of the overall physical status, and a good diet, food supplements, and vitamins are sometimes necessary to provide the vitamins and nutrients necessary for speedy recovery. These concerns are an important part of physical rehabilitation, particularly after a long illness or major surgery.

Restoration of function, re-establishment of motor patterns, and a personalized *exercise prescription* are medical matters of considerable importance preceding or following corrective surgery. The program is precisely planned to meet the needs of the specific individual disability. Injury or surgery can limit the functioning of the individual, and exercise can greatly improve the bodily functions and neuromuscular skills.

Drugs are also medical aids in the rehabilitation process. They are extremely useful in fighting infections, speeding recovery, and serving the individual until improvement has reached a level where drugs are not necessary. Drugs are generally temporary remedies and should not be prescribed if self-sufficiency can be attained without these aids. There are illnesses that require drugs as a permanent part of the rehabilitation program. *Pathological* conditions require constant medical supervision and treatment with modern drugs. Rehabilitation during and after the cure requires the resources of the medical sciences. The individual's condition will determine the requirements.

Exercise, exercise prescription, protection from stress during exercise, and training in exercise patterns are all phases of the medical domain in physical activity. Exercise can be readily applied for beneficial effects in rehabilitation, but ill-advised exercise may be extremely harmful. The healing of a disability can be greatly delayed by improperly prescribed exercise. Factors such as duration, frequency, intensity, and type of physical activity must be determined by the individual's fitness level and the nature of his disability. Exercise and physical activity must be implemented gradually yet progressively for everyone, but this is particularly true for the handicapped. The handicapped require protection during physical activity, and it is the responsibility of specialists in medicine and exercise to ensure that this protection is given.

Educational Domain. The handicapped or injured individual should know the physiological or anatomical nature of his disability and should also be informed of the value of his particular rehabilitation program. Routine schedules are needed for progress in rehabilitation. The value of these procedures must be known, to provide a baseline from which progress can be rated. The individual can increase the intensity of physical activity or modify the patterns of rehabilitation if he understands the program and his disability. The help of the specialist is made available only at intervals in order to review progress and current procedures. Education programs for understanding activity potentials and the personal handicap itself are essential parts of rehabilitation.

The medical and educational specialists in rehabilitation constitute the institutional personnel that provide and administer educational programs. Their background includes knowledge of the developmental potentials of physical activity and exercise and the adaptations of physical activity to suit the individual disabilities. Educational programs for the handicapped must go beyond the handicap itself and help in preparing for vocational or other new pursuits. Clinics help the individual in developing new lifetime pursuits. It is possible to fit the job to the individual and his disability and then provide him with the skills to assume that job. It is fundamental that the handicapped find satisfying work from both an economic and psychological standpoint. Vocational counseling is an integral part of all programs for the handicapped.

The leisure life of the handicapped is also an educational responsibility. A leisure program should assume a large measure of the role of physical activity, as it is adapted to the capacities of the handicapped. Planned physical activity is probably more essential for the handicapped individual than for the generally active person, as disabilities reduce the possibilities for physical activity. Special educational programs are necessary.

Instructional qualifications for educational programs for the handicapped require special skills and knowledge. Program content for the physically fit individual does not apply to the handicapped. The conditions of no two handicapped individuals are exactly alike, and each physical activity must be adapted to the potentials of the individual for learning and development.

Education for the handicapped individual includes changes in personal attitudes, readjustment of life practices, and learning about activities, including physical activity, that lead to a satisfying life. This is particularly true when disabilities come to a previously normal individual through injuries, which can change his life in a matter of minutes. Vital educational programs are then essential.

Helping the handicapped individual to prepare for a leadership role is an important educational goal. Assuming responsibility for one's own destiny is the immediate requirement of leadership.

Professional Domain: The Physical Activity
Content in Rehabilitation

The conceptual structure of physical activity in rehabilitation has been presented in the preceding section. In order to make this meaningful, the content of physical activity is presented for each element or concept. The purpose of this approach is to place emphasis on content or, more specifically, on what results can be achieved by the disabled through precisely designed physical activity. The five categories of concepts given in the preceding section provide the content structure for physical activity.

Physical Content. The role of all therapy is to make physical activity and all other types of therapy valuable to the disabled individual. This means understanding the nature of the disability and the value of physical activity or other therapies in improving functional capabilities.

Neuromuscular skill and efficiency are determined more by exercise than by acute functional residual effects of the injury or disease. If medicine and/or surgery can correct the disease or injury, exercise can restore original movement skill and continue to advance that skill level in accordance with the interest of the individual. Mental factors, such as scars left by the individual's disability, are fundamental to individual progress. The body will generally respond to exercise to the limits of its capacities.

Physical activity or exercise programs must be adapted to the handicap or injury. Exercise can be passive, resistive, or active as well as varying in its degree of intensity, duration, or frequency. The program applied in a specific case is determined by rehabilitation specialists, who understand the physiological implications of the injury and the developmental nature of the most desirable types of physical activity. The proper adaptive exercise program is necessary for the achievement of optimal results. Passive exercise is nearly always scheduled in the early stages of recovery where joint movement should be maintained, yet contractions prevented.

Water therapy permits less external stress on a weakened muscle, because when the body is submerged, gravitational pressure is partly eliminated. This permits more gradual development of muscle movement and strength. Hot and cold water and ice treatments are used to reduce swelling and hasten the healing process. Thermotherapy is essentially employed to prepare the individual for exercise applications. These different types of therapy cannot advance physical development without exercise; they simply prepare the individual to commence exercising.

Sports are generally an important part of rehabilitation programs. They can be used to aid in the rehabilitation of persons suffering several physical disabilities and of those who are mentally and emotionally disturbed.

Prosthetic devices aid in achieving self-sufficiency and are not permanent. They provide support to the injured part so that undue stress is not placed on it, risking further injury until rehabilitation has retrained the neural pathways.

Psychological Content. The psychological status of an individual who has been disabled is perhaps the most important part of rehabilitation, even though the direct rehabilitative process may apply entirely to the physical segment of the problem. Rehabilitation must begin with emphasis on adequate adjustment to the disability. This process requires improvement in physical abilities, but it is also important to achieve psychological stability and acceptance of the disability. A positive frame of mind contributes to adequate adjustment and a speedy recovery. In some instances the physical injury may itself motivate the individual for rehabilitation. The most desirable psychological goal is the development of the will to achieve a recovery. Through the individual's development of a logical attitude toward his disability, a positive program of setting goals and evaluating practices can lead to the achievement of complete recovery. The mentally alert and intellectually competent individual is definitely in a preferred position.

Personal security within an individual's own environment is fundamental to the rehabilitation process. An individual cannot come to terms with his disability if he lacks confidence in his personal environment or the professional rehabilitation process. Personal security then becomes the base from which to launch his rehabilitation program.

Leisure programs, both active and sedentary, play a major role in rehabilitation programs. An individual must develop skills and interests in leisure programs that go beyond immediate rehabilitation processes. These programs should be largely physical, but hobbies that generate intense individual interest should also be included. These programs contribute to the desirable psychological state that is of equal importance in physical rehabilitation. Gains in physical performances greatly aid psychological adjustment by contributing to feelings of self-confidence and personal security. Almost every handicapped individual can become productive and capable of a large measure of independence, but achieving this independence is as dependent upon psychological as on physical adjustment.

Personal attitude is associated with nearly every life activity, particularly during rehabilitation. Psychologists regard the negative attitude of the disabled individual as more important than the physical handicap itself. This is particularly true when judged by the social outcomes necessary for positive rehabilitation.

The health practices of every individual are basic to all the adjustments he must make in life but are of even more significance to the handicapped. The disabled individual can greatly compound his problems through negative health practices (e.g., drugs, alcohol, poor diet). The body cannot respond adequately to rehabilitation efforts if weakened by personal abuses.

Social Content. Social rehabilitation may be a requirement in itself or a phase of physical rehabilitation. No matter what type of rehabilitation is emphasized, the social status of the individual must be fully considered. Persons who have participated in physical activity prior to a handicap usually respond to treatment more successfully than individuals without such experiences. This is probably the result of previously learned skills and past enjoyment.

Damaging attitudes, frustrating settings, and improper self-image are negative factors in rehabilitation for both physically and socially handicapped individuals. These negative factors have a major influence on social rehabilitation. Physical activity, such as sports, can shift the individual's focus and promote positive associations through activity and aid in the development of good relationships with other people. An individual's self-image must be favorable for any significant progress to be achieved in rehabilitation. Physical skills will also aid the handicapped individual to become more socially accepted.

Institutionalized handicapped individuals often become so dependent upon the institution that they cannot adjust to society when treatment is completed; they have not been equipped to meet the demands of the outside world. It is important that the institutionalized patient be given opportunities to gain self-confidence and engage in human relations beyond institutional walls. The societal contacts of these individuals should be frequent and varied and should include competitive sports. Success in such endeavors will encourage the individual to strive for further success and to pursue normal activities despite his disabled condition.

Self-sufficiency, confidence, and personal responsibility are all social concepts essential in rehabilitation. In many instances these qualities are more valuable to the disabled individual than the task of physically overcoming the disability. Handicapped individuals can meet most problem situations if these qualities are positively developed. Sports can aid in this process, because they are dynamic social involvements from which a great deal may be learned about social interaction.

The social involvement of the handicapped individual must be an integral part of every rehabilitation program. Interests, motivations, and personal security should be developed in some particular area. If this area is physical activity, it also aids in the process of physical rehabilitation. The social domain is a part of all rehabilitation. The individual must be prepared to return to his home, community, and former social world adjusted to his handicap. This requires social development beyond normal levels because social pressures will be intense. Sports participation can contribute to societal adjustment.

Medical Content. The medical services required will be closely related to the individual's physical status. If an individual is in excellent physical condition, the effects of injury or disease will be significantly decreased and the period of recovery will be greatly shortened. It has been demonstrated that exercise or physical activity exerts a protective influence against degenerative cardiovascular disease and is an aid in speeding recovery from cardiac disease. The human organism needs physical activity, and a normal heart and cardiovascular system cannot be injured by intense exercise. Fatigue of the skeletal muscles will prevent undue stress from injuring the body, particularly the heart, in any way.

Chronic disease is the major cause of handicaps and disabilities. Disease that continues without cure or arrest will prevent the organism from enjoying the benefits of physical activity and other rehabilitative aids. If the individual can advance his physical status to normal levels, life can continue in spite of disease, and longevity will remain relatively normal. It has been demonstrated that cardiac patients are capable of living a long life with normal activity if they use judgment in their lifestyle and participate in appropriate physical activity.

The ability to relax and the proper prescription of physical activity are both major determinants of successful rehabilitation. The relaxed individual is better prepared to achieve recovery through physical activity and is better able to participate more intensely.

Unwise exercise during medical rehabilitation can further injure the handicapped individual; it is worse than no exercise at all. When healing is in process or the handicap dictates that exercise may be harmful, the individual must live strictly on medical treatment. If the individual is not able to exercise, atrophy is hastened, sometimes resulting in increased disability.

A strong physical base for the organism both before and after surgery is essential. If the physical condition of the patient is good, the effects of surgery or medical treatment will be minimal. In rehabilitation, with the exception of corrective surgery or corrective medical treatment, the physical capabilities of the patient are the essential contributing factors in the restoration of the individual to normal functional levels.

The daily health practices of the individual who is injured or disabled are significant to the rehabilitation process. The alcoholic, for example, will respond minimally during rehabilitation; his body is not capable of physical activity of sufficient intensity to allow him to reach desirable rehabilitative levels.

Rehabilitation programs cannot easily separate medical services from physical activity and its contributions. The cost of injury or disease is generally high. The physical resources of the body, however, can usually sustain the individual if a vital organ has not been destroyed. Specialists in both exercise science and medicine must initially decide the type and intensity of physical activity or exercise rehabilitation to be utilized.

Educational Content. The educational role in rehabilitation is a very large one. Unless the handicapped individual understands the physiological nature of his handicap and understands his rehabilitation program, including the value of physical activity or exercise, he is again handicapped in reaching his goal of optimal recovery. In rehabilitation the handicapped individual is master of his destiny. Each individual is capable of making adjustments in life that can be extremely satisfying. For normal individuals without physical handicaps, there is a huge range of ability, and they must therefore make different adjustments. If program activities are properly selected and adapted, the handicapped can also enjoy a satisfying and constructive life.

The individual who is both handicapped and motivated gives impetus to a rehabilitation program. An individual should understand physical activity and be able to apply self-testing procedures to judge his own progress. Knowledge of the handicap, a program of rehabilitation, and self-testing are especially important for the handicapped individual because of the need to make preparations. The exercise specialist is utilized as a resource person for reviewing progress and administering examinations periodically. Because the effects of exercise are slow and visible only on a long-range basis, the individual should be made aware of the organic changes that occur and how they can be recognized.

The handicapped individual is often unable to perform some motor movements. It is possible through the utilization of carefully planned exercise programs to improve motor mechanisms and to develop compensating responses in motor patterns that can assist the handicapped person to meet daily needs. Normal movement may never be completely achieved, but the individual must work toward the goal of living without assistance, of being self-sufficient. The search for new motor patterns must be constant, and the patient must eventually become a specialist in the rehabilitation of his own disability.

Leisure interests are significant for every individual, but they are particularly valuable to the handicapped individual. They provide enjoyment and a common bond through which to associate with others. The handicapped individual can develop self-esteem and, if needed, recognition as a normal person in any society.

For the handicapped, environmental change has occurred, and educational programs must be planned to teach adjustments to this change. The individual must understand the changes in his environment and be adequately prepared for these new settings. Vocational guidance and preparation are essential in the educational process of preparing the handicapped individual for occupational opportunities that fit his disability. Once they are vocationally trained, the handicapped are often successful in many fields.

The educational application of physical activity is the largest component of rehabilitation. Physical activity has direct value in restoring individual functions, but physical activity, as in sports, has other values in meeting educational goals. Social leadership, human relations, and other qualities important to all of society and especially to the handicapped individual can be achieved through sports programs. These programs become a significant part of rehabilitation as it is planned for educational outcomes.

Preparation for life despite a handicap is the goal for educational rehabilitation. Normal educational programs, in part, apply; however, the life of the handicapped individual is centered around his handicap. His world can be as pleasant and happy as that of any other person, but it will be different in one major respect. Educational programs begin at this point, and all their goals—including vocation, citizenship, and so on—are directed in recognition of this difference. Educational programs must also recognize the differences within the various handicap classifications, whether they be physical, mental, social, or emotional, as well as the differences between these large categories used to delineate handicapped individuals. Program planning is not an easy task, largely because the requirements are considerably more complex than they are for the normal individual.

Physical Activity: A Rehabilitation Profession

This chapter deals with physical activity in rehabilitation. Realizing the requirements of a profession, our analysis is focused on physical activity as a rehabilitation profession or as part of a larger rehabilitation profession. Recognizing rehabilitation as a multidisciplinary profession, it would seem that physical activity is an important and integral part of the total profession. High-level specialization is vital to all professions, and certainly rehabilitation is no exception. From the framework of knowledge and skills, rehabilitation has the qualifications to become a strong profession. Of course, it is professionally recognized and operates in the public eye as a profession. Some consider it a branch or subbranch of medicine, others a social science, a biological science, or an educational discipline. Rehabilitation should, indeed, be considered as a profession, with its many disciplines dealing with the individual who may be suffering from a handicap of any organ or system of the body. It would be inadequate to consider physical activity as a rehabilitation profession in isolation from the other disciplines that make the results of physical activity more valuable and in some cases even possible. The professional goal of rehabilitation should be the development of professional workers who can deal with the total human being in a single coordinated process, whether the individual's handicap is physical, mental, social, or emotional. Perhaps economic rehabilitation should also be included.

Rehabilitation specialists include physicians, pediatricians, orthopedic surgeons, neurosurgeons, plastic surgeons, physical therapists, occupational therapists, social workers, rehabilitation nurses, clinical psychologists, speech therapists, coaches, trainers, physical educators, and many others. All their special skills can be required at some time in rehabilitation. The coordination of rehabilitative specializations is essential to program efficiently the many varying requirements for the handicapped individual.

Chapter 17

Sports Medicine

The most complete presentation of sport sciences and medicine is found in the recently published *Encyclopedia of Sport Sciences and Medicine*.[1] This publication was sponsored by the American College of Sports Medicine at the time of the discipline's infancy in the United States. The American College of Sports Medicine was founded in 1953 by eleven specialists in science, medicine, and education on the premise that these disciplines were essential parts of the discipline of sports medicine. The rationale for this decision was that the basic sciences were essential for understanding the nature of the physical stresses in sports medicine and its various branches; for preparing, correcting, and protecting the human organism under the stresses imposed by sport; and for preparing the athlete to compete in strenuous sports by self-protection and development. The American College of Sports Medicine grew out of the amazing growth of sports throughout the world and the increasing attention focused on physical fitness as a result of scientific research related to the biophysiological changes resulting from exercise in the fields of health and disease.

The *Encyclopedia of Sport Sciences and Medicine* was conceptually structured. This was necessary because only a scattered number of publications dealt with sports medicine, and they dealt with only certain aspects of this potential discipline. Moreover, it was an initial effort at compiling an encyclopedia of sports medicine; therefore, it was deemed necessary to define the full scope of the publication. Conceptualization seemed to be the only possible scientific approach available that would readily lend itself to a full treatment of sports medicine.

Upon completing the conceptual structure of this work, it became

[1] American College of Sports Medicine, *Encyclopedia of Sport Sciences and Medicine* (New York: Macmillan, 1971), 1707 pp.

obvious that sports medicine was more than merely the medicine of sports; it included the physical, biological, and social sciences as well. Earlier views, particularly in Europe, considered sports medicine within the medical domain. It is of interest to note that upon the completion of research on literature and reviews in the field, the major content of sports medicine came from the sciences. Human performance requires interpretations from several scientific disciplines in order to understand and guide performance for the highest positive results.

The term *sport* does not adequately describe the content of the *Encyclopedia*, because the content goes considerably beyond the scope of just sports. To resolve this conflict of terms, the physical activities selected for that publication were those with competitive potentials, whether they were organized as sports or not. The term *medicine* is generally interpreted as referring to the science that treats disease, injury, and malfunctioning of the organism. Sports medicine, however, deals not with the abnormal state of man but with his quite normal or supernormal state, except for injuries and abnormalities that arise from sports competition. It was recognized following initial conceptualization of this field that a large body of knowledge did not fall into the generally accepted definition of medicine. It was later found that as much as 80 per cent of its content dealt with the science of the human organism under stress and other factors associated with physical activity. Because "sports medicine" might be interpreted as including only the medicine of sports, the encyclopedia was titled the *Encyclopedia of Sport Sciences and Medicine*.

Inductive research in the conceptualization stage of the *Encyclopedia* led to the definition of this discipline as the science and medicine of sports. This definition serves the general context of this chapter, although its content differs slightly from that implied by the definition in order to provide a major emphasis on the large scope of physical activity. The scope of physical activity as defined by the *Encyclopedia* includes competitive sports and the science and medicine of competitive sports. This chapter includes physical activity in all its forms in order to judge the professional nature of physical activity in sports medicine. Sports medicine, then, is the science and medicine of all professional applications of physical activity.

In the *Encyclopedia*, physical activity is limited to those activities that are organized as competitive sports, whereas in this chapter it includes the full scope of physical activities. In the *Encyclopedia*, the major concern is competition or competitive sports and encompasses the dangers of participation that result from intense stress, motivations for competition, group pressures on the individual, and spectator appeals. In this text generally and this chapter specifically, physical activity is reviewed for purposes that are considerably different from those in the *Encyclopedia*. The objective here is to study physical activity as a profession, a possible profession, or a part of a larger profession, each within the context of sports medicine. The *Encyclopedia* did not have this objective. The result is that although the conceptual structures are very similar, the overall structure employed by this text differs significantly from that original work. For a professional review, the full scope of physically oriented activity must be employed to serve as the reference point for overall analysis. Sports medicine as a profession must deal with all forms of human movement as physical activity or exercise and need not concentrate only on organized competitive sports. The essential requirement for attainment of professional goals in sports medicine is the inclusion of the sciences and disciplines that are necessary to provide full coverage to all types of human movement.

Professional Status of Sports Medicine

Sports medicine in the United States has only recently been structured as a profession. It was founded as a discipline designed to motivate both the sciences and medicine to joint cooperation in solving problems stemming from sports and sports participation. It was also designed to help apply sports-related disciplines to the protection and development of the average individual involved in sports. This discipline, now just slightly more than twenty years old, has grown into a fully recognized profession.

The Federation of Sports Medicine is an established international profession that includes representatives from most countries who have scientists or scientific organizations that deal with problems related to the scientific aspects of sports. A major limitation of the International Federation is its philosophic emphasis on medicine rather than the more complete view held by the American College of Sports Medicine, which emphasizes that sports medicine is both a science and a medical science, incorporating the principles shared by both.

In the United States, professional associations in physical education deal, in part, with the scientific aspects of sports and sports participation. A major portion of the structure and program of the American Association for Health, Physical Education, and Recreation (AAHPER) is devoted to the scientific study of sports. In the United States there are subgroups or special interest groups, such as coaches, trainers, therapists, and physical education teachers, that deal with individual problems within the scientific study of sports.

In addition to professions that are organized to concentrate efforts on the scientific and medical aspects of sports, there are numerous groups, clubs, local communities, and professional committees from various disciplines [e.g., medical committees on sports from the American

Medical Association (AMA), committees in psychology and sociology, and other such interdisciplinary groups] that are organized to study the problems related to sports and sports participation.

The professional association that is most closely associated with physical activity, which is reviewed in its professional context in this chapter, is the American College of Sports Medicine. Subject areas outside of physical activity are not considered a part of the American College of Sports Medicine (ACSM) program.

The constitution of the ACSM states its objectives, which are reviewed here because of their close relationship with this chapter and section. To quote from the ACSM's constitution on the organization's aims,

> The objectives and purposes of this organization shall be: (1) to promote and advance medicine and other scientific studies dealing with the effect of sports and other physical activities on the health of human beings at various stages of life; (2) to cooperate with other organizations, physicians, scientists and educators concerned with the same or related specialities; (3) to arrange for mutual meetings of physicians, educators and allied scientists; (4) to make available postgraduate education in fields related to these sciences; (5) to initiate, promote and correlate research in these fields; (6) to edit and publish a journal, articles and pamphlets pertaining to various aspects of sports, other physical activities and medicine; and (7) to establish and maintain a sports medicine library.

Over the period since the founding of the organization in 1953, these goals have in most instances been accomplished. Like other established professional associations, the ACSM's constitution defines the various parts of the organization in order to give the organization professional and operational direction and work efficiency. For the purposes of this chapter it is not necessary to present the details of the constitution for the American College of Sports Medicine; it is simply used to cite how this particular organization was structured.

It is interesting to note that the ACSM is the only professional organization in the United States that views physical activity from the point of view of both the sciences and medicine. These two fundamental disciplines are essential in providing the direction of physical activity. The views of other associations are less complete. The AAHPER views physical activity from the educational discipline viewpoint, whereas the American Medical Association Committee on Sports views physical activity as it relates to the medical discipline. Moreover, the American College of Sports Medicine is the only association with an interdisciplinary philosophy that places the full responsibility for the establishment of the profession on physical activity and recognizes its interdisciplinary qualities.

Professional Domain: The Conceptual Structure of Physical Activity in Sports Medicine

The conceptualization of the role of physical activity in sports medicine follows procedures similar to those previously outlined on the conceptualization of sports medicine in the *Encyclopedia of Sport Sciences and Medicine*. The content in both instances is physical activity as it relates to sports medicine. There is a difference, however, in the basis for conceptualization. For the *Encyclopedia*, the concentration is on scientific and medical aspects of physical activity both generally (area I) and specifically as developed through sports, games, and exercise (area II). That text held the goal of sports medicine to be the understanding of the nature of each activity; therefore, conceptualization was planned to promote identification of those concepts that are essential parts of participation in physical activity. For this chapter and section of our text, the purpose is to view physical activity as a sports medicine profession. Of course, a high degree of similarity exists in conceptualization of these two views, because the individual must understand the science and medicine involved in physical activity in order to judge it as a sports medicine profession. The content for judgment of the professional status or potentials of physical activity in the context of this chapter consists of generalized statements rather than the individual details that were necessary for the *Encyclopedia*.

The content of sports medicine is classified into nine categories. In each instance, concepts are listed that fit and define specific elements within the content of each category. This conceptualization will be briefly reviewed simply to provide some rationale for this categorization and the reason for including the element as a part of the profession of sports medicine.

Sociological and Anthropological Domain. Sports medicine includes elements from the disciplines of sociology and anthropology. These elements are important constituents of physical activity in sports, and they vary with each sport or physical activity. They can contribute significantly to performance if positively applied, or they may be deterrents to performance if negative views are held by the participant.

Family life, leisure activities, and health practices are personal choices of the individual. These practices will be reflected in physical activity and sports and may be partially responsible for differences in performance. Personal life-styles can, therefore, have both positive and negative effects in sports.

The individual's mores, race attitudes toward integration, and religion are all personal qualities that may or may not be responsible for differences among individuals. These elements are innately personal and should not be responsible for differences in sports participation. On the contrary, in most instances sports can aid in the favorable development of these qualities.

Social patterns, leisure interests and activities, and customs are elements that are also an integral part of sports. They can be influenced by sports and in turn can influence sports participation. They are then part of sports medicine because of their close association with elements in actual participation (List 14).

List 14. Conceptual structure: The professional domain of physical activity in sports medicine

1. Sociological and anthropological domain.
   - a. Attitudes.
   - b. Beliefs, biases, and prejudices.
   - c. Conflict and cooperation.
   - d. Customs and traditions.
   - e. Economic conditions.
   - f. Environments.
   - g. Family.
   - h. Health practices.
   - i. Heredity.
   - j. Intelligence.
   - k. Integration.
   - l. Leisure.
   - m. Mores.
   - n. Race.
   - o. Religion.
   - p. Sex.
2. Growth, development, and aging.
   - a. Age.
   - b. Body build.
   - c. Caloric restrictions.
   - d. Diet and body intake.
   - e. Differential movement patterns.
   - f. Drugs.
   - g. Epiphyseal development.
   - h. Environment.
   - i. Fatigue.
   - j. Fitness and health.
   - k. Heredity determinants.
   - l. Hormones.
   - m. Maturation.
   - n. Mental and emotional characteristics.
   - o. Physical therapy.
   - p. Rest, relaxation, and leisure.
   - q. Sex.
   - r. Social and economic forces.
3. Rehabilitation domain.
   - a. Drugs.
   - b. Education.
   - c. Environments: social and physical.
   - d. Exercise treatment.
   - e. Health practices.
   - f. Motor habits.
   - g. Nutrition and food supplements.
   - h. Prosthesis.
   - i. Physiology.
   - j. Psychological factors.
   - k. Personal factors.
   - l. Physical factors.
   - m. Relaxation.
   - n. Social forces.
   - o. Surgery.
   - p. Therapy.
4. Environmental domain.
   - a. Alcohol.
   - b. Altitude.
   - c. Automation.
   - d. Clothing.
   - e. Culture and society.
   - f. Diet.
   - g. Drugs.
   - h. Economic conditions.
   - i. Human adjustments.
   - j. Humidity.
   - k. Nutrition.
   - l. Physical factors.
   - m. Pollution.
   - n. Population.
   - o. Smoking.
   - p. Social factors.
   - q. Spectators.
   - r. Temperature.
   - s. Water intake.
   - t. Wind.

5. Psychological domain.
   a. Aging.
   b. Anxiety.
   c. Aptitude.
   d. Body composition.
   e. Cardiorespiratory endurance.
   f. Drugs.
   g. Fatigue.
   h. Interests.
   i. Maturation.
   j. Motivation.
   k. Muscular strength and power.
   l. Obesity.
   m. Perception.
   n. Posture.
   o. Reaction to injury.
   p. Skill.
   q. Somatotype.
   r. Staleness.
   s. Tension.
   t. Tolerance.
6. Prevention domain.
   a. Conditioning.
   b. Body weight.
   c. Communicable diseases.
   d. Diet.
   e. Environmental controls.
   f. Genetic factors.
   g. Health knowledge.
   h. Health practices.
   i. Maladjustment.
   j. Mental disease.
   k. Overload.
   l. Overtraining.
   m. Rest and sleep.
   n. Social forces.
   o. Stress.
7. Personal domain.
   a. Aptitude.
   b. Body function.
   c. Capacities.
   d. Fatigue.
   e. Fitness.
   f. Heredity.
   g. Hypnosis.
   h. Intelligence.
   i. Maturation.
   j. Metabolic function.
   k. Perception.
   l. Physical defects.
   m. Posture.
   n. Reactions.
   o. Sex.
   p. Somatotype.
   q. Speed.
   r. Strength and power.
   s. Timing.
   t. Values.
8. Medical, physical, and physiological domains.
   a. BMR.
   b. Body composition.
   c. Cardiac function.
   d. Circulation.
   e. Drugs.
   f. Energy cost and oxygen debt.
   g. Longevity.
   h. Maximal and anaerobic work.
   i. Mechanical efficiency.
   j. Muscle cramps.
   k. Muscular power.
   l. Muscular strength.
   m. Oxygen intake capacity.
   n. Overtraining.
   o. Peripheral resistance.
   p. Postural effects.
   q. Pulmonary function.
   r. Sensorimotor factors.
   s. Weight control.
9. Safety and protection domains.
   a. Acclimatization.
   b. Age.
   c. Agility.
   d. Altitude and climate.
   e. Clothing.
   f. Conditioning.
   g. Desires and interests.
   h. Education.
   i. Equipment.
   j. Facilities.
   k. First aid.
   l. Intelligence.
   m. Nutrition and diet.
   n. Posture
   o. Protective devices and methods.
   p. Psychological factors.
   q. Static environment.
   r. Transportation.

Personal prejudice, beliefs, conflict, cooperative attitudes, sex differences, and attitudes about differences in general are all social elements related to sports performance. These are the essential factors influencing group morale and status and, therefore, become more significant in sports under stressful competition. Under desirable conditions of play, such negative qualities as prejudice can be favorably affected.

The role of sociology and anthropology within sports and sports competition takes on importance in the determination of the quality of play. Sports medicine is concerned with competition, so these disciplines, in turn, become important components of the overall discipline of sports medicine.

Growth, Development, and Aging. Growth, development, and aging are the biological components of human maturation. They set the limits for the human organism in sports participation. A major responsibility of sports medicine is the proper adaptation of sports to fit the bounds established by these three biological determinants.

The physical status of the organism is the basis for growth, development, and aging. Fitness and health, body build and somatotype, and dietary practices are individual physical conditions that influence all three of these biological factors. They also establish the limits in physical activity. They are part of the set of determinants influencing practices in sports medicine, because activity must fit these characteristics to be beneficial.

The motor and skill abilities, physical movement patterns, and activity interests of the individual are elements that influence growth, development, and aging. The physically active individual is favored in this process. The interests and skills are requirements in sports and can serve to motivate participation; thus they are elements of sports medicine as well.

The individual's mental and emotional characteristics as well as his social and economic status are strong forces in physical performance. They must also be considered when evaluating the results of sports participation.

Individual chemical characteristics of the organism, such as hormones, heredity determinants, drug effects, and maturation patterns are related to sports participation and encompass major segments of the practices in sports medicine. These chemical determinants set limits for growth, development, and aging and are, therefore, fundamental factors in sports participation. (List 14).

Body composition (tissues) and structure also constitute a factor in physical performance. Tissue quality (e.g., lean versus fatty) is an important determinant of human power and strength. The obese individual will generally see his performance suffer, although participation has an effect on reducing obesity. Because individual differences will determine results in sports, they become professional matters included in the discipline of sports medicine.

Social and physical environments, including the traditions and mores of society, are significant factors in health and fitness as well as important qualities in sports participation. They are generally aids to participation, although they can also exert unfavorable effects on the individual's desire to participate. They, however, become essential in sports medicine, particularly at high levels of intense participation.

Drugs to delay the onset of fatigue and as aids to participation are now taken by some athletes. This practice is discouraged by leaders in sports medicine, because it does little to aid performance and has a number of undesirable side effects. Sports medicine supervision is desperately needed in all forms of physical activity, particularly in competitive athletics.

Rehabilitation Domain. Sports participation leads to injuries and resulting readjustment processes. Rehabilitation is a major responsibility of specialists in sports medicine. The effects of injury and disability are social and psychological as well as physical; the services of additional specialists, therefore, are required. The intensity of participation on some competitive levels can also lead to maladjustments (List 14).

The physical factors of rehabilitation are generally of most concern to sports medicine. Therapy and the use of prosthetic devices are both useful in the process of returning the athlete to participation. This work is an important role of the discipline of sports medicine. Major emphasis is placed on therapy, including hydro, light, heat, sauna, and cold therapy, to aid healing and restore normal movement.

Psychological factors are a significant part of sports medicine, just as they are in sports participation. The emotions, intellect, attitude, and social behavior of the individual are all sociopsychological constituents that direct play to a significant degree. The individual must want to regain his normal capacity in order for sports medicine to achieve maximal results. Few individuals are actually motivated to this level. Guidance toward development of this type of positive attitude is part of the discipline of sports medicine.

All social forces and psychological factors are components of sports. Interest, motivation, social practices, and social responsibilities in person-to-person relationships shape our personalities and are important in life activities, but nowhere do these components interact more intensely than in sports competition. They influence the results of sports competition and are, therefore, essential elements in the adjustment process of interest to sports medicine.

Educational factors are also constituents in rehabilitation, because the individual must regulate his own rehabilitation, largely by his own efforts. The results achieved during the rehabilitation process are highly individual. This factor is extremely important in sports, because individual, personal care and protection is foremost in continuing sports participation. Individual practices must be understood to gain the most from participation and to achieve optimal protection from injury.

Applied physiology, surgery, therapy, and drugs are significant facets of sports medicine. Injuries resulting from sports competition many times require corrective surgery. The specialist in sports medicine is prepared for such surgery; of additional importance is the ability to implement the therapy program that follows. Physiology applicable to sports is highly specialized. The specialist lacking this type of preparation would not be fully qualified as a specialist in sports medicine. In sports, drugs for corrective purposes should be used only under the supervision of a physician with an extensive background in sports medicine.

Nutrition and individual health practices are integral components of the overall framework of the discipline of sports medicine and rehabilitation. The results from rehabilitation programs are largely due to practices carried out through dietary programs. These programs are regulated by sports physicians during periods of rehabilitation. These programs include the individual environmental setting, which may either aid or impede the achievements of positive results.

Sports are an important facet of rehabilitation programs, because they may motivate as well as physically produce desirable results required for rehabilitation. For some disabilities sports and exercise programs are planned as the sole component of the rehabilitation program. This is particularly true for those who have emotional disturbances. Sports and exercise are directly related to any rehabilitation program being established for those individuals who are injured during sports competition. They serve as valuable aids in the restoration of normal physiological functions.

Environmental Domain. The environment and its effect on the human organism are significant in normal life and certainly in sports (List 14). The environment contains the social, cultural, and physical forces that establish the requirements for the individual in his life adjustments. The individual must modify the conditions or adjust to them. In sports participation, the requirements are probably more visible and meaningful because of the intense competition. These factors must be understood, and in sports the athlete must be prepared by sports medicine specialists to direct these forces favorably during participation.

The environment can be grouped into three major categories—physical, social, and cultural. Within these three categories are a number of concepts that represent the composition of sports medicine within these areas of responsibility (List 14).

The physical elements of the environment, such as wind, temperature, and humidity, also have an effect on sports participation. They require medical supervision and regulation if there is the possibility of over-exposure. These environmental factors can have various effects on the organism, all of which are the responsibility of the profession of sports medicine.

Life-styles and personal mores have their influence on sports. Diet, nutritional habits and practices, alcohol intake, and overall physical condition of the organism are social environmental factors that influence sports participation and are, therefore, of concern to the field of sports medicine. The participant must be informed about the dangers of unwise practices and must be guided so that he avoids these pitfalls. Under favorable conditions, social mores can contribute to the quality of participation and add to the quality of the individual's environment. Culture and societal settings are important concerns in sports and sports medicine.

There are a number of elements in the physical environment that help to constitute the professional structure of sports medicine, such as clothing during participation, air conditioning in gymnasiums, tobacco smoke and smoking in poorly ventilated buildings, air pollution, and noise disturbances. Regulation and control of such physical factors for the welfare of the athlete are professional responsibilities of sports medicine.

The individual and his attitude about himself and his physical and social environments are of immense interest to sports medicine. Knowledge of environmental effects makes it possible for the athlete to avoid these negative conditions. The sports medicine program strives to provide the individual with a full understanding of physical activity.

Life in an automated society does not promote the physical attributes necessary for the individual to participate adequately in sports. This lack of physical development begins during youth and continues through the early years of growth and development. In order to compensate for this, sports medicine specialists must plan physical activity programs that will aid optimal development during these formative years, when they are most effective.

Psychological Domain. The human mind is the directing force throughout participation in sports and physical activity. An individual seldom experiences complete exhaustion. The mind and the emotions will not allow the individual to drive his body to that point. Unpleasant physical stresses and the resulting fatigue are not easily accepted. Physical activity, unless it is within a pleasant context, will not enlist the enthusiastic involvement of the participant. Until motor patterns become routine, the mind directs each movement of the body and every motor mechanism. Motor performance can come by instinct, but success will seldom be enjoyed without extensive practice. The psychological domain is a professional facet of physical activity as it relates to the field of sports medicine.

The physical condition, fatigue level, learning processes, and physical aptitude of the individual all receive careful scrutiny by sports medicine.

The body structure—its somatotype, posture, weight, and composition—forms the chief limiting factor to physical performance and consequently is carefully studied by sports medicine. The quality and effect of physical activity and sports participation are established to a large degree by these physical structures (List 14).

The motor mechanisms of the organism involving perception, skill, and precision are elements of established motor patterns and the overall mind-body relationship. Success in performance is determined by the individual to the limits of his aptitude and age.

The psychophysical elements of tension, anxiety, tolerance, motivation are constituents of physical activity and can significantly influence ability, particularly at advanced levels. When these elements are negative, they can be a great deterrent to performance. Direction of these elements for positive results is an essential responsibility of the profession of sports medicine.

The aptitudes, capacities, maturation rate, and aging rate and effects are of major concern to sports medicine in the adaptation of physical activities to meet individual needs and abilities. These factors can determine the heights of success achieved by the individual and can be advanced by sports activities properly adapted and scheduled.

Drugs, food supplements, and health habits serve a psychophysical function in sports. Properly regulated and controlled, they can aid the physical organism and provide protection for strenuous continued physical activity and sports.

Prevention Domain. Prevention of disease or injury in sports by securing optimal resources for the individual during participation is a major goal in sports medicine. Losses from injury and disease can, of course, deter further use of undesirable health practices. Losses also have personal effects that can, in some instances, influence personal health over long periods of time. Sports are potentially hazardous, but the individual can gain valuable benefits from participation if he will only strive to protect himself adequately. This is a professional responsibility for sports medicine.

Basic physical conditioning is foremost in any program for the prevention of injury and disease as well as being a preparational requirement for sports. Those who have responsibility for the administration and coaching of competitive sports are most responsible for the physical status of the athlete.

Diet, health habits, rest, and sleep determine, in part, the quality and quantity of sports performance possible for a given athlete. Leadership preparation in sports medicine includes understanding these variables.

Both the physical and social environments are potential hazards to the athlete but can contribute, under acceptable conditions, to both his performance and well-being. Certain elements of the physical environment, such as pollution, temperature, humidity, terrain, clothing, and equipment, will affect the individual. Their effect should be favorable. The social environment, which includes tension, prejudice, and frustration, can also influence participation unfavorably. An attempt should be made to control each of these factors under the supervision of specialists in sports medicine.

Health knowledge and practices, housing and living conditions, and mental health status all influence the quality of physical activity. Properly directed and with adequate practice, these factors can add to the health-fitness level of the individual and, therefore, his performance. Additional success is the result of favorable preparation.

The overload principle, training procedures, individual training regimen, and overtraining exert their own particular influence on physical activity as it relates to sports medicine. The training programs for each sport have specific requirements and must be designed to meet the objectives of each sport, as must overload practices. It is possible to elevate physical loads beyond the requirements of the individual sport. Additional loads are placed on the organism and its specific related functions in order to reach higher performance levels. Participation in sports alone will not stress the organism beyond requirements of that sport, so that results will not be greater than the stress placed on the individual through participation in that activity.

Personal Domain. The personal components of physical activity and sports are closely associated with participation. This fact is probably more visible in sports than in any other human activity. No two individuals are alike, and no two sports have identical requirements.

The physiology of the human organism takes its structure as a result of the individual's life habits and has some common bond or association with others with similar life habits, but they are not identical. This difference should be taken into account in preparation for sports participation.

Maturation, hereditary factors, aptitudes, and individual capacities are personal qualities that are related to preparation for sports participation and participation itself. The specialist in sports medicine defines and establishes practices specifically for individuals in order to achieve optimal results. He is aware of the wide ability range, which extends from the individual almost devoid of aptitude for a particular sport to the champion in that particular sport.

Individual sex differences and differences within each sex also play an important role in determining suitable activities for an individual. These differences are recognized by sports medicine specialists in order to plan sports activities appropriate for these differences. These differences are evident in maturation periods, body types and body structure, and physical capacities. Sports generally take account of sex differences (e.g., American football is not necessarily desirable for women because of the violent physical contact).

Individuals differ in motor responses, perceptual abilities, motor capacities, and specific motor elements within the sports framework. Qualifications for participation in sports and the results from such activities will be determined to some degree by these perceptual and motor characteristics.

Personal heredity, somatotype, aptitude, and physical capacity differ with the individual. The sports medicine specialist must fit each individual and his abilities to the sport or activity that will prove the most productive and satisfying.

There are numerous other individual differences to be taken into account in participation and they should never be disregarded in organizing and directing a sports program. This is true both when an individual is selected for a professional sports team or when he is simply directed into sports activities for the overall personal benefits so important to achieving good health and fitness levels.

Medical, Physical, and Physiological Domains. Medicine and physiology are sciences basic to sports. They assess the participant's qualifications for participation. Motor skills and patterns will determine an individual's efficiency in applying his physiological resources. Physiological requirements will differ in each sport. Some activities or sports have only minimal physical demands (e.g., golf).

An individual's physiological status and medical condition are reference points for determining initial levels for sports participation. The individual who is unprepared medically and physiologically must be first conditioned in order to reach a fitness level adequate for sports participation, or the sports must be adapted to fit his present health and fitness status (List 14). It is possible, if the organism does not have an organic defect, to prepare the individual through appropriate progressive physical activity until he is ready for more strenuous sports competition. It is possible to alter slightly the requirements of a particular sport so as to gain progressively from participation.

Physical powers, such as muscular strength and endurance, circulatory and respiratory endurance, and body composition, are necessary in all sports in widely varying degrees. The normal individual can meet normal fitness requirements by stressing activities that develop the necessary skills; this can be done through exercise organized as a satisfying play activity. Specialists in sports medicine guide and prepare the individual toward these ends.

Weight control, drugs, nutrition, and *food supplements* are elements of sports medicine that have a direct bearing on physical activity. These factors are regulated largely by specialists in sports medicine.

Reference should be made to List 14 and the *Encyclopedia of Sport Sciences and Medicine* for a more complete listing of these medical, physical, and physiological elements that constitute the discipline of sports medicine. Specialists in sports medicine provide supervision for participation, because both the dangers and benefits achieved from sports are determined by the method each individual uses. Death can easily result for individuals who exercise without physiological and medical preparation.

Safety and Protection Domains. Without safety and protection controls, sports could result in more losses than gains. Each sport has specific safety requirements, and each requirement should be determined by specialists in sports medicine.

Equipment and facilities are basic to most sports. They must meet standards for safety in order to ensure the sport participant against injury. Unsafe equipment and facilities have been responsible for numerous serious accidents and many deaths. Safety standards must be supervised and controlled by sports medicine specialists in order to ensure the greatest possible protection for the participant.

The education of all sports participants is essential for safe participation. The coach, teacher, or recreation specialist must instruct the participant of the dangers involved in each activity and the necessary protective procedures to ensure safety.

Avoidance methods, safety devices, first aid procedures, and protective clothing are all necessarily associated with sports and sports participation. Each procedure is specialized in its application and, therefore, becomes an integral part of sports medicine essential in protecting the participant and preventing injuries. They also provide assistance in the process of rehabilitating the individual following injury and, as such, are important functions of the sports medicine specialist.

Professional Domain: The Physical Activity Content in Sports Medicine

Sports medicine is defined in the previous section by a conceptualization process. The work of identifying all the concepts within sports medicine is not intended to be complete; rather, it is simply an identification of the nine major categories and a listing of a sufficient number of concepts in each of the nine categories to establish the nature of sports medicine. This conceptual procedure is considered sufficient to define sports medicine and to serve the purposes of this section of the text in reviewing the ten applications of physical activity in their professional roles. These applications are now operational as professions, each employing physical activity as the major component of its implementation program. Sports medicine is one of these applications. This section gives reasonably representative examples of content in order to judge the value and potentials of sports medicine for sports participation and in service to society. A strong profession arises only when its services are needed and it renders worthwhile, high-quality programs.

A historical review is made of sports medicine by Ryan [2] in the *Encyclopedia of Sport Sciences and Medicine*. This review is worldwide in its scope and investigates the status of this profession. In most countries, sports medicine is a branch of the medicine profession and deals with the medical aspects of sports. In the United States it is an interdisciplinary profession that applies the services of numerous professions besides medicine to problems that result from an individual engaging in physical activity. The full range of historical developments in sports medicine is investigated from simple general exercise movements to the highest-level, most stressful professional sports.

To provide more understanding about the nature of sports medicine, brief summary statements and some comments about each content category will follow in this section.

Sociological and Anthropological Content. Sociological and anthropological content in sports medicine has come largely from clinical judgments made by scientists in these disciplines who have attempted to apply basic research findings to the medium of sports and sports competition. During the past decade in the United States research studies have been under way to generate procedures for applying these two disciplines to sports.

The attitude of the sports participant is indeed related to the outcome of his participation. An attitude that views sports as valuable and personally worthwhile will result in more intense participation and better results.

Sports medicine is a relatively new profession in the United States, and it is harassed by unfounded bias, beliefs, superstitions, and fads. Misinformed groups include not only the general public but athletes as well. Practices that have long since been proved false are still followed by many individuals. Food, diets, and drugs often involve misconceptions. The concept of athletes being "muscle-bound" is still popular, though false, as is the idea that women who participate in sports become "muscular." It is essential that sports medicine specialists include the rationale for each practice or treatment they administer to an athlete in

[2] Allan J. Ryan, "History of the Development of Sport Sciences and Medicine," *Encyclopedia of Sport Sciences and Medicine* (New York: Macmillan, 1971).

order to gain his complete cooperation. Without it the results achieved will be less than optimal. Programs planned by specialists must be continued on an individual basis if corrective results or developmental goals are to be achieved.

Knowledge, understanding, and intelligence are positively related to sports interests and participation. These intellectual characteristics are related to the quality and level of performance. Unless the athlete is overwhelmingly overendowed with ability, championship-level achievement cannot be reached without a clear understanding of the sport and its personal requirements.

The social status and cultural status of the individual are influenced by sports. The athlete can improve his social status through an understanding of the nature of social status and a personal desire to be a part of a desirable social order. The strength of social forces in the integration of race and cooperation among nations has been demonstrated over only the past few years. In the United States, sports are one of the most valuable tools in integrating the deprived and those who are victims of discrimination into the mainstream of society. In sports, opportunities have been significantly equalized. The cultural and social structure of society can also be influenced through sports by participation that includes individuals from various levels of the social structure. Most religions are aware of the importance of sports in social character development. Because the results of such integrating processes can be both good and bad, church supervision represents a valuable setting for such interaction.

Societies are stratified economically, and the successful sports performer is generally found in the higher strata.

In some societies the results of poor nutrition are readily seen in sports, because an underdeveloped body structure generally manifests a generally low level of ability. Overindulgence, on the other hand, which is evident in many of the affluent countries, also has negative consequences in sports.

Growth, Development, and Aging Content. Growth, development, and aging and their relationships to sports are an important part of the content of sports medicine. These factors affect sports participation and the results from participation. They generally establish participation limits; these limits, however, can be positively affected through the proper selection and application of physical activity. This becomes the responsibility for the sports medicine specialists.

Work capacity and physical activity potentials increase with age up to a certain point and then decline again. Growth rates account for differences and variability in muscular strength, motor abilities, and working capacity. Work and physical activity must fit the individual's capacity level at each age in order to achieve effective participation results.

Little evidence exists that food supplements, except in case of vitamin or nutrient deficiencies, can advance the muscular growth and development potentials of the individual. Drugs and chemicals have demonstrated a little effectiveness on normal growth and development (e.g., anabolic steroids) and must be administered in conjunction with vigorous exercise programs.

Smoking is regarded as extremely undesirable by sports medicine specialists. This opinion is based on performance experiments and general health information on smoking practices over a period of years that show a definite link between cigarette smoking and lung disease.

Growth, development, and aging processes are correlated with changes in psychological security and status of the individual. Normal patterns can be observed and are meaningful to the individual, particularly if security or status deviations are noted. Sports and physical activity contribute to normal psychological growth as well as physical growth and development.

The growing child needs a good deal of physical activity. The growing child sometimes shows abnormal conditions. When this occurs immediate attention should be given by the sports medicine specialist and other appropriate specialists.

The aging process is significantly influenced by physical activity. The individual who has had an active physical life and continues to be active through later stages of maturity will be able to maintain his body at normal physiological levels. Such an active physical life is responsible for maintaining the individual's physiological age at a level lower than his chronological age. There are many young people whose bodies reflect advanced chronological age, because they are physically inactive. The process of atrophy is a negative factor in the maintenance of an individual's physiological age, and this condition should be avoided. An organism's posture and organic composition are highly influenced by physical exercise, in addition to health practices that aid overall individual fitness levels.

Rehabilitation Content. Rehabilitation, particularly as it applies to sport injuries, is a large part of the overall sports medicine program. Specialists in sports medicine are particularly needed.

The proper adaptive physical activity is individually determined in rehabilitation. It must be based on individual capacity. Such a rehabilitation program must be fully understood by the patient, so that the program can be continuously applied even upon release from direct medical supervision. This will further ensure program results that follow the overall plan as designed by the rehabilitation specialist.

Sports have therapeutic value for the normal, retarded, and injured individual. For the injured individual, the physical function of sports is to aid healing through appropriate therapeutic applications of a particular activity. For the retarded individual, the physical abilities and experiences gained through physical activity will provide learning experiences that promote adaptation to life activities. These therapeutic effects represent an outlet for normal drives and serve to counteract tendencies toward neurosis. For psychotics, physical activity must be prescribed according to the needs of the individual and the potential value of a particular physical activity in meeting those needs.

Cardiac rehabilitation is becoming an increasingly large segment of sports medicine programs. The goal is to normalize physiological functions through progressively planned exercise in order to sustain and develop the organism and gain additional power with a minimum of physiological stress. For individuals with muscular defects, physical activity will aid in the process of making normal physical adaptations.

Regulation of body weight falls within the realm of sports medicine. Overweight and underweight physiques have an effect on sports participation. Properly planned physical activity in conjunction with the development of good health habits should be the major part of any weight-control program. An active individual can consume more calories, which is favorable to human development and health.

Rehabilitation and adaptive physical exercise are closely related fields and are both functions for the specialist in sports medicine. Disease or sports injury may cause permanent physical handicaps. Adaptive exercise will aid the individual toward rehabilitation to the limits of his particular handicap. This program applies to the effects of any disease or results of any injury whether in sports or other life activities.

Rehabilitation and sports medicine are almost completely integral components of the same overall field. The specialist in sports medicine understands exercise; of equal importance, he understands the stresses and requirements of sports that he utilizes as his rehabilitation goal.

Environmental Content. The physical and social environments affect the performance of the individual in sports and physical activity. Environmental protection and control are of major consequence to the field of sports medicine.

Drugs, as an aid to physical performance in sports, are ineffective, and some drugs have side effects, in addition to constituting an unethical sports practice. No constructive results have been achieved through the use of drugs by athletes. This makes a broad drug education program necessary by sports medicine specialists. It is also important to note that stimulants of the central nervous system are dangerous and can seriously impair human performance.

The dissipation of heat through perspiration while wearing excessive clothing can have serious side effects. In extreme cases where nonporous clothing is employed in an effort to increase weight loss, death could result if the temperature climbs too high or if exercise is too strenuous. Water lost during strenuous exercise must be replenished.

The athlete or the individual exercising at high altitudes must recognize that the oxygen pressure is reduced, which will, in turn, reduce oxygen availability and consumption during exercise. One must become acclimatized before strenuous exercise is tried. Peak performances usually occur under conditions that are normal for the individual athlete in both temperature and altitude. At normal altitudes, the oxygen pressure is more favorable to the physiological system. It is also recognized that the well-trained athlete can tolerate higher temperatures, with less discomfort, than can nonathletes. The physical environment, with its physical and chemical contamination, has a definite effect on the individual. If the environment is polluted, it will have an unfavorable effect. For example, pollution may not influence the high jump, but on maximum respiratory efforts such as the 440-yard dash, it may have a significant unfavorable influence.

An individual's social setting is many times related to his performance. Enthusiastic spectators, for example, can motivate individual performances far beyond normal levels. Physical activity in an isolated setting functions largely through self-motivation. Social environments do influence the emotions and can be an aid in utilizing the individual's full resources.

The psychologically secure individual always has an advantage in dealing with unknown factors in both the social and physical environment. The frustrated individual will generally not perform optimally. Security includes all factors that can make an individual insecure in daily life from personal finances to confidence in one's performance. Moreover, the individual's emotional state can be impaired by unacceptable noise or unfavorable comments. More than one athlete has allowed spectator comments to "get his goat" and lower his performance level. The athlete that concentrates his attention on spectators soon loses his concentration on his own performance and his performance suffers greatly.

The specialist in sports medicine should give a careful briefing to the athlete of the possible effects the environment may have on him.

Psychological Content. Participation in physical activity involves psychological factors. Emotional and mental stability and adjustment are factors in an individual's ability to relax during physical activity and enjoy it. Mental and emotional adjustment are more closely related to performance and the avoidance of injury. In this connection physical activity reinforces mental and emotional stability and serves as the basis for continued mental health. Strengthening the individual's psychological image of himself through intense play adds to emotional health and stability.

Staleness has been a subject of extensive study for a number of years. Teachers and coaches have believed that it is largely due to physical factors prevalent in overtraining. This, of course, can be true in some instances, but it is now believed that psychological attitudes—lack of motivation or other psychological variables that lead to boredom—are probably of equal, if not more, importance.

The relationship between exercise and senescence is a topic that is under constant study. A delay of senescence appears to result from consistent exercise regimens coupled with acceptable health practices. Dietary practices and body weight also appear to have a psychological influence on exercise. The obese individual has usually reached an excessive body weight by eating constantly, and the volume of food intake then provides a psychological hunger to continue eating for eating's sake. The emotions resulting from this traumatic situation can be regulated by the mind if the individual is capable of looking objectively at his problem, making a commitment, and then sticking to that commitment.

Fitness levels of the circulatory, respiratory, and muscular systems are determined by stress placed on the organism through intensive exercise. The drive to maintain exercise stress is, in part, influenced by the individual's psychological makeup, which allows him to drive his body to stress levels beyond the pain threshold. Determination is a potent psychological force. It is the display of a strong desire to achieve positive results even at a high price. Its effects are also noted in the posture, for it is possible to read the mood of the mind by viewing postural variations.

The psychology of sport and physical activity is now a part of sports medicine. Its content, based largely upon applied psychology, has not yet reached a high supporting role for physical activity, but studies and papers are reported regularly at scientific meetings dealing with the psychology of sports.

Prevention Content. Prevention of organic losses to the individual from sports participation is a major goal of specialists in sports medicine. Under unsupervised conditions, losses resulting from sports participation can be greater than the gains achieved.

Glandular activity of the endocrine system is stimulated by physical activity and is an aid to both physical performance and human development. After strenuous physical activity, it is generally desirable to assist the body to achieve toxic relief through supplements, of which water is most beneficial, although glucides can also be helpful.

Appropriate physical preparation for sports is one of the most important requirements in prevention of injury and other organic loss. Each physical activity or sport has specific preparation requirements. An individual should not participate intensely in a sport without prior conditioning for it.

Bad eating habits or a poor diet constitute one basis for injury and organic loss in physical activity. Inadequacies in an individual's diet result in organic deficiencies with a corresponding loss of resources necessary for strenuous sports that can be extremely dangerous.

The well-conditioned individual has many advantages. These advantages go beyond the ability to participate in sports with minimal demands on the organism. There is some reason to believe that the conditioned individual is also more resistant to disease and less susceptible to aging. If aging involves the slowing of organic functions, physical activity can, indeed, serve to delay this process. An individual's normal physiological status, barring disease, can be sustained until the very late years of life, if he continues to exercise and remains physically active for a significant portion of his life. It is the belief of many experts that after retirement, the major portion of the individual's time should be spent in physical activity of varying degrees of intensity, just as in the early years of life. This serves as a deterrent to many ills during the later years of life.

Personal Content. The individual is, indeed, an individual in every sense of the word in sports and physical activity participation. The abilities and results derived from physical activity are, indeed, personal. No two individuals are alike and no two can gain the same results from the same activity, even though they participate on the same team and in the same sport. The differences in results will be reflected in various individual systems, organs, and functions; differences are also found between sexes. These are primary reasons for the planning of sport programs by sports medicine specialists.

Aptitudes are also specific. Each individual varies in ability to perform an activity and in the result he will obtain from that particular activity. There is hardly an individual who can exhibit a consistently high level of abilities in every activity. An individual generally can participate with ease in one activity while he is under great stress in another. The qualities and requirements differ among activities. In some activities, for example, muscular power is foremost, whereas in others it plays only a minimal role.

Personal fads, superstitions, and beliefs are found among most individuals. This is particularly true in sports. For example, some coaches will cling to certain customs of dress if they were successful previously while wearing that same attire. When beliefs are strong, such superstitions will influence individual attitude, motivation, and play interests. The popularity of fads is, of course, completely without scientific foundation. Among other things, the sports medicine specialist must be a psychologist in order to combat such nonscientific practices.

Intellectual abilities are not clearly associated with sports participation, but they appear to have an influence on motor learning, particularly when viewing the full pattern of a motor performance. This establishes the direction for physical performance and should facilitate learning and achievement. In team play, the active and qualified mind should be able to perform more successfully through the development of anticipatory responses and sensitivity to certain cues within the myriad possibilities during play. The retarded individual, on the other extreme, is greatly handicapped in his performance because of an inability to learn to recognize such cues.

Considerable interest has been placed on motivation, interest, hypnosis, and other factors that provide impetus in the sports context. Each of these factors appears to aid the individual by sensitizing him to appropriate cues during performance that will assist him in applying his full resources.

Body structure, posture, and somatotype are factors in the individual's aptitude in sports. They will establish the limits of success and even of the play itself. The heavy-boned individual is not likely to be successful in the pole vault, high jump, or swimming because of a disadvantage in body structure. Achievements in physical activity are influenced by body structure. The heavy-boned individual must expend more in calories and organic resources than his slender-framed counterpart.

The specialist in sports medicine begins his analysis with the individual; examinations and tests will determine individual qualifications for sports and physical activity.

Medical, Physical, and Physiological Contents. The basic foundations for sports medicine are in the biological sciences. The medical aspects as well as the physical and physiological content of sports provide an understanding of physical activity and its effects on participation.

Physical activity is a physiological phenomenon. The response to physical exercise involves several mechanisms of the body, including the physiological, structural, and mechanical processes. Body weight itself can be a factor in the degree of success or the results achieved through sports. The cardiorespiratory capacity of the individual for physical activity can be significantly improved by training and participation in strenuous sports.

Physical activity involving mild stress or intermittent participation is of little physical value except for personal or psychological refreshment. These benefits arise from the removal of stress and frustration that can have negative psychological effects.

Exercise of high intensity continued over a prolonged period of time can achieve significant improvements in overall fitness. These improvements involve the heart and circulatory-respiratory systems as well as muscular power if the activity is dependent upon these physiological systems.

Sports medicine specialists recognize the importance of regular exercise and therefore support programs that provide skills and recreational activity interests that can continue at all ages and in all geographical locations. It is recognized that continued activity will significantly aid in retarding the degenerative process of aging and will serve to maintain a healthy cardiac system.

Training is essential to avoid cramps, muscle soreness, muscle injury, and to protect the individual during physical activity. Typically, there is no danger of overtraining, but an individual can reach a point of diminishing returns for his efforts that may cause disinterest in routine training procedures. This is particularly true if formalized training procedures are strictly followed. Such procedures are most economical as well as productive, because exercise can be directed at the specific system that is deficient.

Physical activity is essential for everyone. It is needed to maintain a constant weight if one follows a desirable diet, and it is necessary to maintain organic functions at a normal level. If physical activity is planned in an enjoyable sports context the effects are more worthwhile than if the exercise is routine, formal, or individual.

Sports medicine is an interdisciplinary profession and includes all the disciplines necessary to develop sports for the greatest possible benefit. A single discipline cannot provide the knowledge and skills needed for a full range of sports activities.

Safety and Protection Contents. Safety and protection in sports and physical activity have significant roles for the sports medicine specialist. Every sport, in varying degrees, is hazardous and must provide adequate protection for its participants.

Relaxation is vital for protection from injury. The tense individual does not enjoy the movement efficiency or skills of a relaxed individual and this is likely to result in injury. The highly skilled and relaxed individual can move powerful forces during activity with fewer risks of accidents. Skill preparation and appropriate safety measures are important requirements for personal protection.

Drugs are hazardous in sports, both to safety and to health. Little evidence exists substantiating the fact that drugs aid performance, but they may have side effects that increase the likelihood of accidents. Extreme noise is also hazardous to the individual and can lead to accidents.

The physical environment is related to safety and protection in sports. Extremes in temperature will affect performance.

Motivation in sports is also a factor in safety and protection. The poorly motivated athlete is prone to accidents in sports that require physical contact. The motivated individual takes the initiative in body contact and thereby redirects the impact of the contact. This protects the aggressor, whose body is in readiness because of tension in his muscular system, and makes him less subject to injury.

For endurance activities, the effects on the individual should be monitored under varying degrees of stress to establish individual reactions to specific exercise stresses. Exercise in progressive stages should be planned from these results.

Each individual has his own personal and genetic qualities. Each person also has potentials for development and learning in certain defined and sometimes limited activities. There are only a few individuals who are endowed with the capacity to become champions in an activity. There are very few individuals who can become champions in two different activities. For those who simply use physical activity for leisure or recreational purposes, aptitudes are not essential, although if one has the natural capacity, learning and development are less stressful. If a sport is properly adapted to the individual, the risk of injury or accidents in sports is severely reduced. It is a professional task for specialists in sports medicine to adapt sports to individuals according to their abilities in order to provide protection against injury and against body malfunctioning.

It is recognized that the sports medicine specialist directs a major part of his services at protecting the individual during physical activity. The need for the sports medicine specialist is increasing because of the huge numbers of individuals engaged in sports and the lack of knowledge by the participants. Most accidents in sports could be prevented with sufficient time devoted to training, protection, and supervision in play.

Physical Activity: A Sports Medicine Profession

Sports medicine as it is designed in the United States is a multidiscipline profession. It functions within several disciplines in sports requiring specific scientific and medical services. This facet of medicine renders special services; physical conditioning for sports is guided by qualified scientists in both physiology and physical education. Conflicts, morale problems, and prejudices that influence participation are the responsibilities of the psychologist and sociologist who are also specialists in the discipline of sports medicine. Sports medicine, then, include specialists from medicine, the sciences, and education. This is because of the requirements for physical activity and sports participation. Special services are required from medicine, the sciences, and education in order to provide knowledge and understanding to sports and physical activity participants and to the profession as a whole in order to plan suitable educational programs. The profession could not function without these three disciplines, which intermingle and help make sports a vital and positive part of the lives of every segment of society.

Sports medicine in other countries around the world is not viewed in the same context as it is in the United States. It is almost always considered a facet of medicine. This view cannot be accepted by the fast-growing profession of sports medicine. It was noted that in the development of the *Encyclopedia of Sport Sciences and Medicine* it was found that most of the content in sports medicine comes directly from the sciences.

The future of this newly developed profession is very bright indeed. Preparation for this discipline is now beginning to draw people interested in sports from the sciences of psychology into the field of psychology of sports, from sociology into the field of sociology of sports, from physiology into the field of physiology of exercise, and from the physical sciences. From medicine, doctors interested in retraining in sports-related studies have been accepted from preventive medicine, cardiology, internal medicine, and other branches. From physical education, many university students are now indicating interest in the "science of physical activity."

Preparation for this new profession is in the planning or implementation stages at several institutions in the United States. The number of new sports medicine specialists in fifteen to twenty years will be considerably beyond current estimates. These young scientists will understand the stresses of physical activity from the viewpoints of science, medicine, and education and will serve as specialists in one of the three facets of the field or, as specialization increases, in one of the facets of an individual discipline.

The understanding of the relationship to other physical activity disciplines is of major importance to the specialist. One cannot work alone in this new profession of sports medicine. It requires a team of specialists to work together on a specific problem.

PART IV

The Perspectives of Physical Science

This section of the text on foundations deals with perspectives. In Chapter 18 the perspectives are viewed within the social and cultural contexts of physical activity. In Chapter 19 the social-cultural perspectives are applied to physical activity as disciplines and professions. The design for these two chapters is founded on two premises: (1) physical activity is an integral part of the culture and, therefore, must be studied within this context and its internal relationships and (2) because of its cultural roles and relationships, physical activity is influenced by social and cultural conditions and through them can contribute to society and the culture.

This text begins with a discussion of the modern world in Chapter 1 and references will be made to this chapter in reference to sociocultural status. Chapters 18 and 19 will provide brief reviews simply to establish a basis for these projections for the future. The entire text on foundations is founded upon the setting established in Chapter 1 based on the two premises cited in the preceding paragraph. When dealing with status and projections, it is impossible to review a single aspect of the culture; one must view the culture as a whole. The essential emphasis in this section is on the American culture, with only minor references to the wide cultural variations of people throughout the world.

Sociocultural reviews require limitations. For this text the conceptual structure will contain those facets of the culture that influence or can be influenced by physical activity. To initiate this discussion, physical activity is conceived and directed to meet the needs of the human being and society. This includes both the physical and social environments but is limited to resources as media for human development. Any other within the environment will not be included. It will be possible to view the current status and projection for the future of physical activity as a sociocultural phenomenon.

It is appropriate to begin and end a text on the foundations of physical activity within the framework of its societal and cultural contexts. Foundations represent the sustaining base and are the structure upon which one can build with confidence and security. Strong foundations are an essential requirement for physical activity. The structure of this text rests, therefore, on the sociocultural content that defines the developments and results of physical activity in its many roles.

Chapter 18

Social and Cultural Perspectives

Man can, through technological manipulations, control many of the conditions of his life. He is the central figure in his environment. Whether he is cloistered in a laboratory in the great depths of the ocean, in a skylab near the moon, or in the jungle, the environment is a crucial factor in determining the quality of life. Man is influenced by where and how he lives, and these influences he can control to a large degree.

The environment is not a single facet of the culture; it is a synthesis of all parts of society and the culture required for life and desirable for satisfactory living. This represents the position to be taken for a review of the social-cultural references for specific physical activity perspectives. Social-cultural forces for maintaining physical activity today will change in the future. It is quite possible that these changes will be more favorable to physical activity or research, and social changes may place less value on this facet of the culture.

A review of the conditions of the modern world is presented in Chapter 1. Conditions in the modern world range from those of relative comfort and abundance to those of filth and starvation. Political leaders in the United Nations recognize that to save nations from war it is necessary to improve conditions in many countries in the world. Major programs are under way in the more affluent nations to aid in the development and improvement of living standards elsewhere in the world. The United Nations, which was developed as a deterrent to war, now occupies more than four fifths of its men and funds in the effort to improve underdeveloped nations. In addition, there are numerous public and private agencies that devote funds and manpower to the solutions of world problems.

The modern societies of the world have social-cultural conditions with both favorable and unfavorable effects on their people. In every case, the conditions are modern and are different from those of several decades ago. These conditions represent changes within one generation of mankind.

Population Growth. Population growth is the greatest single factor influencing the economic and social advancement of most people in the underdeveloped countries of the world. The continuation of population growth at the current rate would lead to economic and social disaster not only for underdeveloped countries but also for those countries that now have abundant resources.

Technological Advances. During the period encompassing the past two or three decades a technological revolution has occurred. It is now extremely difficult to find work that has not in some way been automated. This revolution has been greatly influenced by the computer.

Social Mobility. The class structure of the world is now indeed a modern one and differs greatly from that of the past. Movement from one class to another is now easier.

Advances in Knowledge. Modern technological advances certainly constitute an explosion of knowledge. Technological advances are found in nearly every discipline and profession. Such knowledge provides an understanding of our world and its people.

Cultural Differences. The people of the world who live in nations with differing traditions and ways of life also differ significantly in social-cultural practices and beliefs. These forces influence daily behavior and attitudes; it is not possible to separate the social-cultural experiences of people from personal experiences; both have profound effects.

Work and Leisure. The modern world is certainly different in its work-leisure relationships than was the period of only two and three decades ago. Major changes have occurred as the long workday of hard physical labor for most people has been reduced to the short day with little physical effort. Through automation work production has significantly increased, utilizing less manpower but with improvements in both quality and quantity. A significant social fact that now underlies every social institution is that man often now has more leisure time than work time. To add to this social condition, the number of people retiring before sixty-five is increasing. The retired population is large and rapidly increasing.

Government and Politics. Modern world governments and politics vary significantly today, and the political world is different at this period from that during the earlier years of the twentieth century. The major change in both autocratic and democratic governments is the rise in the involvement of the people in government and politics. The people now regard government officials as their representatives. They insist that officials represent the people, not just themselves. Representation of the people is now rapidly increasing and will lead to carefully planned policies with which the official must comply. A more complete governmental setting in this modern era is presented in Chapter 1.

The Changing Society

In a recent text [1] by this author on curriculum foundations for physical education, one section presents a review of the changing society (pp. 4–8). Conditions within a society are considered as references for the physical education curriculum and in the establishment of foundations for this program. This reference becomes increasingly important when physical activity is considered in all its present applications. These applications are made within a society and culture and they therefore start with this base and plan programs to change those attributes that are discovered as undesirable.

Social-cultural changes that appear to be foundational to curriculum interests of physical education were identified and summarized into ten components. These ten social-cultural components are also the foundations of other physical activity professions and disciplines. These influences and effects are chiefly concerned with physical activity, but additional favorable or unfavorable influences will occur with physical activity organized as disciplines and professions. These elements of our changing society will be briefly reviewed and additional content will be found in the text cited in footnote 1.

The World Is Shrinking. Because of communications, both through transportation and the communications media of radio, television, newspaper, telephone, and so on, the world is smaller than ever before, and getting smaller still. It is also possible today to travel to any part of the world within a matter of hours. Overnight travel can take an individual to nearly any country in the world without losing a single day of work.

---

[1] Leonard A. Larson, *Curriculum Foundations and Standards for Physical Education* (Englewood Cliffs, N.J.: Prentice-Hall, 1970).

Physical Effort in Work Is Reduced. Scientific and technological advancement have removed much physical effort from nearly every industry. This means fewer unskilled workers and fewer overall employees are necessary in a given industry. It is a pleasant experience to see drudgery removed from work, but the removal of physical effort will also have negative effects on the individual. If physical work is not found in sports or other forms of physical activity, its effect on mankind over a long period of time will be deleterious.

Longevity Is Increasing. Advances in the sciences and medicine have resulted in longer life for the individual human being. For Americans, chiefly during this century, the life-span has increased from an average of thirty to forty years of age to an average of seventy to eighty years. The change in longevity to the middle seventies is indeed of major social consequences. The elderly population has significantly increased and has brought with it increased social needs.

Benefits Are Shared Unequally. With modern developments and especially modern technology, it is surprising to note that at least one half of the people in the world are living in ignorance, poverty, and misery.

People Are Abusing Leisure, Wealth, and Technology. Technology has given people more leisure. Working a ten-hour day, six days a week is rare today. This change has occurred within the twentieth century, a period of less than seventy-five years.

Leisure time must be planned constructively. If it is not so planned, the individual and society will deteriorate and finally be destroyed. Leisure time is often used for sedentary, health-damaging activities. Many people, especially Americans, are physically soft, overfed, and overweight. With increases in technology, less work and more time, what will happen to the individual and society? Preparing the individual for leisure is now as important as preparing him for a profession.

World Population Is Increasing. The population of the world is increasing rapidly. The rate of increase is estimated at 100,000 per day, largely because of the decreasing death rate and the increasing birth rate. In the more heavily populated countries, this problem is now acute. The current emphasis (and its increasing success) on birth control is having some effect on growth rate.

People Are Becoming Urban-minded. With advances in technology, less manpower is needed in rural areas. Land has become less fragmented and land management requires fewer people.

The number of farms in the United States is continuing to decrease.

By the year 2000 the present rural population may shrink another 85 per cent. The movement trend is definitely toward the urban areas. Can industry manage employment to meet these increases? During the past two decades, moderate-sized cities (approximately a population of 100,000) have doubled in population. Employment has remained fairly constant, but will it be possible to prevent unemployment from rising?

Attitudes Are Changing. The American people may be considered secure largely because they experience the highest standard of living in the world. Although slums and poverty do exist, few need to go without food or shelter.

Man needs to be challenged; if he is not, he atrophies. He must work toward something and not just maintain a status quo. The struggle for existence has many positive values and only a few negative ones. Success through persistence leads to such qualities as joy, happiness, and personal well-being.

When he is secure, an individual tends to be against change. Anything that threatens the status quo is then viewed negatively, since the possibility of losing security is too great.

Values Are Changing. Many basic individual values seem to be shifting. The shift has been from the home and the family-oriented and community-related life to one that is highly materialistic and urban. Other human values are, to a large extent, determined by this setting.

People Are Getting Physically Soft. It is predicted that by 1980 the majority of the working population will be employed in what is today described as a "white-collar" job. Those individuals still in "blue-collar" work will be largely technicians and machine operators. Unless physical work or exercise is found outside industry, the future holds only physical decline for the individual. Unfortunately, physical development in the past came largely from an individual's work and not from a cultural pastime within society. It is feared that people will choose less physically strenuous leisure patterns to avoid physical work or exercise rather than place this human requirement in a daily regime.

Foundations for Perspectives

Physical activity as a discipline and profession is designed to meet the needs of the human being. We want to understand physical activity from a scientific point of view, as well as to understand the nature of physical activity. There are six disciplines within the established scientific disciplines. These are combined into four specific disciplines for this text. For example, the purpose of the discipline of physiology is knowledge of the physiology of physical activity. This includes all facets of physiology and all facets of the organism that are influenced by physical activity.

Professions are organized from physical activity for individual or societal objectives. There are ten physical activity professions that are sufficiently organized to be recognized as professions. These foundational disciplines come from the value of physical activity in these ten professional roles, which differ in objectives and, therefore, in uses of physical activity.

For a brief review of foundational settings for physical activity in perspective, reference will be made to Chapter 2 of a recent text [2] by the author. This chapter reviews the basis for physical activity within two categories that significantly influence the value of physical activity in all its roles. These two categories include (1) those factors that delay or negate the effects of physical activity and (2) those factors that contribute to the effectiveness or value of physical activity for the individual and society. These two categories will be briefly described; for more information see the text cited in footnote 1.

Physical activity under unfavorable conditions will reduce its value and may be extremely harmful. It is essential that negative factors be corrected. In some instances physical activity will serve only as a corrective action without any normal physical advancement for the individual.

Stresses and Fatigue. It is recognized that modern life causes stress, which results in both physical and emotional fatigue. An individual has two methods by which to benefit from physical activity. He can reduce stress and fatigue through personal planning and, if this is not possible, he can increase the amount of physical activity in order to neutralize the effects of stress and fatigue as well as establish a physical organic basis by which to counteract the negative effects of stress and fatigue. If continued, these stress factors will eventually lead to ill health and poor physical fitness.

Unacceptable Health Practices. The body cannot constantly be abused and still retain good health, nor is an abused body capable of instigating counteractions when that is necessary. A person must be physically active in order to achieve optimal health. The drains on the organism are numerous and include disease; physical defects; constant stress; lack of proper rest or sleep; poor diet; overindulgence in food, alcohol, or tobacco; accidents; constant use of self-medication and drugs; poor human relations leading to tension and unhappiness; unwise or no exercise; and chronic fatigue.

[2] Ibid.

Self-medication and Drugs. The faith of people in many self-medication and drugs is largely unfounded. These range from self-treatment of serious disease to the use of narcotics to elevate individual emotional levels.

Drugs in the hands of physicians have saved numerous lives. Today nearly 50 per cent of all medical prescriptions are written for antibiotics. Their use to combat disease has saved more lives than all other remedies combined. Penicillin alone is our most effective drug for the prevention of disease. On the other hand, marijuana and heroin have caused additional injury and sometimes complete deterioration.

The Unprotected Individual. Often the individual does not protect himself from his environment. Home accidents alone injure some 5 million individuals per year, kill another 30,000, and cripple 100,000 more. There are routinely 500 to 1,000 or more deaths on long holiday week ends.

Emotional instability, hostility, frustration, and aggression are some of the factors that may lead to accidents, injury, and death. The assumption that self-preservation is sufficiently strong to control the individual's actions has proved false. The emotional status of man seems at times to override his intellectual control and render his reasoning and thinking powers ineffective under stress.

Unwise Exercise or Lack of Exercise. Exercise is one of the essentials for life. Without it the body will deteriorate. Through exercise the vitality of the organism can advance considerably beyond the needs of daily life and normal activity. No one has to be fatigued or unable to meet normal daily living requirements, with the singular exception of the individual who is structurally deficient.

Unsatisfactory Human Relations. Unhappiness, tension, social isolation, and constant rejection are not the ingredients necessary for positive human development. On the contrary, they cause poor health, poor development, and functional destruction. The mind and the emotions become the destroying agents, and the physical body assumes the role of the target. This requires that the condition be corrected, and physical activity can be designed to emphasize the social values of physical activity, thereby helping to remove negative emotions.

Boredom. Unfortunately man has difficulty breaking from routine, and routine is demanded of man for a good portion of his life. Nearly all of the essentials of life take place within a routine. The result is that life becomes dull. Motivation for new learning and new experiences is reduced in such an environment.

Boredom, then, is a major concern in physical activity. It is possible to develop interests in sports that are satisfying. An individual is challenged by competition, and this provides new interest and the positive values that are necessary for nearly everyone.

Nutrition. Proper nutrition is essential for proper growth. The size and physical vigor of the organism are, in part, determined by the quality and quantity of food. The effects of starvation and inadequate diet clearly illustrate the importance of good nutrition. Undernourished children, for example, are underactive and because of this and related factors become underdeveloped. Nutritional requirements are determined by an individual's exercise and activity level, skeletal development, muscular power, adipose tissue, and energy requirements for daily activity. To fulfill his nutritional requirements, the individual must have a proper balance of carbohydrates, proteins, and fats that include the essential caloric, mineral, and vitamin content.

The result of exercise and adequate nutrition can be seen in an organism with appropriate symmetry, acceptable posture, muscular strength, endurance, and abundant vitality.

Work and Exercise. The foundations for physical activity are basically physical work and exercise. The organism needs stimulation for work and exercise to attain its normal functioning and physical development. Properly planned exercise programs can mold and establish potentials for the individual, particularly during his early growing years.

Leisure and Recreation. Wholesome and enjoyable play is as important for individual growth and development as exercise and nutrition. Physical recreation provides a setting for social and emotional development and adjustment in addition to the physiological outcomes that are valuable to the individual.

Security. In order for the individual to grow and develop properly, he must acquire a feeling of security that is an integral part of his life. Security is essential in itself and it is important to the organic processes of the body. In contrast, insecurity leads to a complete loss of self-confidence and often to a complete loss of physical health. Personal security is promoted by success and achievement. Physical activity can contribute to an enhanced feeling of security.

Health Practices. A well-rested and adequately nourished organism is a prerequisite for physical activity. This provides the basis for more intense participation results and further improvement and development of the organism.

A significant part of the foundations for physical activity rests upon health practices. With planned physical activity, negative influences will cause less damage; if there is no physical activity, ill health will result.

Personal Attitudes. The individual who has personal interests in various activities is generally enthusiastic about his life and welcomes challenges and has the personal qualifications necessary for participation in physical activity. With the necessary physical development levels required for participation, the individual will benefit from activity. Sports and physical activity require enthusiasm, because satisfactory participation in sports comes from a deep interest and strong desire for participation and competition against oneself and others. The individual must always be reaching out for new experiences. New skills, new experiences, and new interests are the pacesetters for active living, and the larger the range of interests, the more effective the results.

Perspectives: Sociocultural Modules

The introductory part of this chapter is a setting for perspectives. This is represented by the fundamentals that underlie physical activity in its various roles. This setting is recognized within many societies and cultures, which range from an almost infinite number of local communities to the more complex societies represented by larger population areas and by the cultures of the various nations in the world. Each of these is influenced by physical activity, and physical activity influences these social groups, from the single family to world cultures. The stage is now set through this brief introduction of sociocultural conditions to deal directly with the perspectives that bear directly on physical activity. The beginnings of this discussion will be presented in this chapter on structural organization for review and analysis. The modules will include the structure of these concepts in the contemporary world (Figure 1) and the conceptual module as the basis for perspectives and projections of physical activity as disciplines and professions (Figure 2). This chapter will deal essentially with the foundations for these projections and Chapter 19 will deal more specifically with the disciplines and professions of physical activity.

Physical activity in all its forms must be considered in an environmental setting. Physical activity is influenced by its location. Physical activity and sports, therefore, will differ by the influences exerted on them. This conceptual module is presented in Figure 1. The setting for physical activity lies in three relationships:

1. Forces that are in dynamic interaction. These are the cultural, societal, and individual forces that characterize the individual. The reactions to

physical activity are determined by social needs and interests and, in return, by physical activity as it exists in relation to each of these social constituents (Figure 1).
2. Forces that represent the shaping functions of physical activity.
3. Controlling forces that advance or limit physical activity in service to the individual and society (Figure 1).

In Figure 2, physical activity is structured in relation to its functional roles. This constitutes physical activity as representative of the potential for change in the individual and society and the effects on the culture over a period of time. These roles affecting change will be influenced by the various forces operating in society and the culture. Whatever the goals for change, physical activity is designed as a medium for people. The nature of the direction taken will be determined by the discipline and by the profession. In another section of this chapter, the effector functions of physical activity will be reviewed in more detail.

These structures represent the content organization for this chapter. Because of the size of such a review of sociocultural perspectives, it is necessary to limit the scope of the discussion and to analyze perspectives in modular form.

Conceptual Analysis of the Contemporary World

Physical activity as disciplines and professions has its roots in the contemporary world (Figure 1). These settings are provided by an infinite number of environments, ranging from local to worldwide. The contemporary setting for physical activity incorporating its various influences takes on three basic aspects (Figure 1). These include the shaping, controlling, and interaction forces that act on people and physical activity to establish individual and group needs and roles.

Dynamic Interactions. Social institutions, programs, and people are involved in constant interactions. These interactions do not maintain an established influential system. In Figure 1 this fact is reflected by people as individuals, societies, and cultures. These forces interact with physical activity and will establish the nature and form of physical activity as it is designed for the public. Environmental forces exert control on the roles physical activity can play in service to the community, although physical activity can be effectively planned in spite of handicaps placed on it by the various environments.

The individual is a person with needs and desires that may or may not include physical activity. He has varying levels of knowledge, health, and fitness, and so on, which make him unlike anyone else. The individual will strive for his needs, and these may, of course, include physical activity. It is possible that this drive for need fulfillment can be accom-

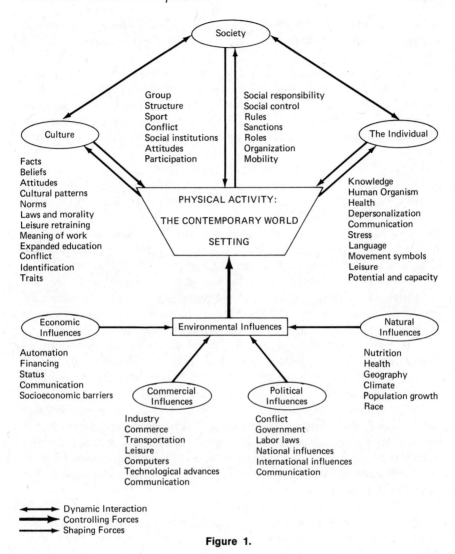

Group
Structure
Sport
Conflict
Social institutions
Attitudes
Participation

Social responsibility
Social control
Rules
Sanctions
Roles
Organization
Mobility

Society

Culture

The Individual

Facts
Beliefs
Attitudes
Cultural patterns
Norms
Laws and morality
Leisure retraining
Meaning of work
Expanded education
Conflict
Identification
Traits

PHYSICAL ACTIVITY:

THE CONTEMPORARY WORLD

SETTING

Knowledge
Human Organism
Health
Depersonalization
Communication
Stress
Language
Movement symbols
Leisure
Potential and capacity

Economic
Influences

Environmental Influences

Natural
Influences

Automation
Financing
Status
Communication
Socioeconomic barriers

Nutrition
Health
Geography
Climate
Population growth
Race

Commercial
Influences

Political
Influences

Industry
Commerce
Transportation
Leisure
Computers
Technological advances
Communication

Conflict
Government
Labor laws
National influences
International influences
Communication

Dynamic Interaction
Controlling Forces
Shaping Forces

Figure 1.

plished individually outside the societal environment or in such a way as to be contrary to the cultural mores of the community (Figure 1). In every instance, however, there are forces interacting with society and the culture that will have a direct influence on the individual and on the physical activity chosen.

Society is a collection of people and social institutions. Societies are groups of people organized around interests, social institutions offering programs and services, and every other element needed by people living as a group (e.g., government, schools, hospitals, and so on). Physical activity as sports, for example, is considered one of these program com-

ponents. It interacts with every other social element and with society as
groups and as individuals. This is indeed the contemporary nature of
physical activity.

The culture of a community is the sum of all the activities and people
within a given setting. Culture is described by what people do and how
people live within a community and world setting. Language is only one
example. There is a cultural change under way as people and nations are
changing to the English language as a means of communication (Figure
1).

Controlling Forces. Controlling forces are found essentially in the
environment. They comprise largely the physical environment but include the social as well. The economics of a community or nation is
indeed a controlling force. This does not mean that economics exerts an
absolute control of sports or physical activity, but it may have a strong
influence on development (Figure 1). Conflicts, labor disputes, strikes,
graft, and many other factors influence people and programs. In most
countries the government has a very favorable and strong influence on
physical activity as sports. At the current time, physical activity is
stressed in order to maintain the fitness level of society.

The natural setting of a community or nation has an important influence on physical activity and society. This includes the way people
live, their health, their occupation, the climate, and all other elements of
an individual setting.

Man is indeed limited in what he is able to do. The environment
establishes certain limits. Within these limits, however, many choices
are still freely available for the individual. Sports and physical activity
are certainly viable choices for many individuals. The physical limitations influence individual activities but many opportunities exist within
these limitations.

The Shaping Forces. The most valuable forces within sports and
physical activity are the shaping forces. These forces include the environment. These forces, although they influence and limit physical activity,
do not have a relationship that determines changes in sports interests
and forms. They are essentially limitations in relationships. Forces within
the culture, society, and individual determine needs, interests, programs,
facilities, and all the other requirements for sports needed by society.

In viewing Figure 1 and the concepts within the culture, society, and
individual, one can easily realize the many relationships possible in association with physical activity. Each relationship will have a definite influence in shaping the life-style of the individual. For example, individual
knowledge about sports will influence social institutions within a society
and also will eventually establish a cultural setting as a result of these
relationships.

Thus a brief review has been presented of the conceptual structure of physical activity within the contemporary world as a basis for establishing perspectives and projections.

Perspectives and Projections: Conceptual Analysis

The central purpose of this chapter is to view physical activity as disciplines and professions for the future. It is physical activity in perspective as well as the projections that can be made from these perspectives. The scope of these analyses is extremely wide-ranging and essentially starts with physical activity as disciplines and professions that have scarcely progressed past their beginning roles. The only exception is physical activity as education, but this field too is far from what it should be in professional development.

In the preceding section of this chapter, the conceptual analysis deals with the influences exerted on physical activity as disciplines and professions. This establishes a definite setting within the contemporary world as well as the forces that act on physical activity in order to benefit the individual or to limit his activities. This will always be the case, but an individual does not need to accept unfavorable environmental influences. It is possible to change environmental influences in order to benefit any program essential to society. This is the role of physical activity as well as the initial reference point for perspectives and projections.

The starting point for perspectives and projections can, of course, only be the people. Physical activity is designed for the human being within the social constructs of life and living. Physical activity as disciplines and professions also begins with the individual as the fundamental base reference. An individual is unlike any other, and it is the individual who must initiate the considerations necessary for benefits gained from physical activity as disciplines and professions. It is also recognized that the individual does not and truly cannot live alone. If isolation is attempted, it leads to distortions of both the mind and the body. Physical activity perspectives and projections must then be related to a group of at least two people. This social range may be extended to the appropriate community, region, state, nation, and society of the world. This focus deals with a collection of individuals that in each case becomes single units of individuals who must live together. They have no other choice.

In the final analysis, people as individuals and societies become the culture, which is the result of all activities of man. The culture represents the traditions, ways of life, and mores of man within the life of the home, the nation, and the world. This concept incorporates all of what society is today and provides the base for what it should be in the future. The culture is a strong force on society because it is the result of life as it has progressed from past generations. This heritage is not easily changed. Perspectives and projections for physical activity based on these references begin with a conceptual analysis that provides sufficient detail to give understanding to these projections.

The Individual. The individual initiates the process of analysis of perspectives and projections (Figure 1). This analysis becomes a matter of deciding what benefits for the individual are attained from physical activity as disciplines and professions. This role must be extended to its larger societal context and a decision must be made on its role. This analysis must also be conducted within a framework of the desire to recognize individual differences as well as provide freedom for individual development. The strongest society is the one with the greatest individual freedom, which lives within the rules and laws of society and provides protection to all other individuals. This is the basic foundation for democracy.

The conceptual structure for the individual is illustrated in Figure 2, which provides some of the important concepts of physical activity as they apply to the individual. This approach is predominant today and is the basis for judgments about what such projections should be.

Human values and fitness are needed by every individual. All experts realize their importance for a life that leads to health and happiness. Physical activities are applicable to the individual as a learning discipline and as a profession. Physical activity is also applied in its various forms for leisure activities, which result in improved health and fitness. Realizing the existence of many individual differences, the true value of physical activity is in its many combinations as sports, athletics, recreation, and so on, which will cover everyone's needs who has a basic interest in physical activity. Children begin their lives naturally enjoying physical play. This role can be continued into adult life under proper instruction and provisions for each individual.

The freedom of communication between individuals is found in physical activity and is important to most individuals. In fact, this freedom is most important as young individuals seek to master the ability to communicate (Figure 2). Physical activity is increasingly becoming co-recreation as a setting for both sexes to meet within an informal goal-oriented setting.

Interest in creative experiences, self-expression, and adjustment to others is important to the individual. The learning of skills in physical activity and their expression through sports have infinite potentials for the individual. If an individual becomes successful, he establishes a firm association with the sport.

The objectives that can be accomplished through sports and physical activity are most valuable to the individual. Physical development of the

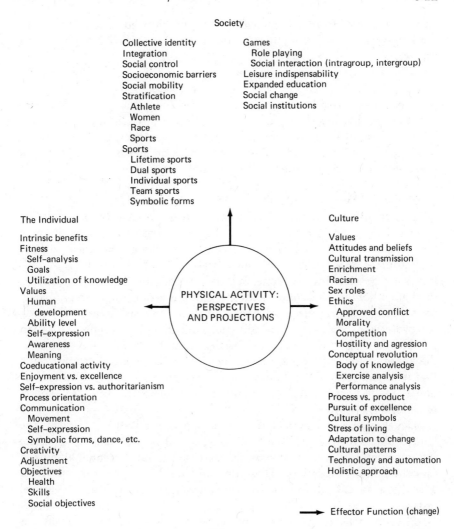

Figure 2.

body aids not only in achieving good health, but also in attaining a pleasing appearance. Starvation diets to hold weight constant are usually not medically sound, but through physical activity one can maintain body symmetry and weight while consuming a sufficient amount of food to provide for an adequate diet.

Learning sports skills can lead to deep personal satisfaction. Play alone can be the only purpose, but sport also provides deep physical and emotional satisfactions, which, once experienced, will generally continue to be desired by the individual. The social goals of sport are a valuable part of physical activity. If physical activity is utilized in sports that are high in social potentials, their value to the individual becomes even greater.

Thus the first reference for perspectives and projections is the individual. The individual is the most valuable and the most basic reference for physical activity because of individual differences. It is also important to note that physical activity ranges from activities that are indeed individual to mass performances structured for the group. The scope of physical activity provides activities to meet the needs of all. Everyone needs exercise, but some individuals do not recognize this need.

Society. The individual must live in a group and/or society. It is difficult to live without the help or resources provided collectively by other people, such as hospitals or schools. It is hard to identify a single item necessary to the life of the individual that can be provided without the resources of society. A few individuals can raise their own food, but this is not possible for everyone. Society incorporates collective planning. Provisions for the individual within a discipline can, for example, come only through the resources of educational institutions. This is also true for professions. Education as physical education is presented through schools, colleges, and social agencies. Through these collective agencies, the needs of the individual can be met, including financial requirements that will make the services possible. Physical activity as physical recreation is made possible by community possession of facilities for sports of all kinds (Figure 2).

Development of physical activity as sports has been so rapid in the United States during the past two decades that it is difficult to estimate the financing involved. Expenses of professional sports teams alone run into the billions of dollars. These developments have elevated sports to a position as one of the major components of society and the social order.

Physical activity, as a societal component, has made significant advances as disciplines and professions. There are six long-standing disciplines (e.g., sociology) that are now applied to physical activity. Physical activity has also been developed into at least ten professions within society. In both instances, applications should grow in strength and number.

The effective roles and functions of physical activity have resulted in sports becoming a chief interest of most people. The value of physical activity has been noted by citizens, and their financial support has been given. There has been increasing emphasis on physical fitness and exercise, as evidenced by the jogging programs found in nearly all communities.

Physical activity has numerous potentials in enabling society to provide service to the people (Figure 2). Some roles of physical activity are not only health-centered, but also contribute to the status of society as a desirable social order. The contribution of physical activity to social integration over the past two or three decades is, in itself, one of the major aids to the social order of any societal program. This includes education for social integration. Integration through sports has not completed this process, but maximum contributions have been made.

Culture. The culture is the result of human activity and includes sports and physical activity. Culture not only is the result of events, but exerts its effect on those events. Cultural forces are usually strong. They influence what people do because the culture is generally recognized as the result of individual and group accomplishments. In a democracy, it is surprising the extent to which one individual can change these cultural forces. This is not easily accomplished, but with strength, determination, and perseverance it can be done.

In recent years cultural changes have been significant. The knowledge revolution alone has changed the ways of life for all. Knowledge about the effects of exercise has provided a different view to the citizen. Physical work and exercise a few years back were considered menial and undignified. This view has changed because of recognition of the need for physical work by the organism.

The stresses of life, the adaptations to change, and improved technology and automation are all elements of the culture that directly influence programs of physical activity. The status of physical work as exercise is almost completely opposite from what it was only thirty or forty years ago. Cultural changes are indeed of major importance. The role of the culture in physical activity must be considered both in planning and implementing various programs.

Perspectives and Projections: Foundations for Physical Activity

This section deals with perspectives and projections as a foundation for Chapter 19. We shall consider physical activity as a whole, with no immediate reference to disciplines and professions. The content statements will be interpreted in Chapter 19 as bases for projections of physical activity into the various professions and disciplines. Perspectives and projection foundations are organized in two parts: (1) the contemporary world setting for physical activity, and (2) perspectives and projection foundations of physical activity.

The Contemporary World Setting

The first part of this review deals with the contemporary world setting for physical activity applied to the individual, society, and culture. Physical activity as sports and games is an established part of the culture. It can help shape the culture as well as be shaped by it. The attitudes and interests of the individual and society are influenced by the social position of sports in a culture. Physical activity, particularly as sports, is programmed to maintain cultural patterns and particularly to establish youth roles in a sport-centered culture based on the premise the attitudes and beliefs originate through social interaction. It is also believed that sports provide for such interaction, and they therefore will influence society. It is the strong belief of some experts that sports and games have the potential both to reflect and to structure a society. As an example, sports provide an opportunity for expression of moral behavior, and society will endorse the potential of sports for directing moral behavior.

The concern about leisure and its use is a matter reviewed by every community. In this era of automation it is recognized that man has more free time. Communities now plan for recreational facilities. In some instances, guilt about leisure still prevails and is applied to sports; instead, of course, one should view participation as essential for well-being and health. A mature view of leisure is needed by youth not only in learning skills but in preparing for adult life, when physical activity needs will continue to be essential parts of daily life.

Social integration between races, sexes, and other minority groups is a concern for any community. These problems, of course, range from minor issues to those of major international consequence. Racial integration is far from fully achieved in the United States, but sports have been helpful in moving toward that goal, particularly in the huge metropolitan areas. Sports also have a role in the fulfillment of women's equal opportunity goals. The application of sports in improving social mobility is an accepted norm with few barriers. Excellence in sports participation facilitates upward social mobility; this may be the only way open to many individuals in a society. In some societies, although they are rapidly changing, sports for women is low on the social value scale. The social gains for women in sports have been phenomenal during the past few years. Styles in sport clothing, especially for women, have reflected increased interest in sports and their attraction for women in particular.

The second part of this review on the contemporary world setting for physical activity deals with relationships with the physical and social environment. These references are essential to any review dealing with perspectives and projections, particularly for sports and physical activity.

Some of the most influential environmental forces are technological changes. These changes improve man's efficiency in both time and energy and have therefore changed man's schedule correspondingly, with more free time and less energy expended in work. Because physical work is often no longer required in one's work, the individual must turn to sports for fulfillment of health requirements. Physical activity also aids morale. Sports are both socially and emotionally demanding. They can command people's interest. Fitness would soon decline if physical work or sports were not substituted.

The physical environment is a part of the life of society that cannot escape environmental conditions. The compatibility of the social and physical environments is basic to the adjustment of the individual. If he can use the environment as a natural facility for physical activity, he has achieved a major accomplishment. This places him in harmony with his environment, while providing beneficial physical activity. It also reduces the need to plan man-made facilities, which are always built at a tremendous cost to the public and cannot always be made available. The immediate environment will influence the selection of the activity (e.g., lakes and rivers for water sports), will determine the cultural patterns in the sport, and will influence societal patterns as a whole. It is recognized that man can change both his physical and social environments. The challenge can be in conquering the physical barriers and in providing shelter and conditions necessary for a particular sport (e.g., indoor artificial ice in tropical climates). It is desirable, however, to plan physical activity within a local setting to fit the sport to the conditions. Facilities will then be available when needed.

Economic conditions influence sport and physical activity. During periods of prosperity, sports tend to flourish. Socioeconomic status also influences sports. The golf club and other such exclusive associations have always been a center for people who could afford the costs of membership. Because local communities have attempted to meet the needs of all its people, there are, for example, numerous public golf courses available to everyone, regardless of economic class.

Perspectives and Projections

This section deals with perspectives and projections as they more directly deal with physical activity and its changing nature. This step is necessary prior to the discussion in Chapter 19, which will deal with physical activity organized directly as disciplines and professions.

The leisure concern, as reviewed in the preceding section, continues to be the basis for further projections in physical activity. The true question in this regard is whether man will use constructively the free time he is rapidly gaining. Will physical activity play an important part in his life? It appears that there is increased interest in physical activity, and this is favorable. Educational programs must continue, however, to emphasize the importance of leisure and prepare one for this type of life. Sports and physical activity, including physical work (e.g., gardening, mowing the grass, and so on), must play large parts in an individual's daily life. For most, creativity does not come with birth; it must be stimulated and developed within schools and social agencies.

For projections in planning physical activity for society, research is necessary to identify the cultural patterns that influence sport and physical activity. If man is to benefit from sports, he must be free to choose those activities that provide optimal results for all potentials provided by physical activity. The nature of stressful competition and hard play should be understood by the individual. The effects should contribute to his social well-being and not be destructive. The role of sports must be accepted by society and directed as a valuable phase of cultural life. Sports in proper cultural focus provide the basis for study by the various disciplines and professions that deal with human movement and physical activity as a part of man's life. With further understanding their value to the individual will further increase. This certainly is the basis for directing people into physical activity, which represents the answer to a basic human need.

Physical activity has an amazing performance range. It can be applied simply as play in a sport, with little skill or understanding, or it can reach the loftiest heights of world title competition. It is also amazing that the personal satisfactions that come in each case can be so deep. However, an individual can gain more from sports when he possesses skills and understanding than when his participation is inadequate.

Sports have unique qualities and potentials because the participation process can be as important as or more important than the physical process itself. Such benefits will be determined by the objectives or purposes of participation. Golf, for example, may be planned entirely for social communication and play itself may be completely incidental. Mistakes in technique are overlooked or may not be recognized. Scores may not be kept; if they are, they are simply for conversation following play. It is truly a mistake in any sport to regard the social aspects of play as equal to the physical aspects. By emphasizing the process, the value of sports will be significantly increased. These values are beneficial to society in the preparation of a social order that also fully regards the process of human associations. This also focuses attention on the development of the "whole man" in preparation as a citizen. In sports there is no dichotomy of man. If the whole mental, social, physical, and emotional man does not participate, play achieves less than optimal results. When this occurs, the changes in these qualities will be equal to their involvement in play. Sports can cause changes, but the quality to be changed must be part of play if it is actually to be changed. This situation is analogous to that of a muscle. If not used, the muscle cannot be built up and, in fact, will atrophy.

It is most essential in sports not to lose sight of the individual himself. The current interest in national and international sports may emphasize the team as a whole and the country that wins or loses. The individual can be completely lost in this process, which is unfortunate, because, of course, without the individual there can be no sports.

An Overview

Social and cultural perspectives are foundations for the growth and development of all social institutions. An institution designed to serve the public must be able constantly to view immediate and long-range changes. When you no longer understand the people you are serving, this is the beginning of failure. There are many examples of this principle in the social and business worlds, and it also includes institutions in sports and physical activity.

The setting in this chapter is a preparation for Chapter 19, which will deal essentially with projections. The analyses in Figures 1 and 2 provide the foundation for development of these physical activity projections as disciplines and professions.

Chapter 19

Perspectives Applied: Disciplines and Professions

In the preceding chapter we reviewed physical activity in terms of current practices and philosophies. In this chapter we attempt to project physical activity into the future by a process of extending existing trend lines.

This text is structured in four parts, which denote the foundations for physical activity that describe its various roles and applications. The reasons for the applications are found in this structural presentation. The foundations of physical activity are based on the premise that physical activity is rooted in society and culture, as is developed in Part I. The content of physical activity stems from its setting in the modern world and its potential value within society and culture. Physical activity is developed as various disciplines (Part II). Study of physical activity from a scientific and philosophic standpoint is only of recent origin. This development has covered six disciplines in various degrees of advancement (combined into four for this book). In Part III the current professional applications of physical activity are reviewed. There are at least ten professions that use physical activity as a medium, either in part or in whole. In each case physical activity is planned toward the achievement of objectives desired by the individual or society. Because these objectives represent pragmatic goals, the validity of the profession is derived from the results of the applications and directions for physical activity obtainable through professional organization and development.

348

The final section (Part IV) is on the perspectives of physical activity as disciplines and professions. These are the projections into the future of what appears to be the role of physical activity in the years ahead. It is most encouraging to note the trends for physical activity. The advancements have been so rapid over the past few years that favorable projections for both the continued development of disciplines and professions are prevalent.

The Changing Focus

Physical activity has evolved through three stages in the United States and is now rapidly entering a fourth stage. Such stages and the changes they have brought about are not unique to the United States but have occurred in most countries. The last two stages are significantly more advanced in the United States than elsewhere but the fourth stage of physical activity has been developing rapidly in many countries.

In the United States, organized physical activity first appeared in schools and communities as *physical culture*. This period began during the late part of the nineteenth century and continued to about the 1920's. The term *physical culture* is still used by some to represent physical activity. This pseudoclassification for physical activity was discontinued soon after World War I.

Physical activity was applied as physical culture in a formal context. It was designed to develop the human organism in symmetry and balance, with improvement of the exterior lines of the human body as the major objective. Anthropometry (the measurement of man) was an important facet of physical culture, and gymnastics was emphasized because it could be specifically applied to develop different segments of the body.

The second period or stage was that of *physical training*. This classification was derived during World War I and continued through the early 1940's. It was also the designation for physical activity in the various services during World War II and to this day is occasionally used by newspaper reporters and some commentators. The term was properly applied in the services because personnel were being trained or conditioned for work, an objective that stressed and required physical preparation for its attainment.

Physical training had a much broader interpretation than physical culture. The individual was trained and physically developed for more functional types of activity, ranging from sports or athletics to other applications of physical activity, such as recreational sports of all kinds. In schools, programs consisted of formal gymnastics for the direct purpose of training the performance capacity of the individual. Indeed, its fundamental aim was to train the body physically.

The third period overlapped the second to some extent, beginning in the middle 1930's and continuing to the present time. The evolution of *physical education* enlarged the scope of physical activity to include all qualities of the human being that could be changed or influenced by education through physical activity. The objectives for physical education, as a profession, are presented in Chapter 11, as one of the ten professions that have been developed for physical activity. The goals for physical education are the same as for education, the only differences being in the contributions made to the goals. Significant progress has been made in the integration of education and physical education, both philosophically and through its implementation as seen in the preparation for leadership.

Physical education in current programs includes as important facets both the product coming from physical activity itself and the process of leadership necessary for the achievement of desired goals. The value of physical activity has been significantly increased by its integration with education and by its own autonomous associations. In the United States it is now a part of all educational programs. Colleges and universities schedule sports and athletics as an integral part of their programs. Social agencies—both educational and commercial—also provide programs of physical activity designed to meet institutional goals.

The fourth period in the evolution of physical activity is currently in effect. Professional groups in physical education and sports have attempted for several years to find an appropriate name for this development, but have failed to come to any concrete agreement. All insightful professionals recognize this development and can describe it, but, ironically, cannot find the appropriate designation. This phase goes beyond physical activity as education per se in emphasizing the other professional applications of physical activity. In addition, there are six basic academic disciplines involved with physical activity. Physical activity is now viewed as a *movement science,* with accompanying scientific terms, such as *kinetics, kinesiology,* or *biodynamics,* and other less-defined terms that refer to its new applications. In this book we have simply used the term *physical activity* within the context of each discipline and profession without any attempt at new terminology.

These developments involve all who are concerned about the roles of physical activity in both personal and professional well-being. The public and professionals view physical activity differently today from the way they did during the physical education, physical training, and physical culture periods.

To bring new developments in physical activity into practice, the public must be provided a rationale. What does physical activity do for the body and personality and why is it a necessary part of life? This question represents the inquiring attitude of the thinking and receiving public. Physical activity is founded on well-established basic sciences and philosophies, and considerable knowledge has been obtained from direct research on physical activity in its applications. It is now possible to support, not always fully but at least to some degree, the nature of physical activity, with its potentials for health, fitness, and general development.

The biological sciences have been applied to physical activity for many years; in the United States this constitutes about seventy-five years of study. More recently the sociological and the psychological sciences have entered into the study of physical activity. The discipline of history is actively recording physical activity as sports and games during the various historical periods. The engineering sciences and physics have also contributed to the study of physical activity. Medicine has recently entered into research on physical activity in rehabilitation, weight control, disease relationships, and other areas of medicine, where it is believed that physical activity plays an important role. Sports medicine combines medicine, science, and education as three disciplines essential for the understanding of sports and physical activity; and, in addition, it assists participants in physical activity to obtain optimal results with a minimum amount of risks and losses.

The Modern Societies and Cultures

Specialization has always been an integral part of civilizations. The great Roman Empire, for example, with its art, music, military skills, and government represents one such culture. Specialization is accountable for the twentieth-century developments in science and technology that have progressed so rapidly that hardly a job exists that does not require the use of some technical device. Specialization in the technical sciences is no different from that necessary for the solution of social, educational, and political problems. Society is highly complex and, as in technology, one must strive to understand the parts in the system in order to understand the whole.

Specialization occurs in all fields that require technical knowledge and skills, especially those dealing with human development, which involves specialization of the highest order. The bases for knowledge come from and are developed by science and philosophy.

Advances in the various fields of science today are the result of a problem-solving approach. One investigation leads to another, which in turn leads to many new lines of inquiry. The process of classifying types of scientific investigation has led to a differentiation of the various sciences. The field of sociology is composed of several subareas representing different approaches, for example, to the study of man within his social environment.

A complex phenomenon needs to be analyzed in parts. The human organism is not merely physical, but is also characterized by social, emotional, and intellectual qualities. The organism functions as a whole in nearly every action or movement. Although the individual components of human movement have unique characteristics, all are highly inter-related. For complete understanding, it is necessary to concentrate initially on the parts and then focus on their relationship to the whole person and his personality. As knowledge increases, the approach becomes more molecular, and further subdivision is necessary. The most rapid develop-ment is occurring in the applied sciences, which include physical activity, and new specializations are also being developed, of which sports medi-cine is a prominent example.

The human organism and how it develops, adjusts, and changes with physical activity and the environment represent most complex phe-nomena. The study of this interaction requires, for each problem, a carefully planned interdisciplinary approach with contributions from several of the basic sciences. Such a research approach is undertaken in studies related to physical activity representing a range from education to the prevention of cardiac failure. The content of this work represents a field of science that is indeed unique and of major significance.

Physical Activity: Disciplines and Professions

Physical activity has two channels for development that take dis-tinctly different routes and result in different functional operations. These two channels, physical activity as disciplines and as professions, have developed during the twentieth century, and in fact, principally within the last three decades.

The most prominent role for physical activity at this time is in the professional domain. Physical activity developed as a profession has practical roles for achievement that are tested by their ability to ac-complish organismic change. For example, physical activity within its professional role as sports medicine must, in order to be accepted as a profession, aid in the process of preparing the individual for physical participation so that optimal individual or team results can be attained. If contributions are not made, the profession cannot survive.

The second channel involves physical activity as developed by disci-plines. Currently there are six basic disciplines. With the possible ex-ception of physiology, all are in the initial stages of development. The former, however, acts more as a basic resource for physical education in the other professions than as a physiological discipline per se. The disciplines of physical activity provide knowledge from the scientific viewpoint, providing the professions with information useful in achiev-ing professional goals. The relationship between the researcher and the practitioner is needed because the daily activities of the professional do not allow for the depth and objectivity possible in research programs. Constant research in physical activity is needed to provide information on current concepts that will influence and improve practices. The relationship between the disciplines and professions in physical activity is not old, having been developed within the past few decades. A mutual relationship exists; each, in order to survive, is dependent on services provided by the other.

Physical Activity as Disciplines: Projections

It is established in this book that, on the basis of current practices, physical activity is presently developing within six disciplines. The basic disciplines being applied to physical activity are sociology, psychology, history, philosophy, mechanical physics, and biology in its subdiscipline, physiology. In the present context sociology and psychology are applied as sociopsychology, with physics and physiology being subsumed under the biophysical sciences. The principal reason for these combinations is to accommodate common practices in the disciplinary and professional domains of physical activity as they exist today. Work in the development of the applied disciplines of physical activity is now primarily at the university level, and the research going on within each of the basic disciplines is applied to physical activity and sport.

This review will be presented in two parts: (1) briefs on the current status of the disciplines, and (2) projections. The briefs are derived from the more complete discussion on the current status of the disciplines. Our projections are based on perspectives presented in Chapter 18 and on the content of the entire book. Developments are reviewed for content that appears to be supportive of continuing and advancing practices in physical activity.

Current Status Briefs on Disciplines

The application of physical activity in a professional context requires knowledge about its effects. To understand human behavior and organismic changes as a result of physical activity, within the ten current professional applications, requires research on the functional status of the organism, including all its characteristics. Our primary source of information is the basic sciences and philosophies that obtain their content from extensive studies of the human personality and organism. This body of knowledge is then applied to the individual or group in physical activity, thus providing basic information for professional program planning and eventual achievement of goals. Such is the role of the disciplines and the rationale, to a large degree, for their development. However, even though the disciplines propose knowledge and understanding as their goal, they must also have some social or cultural value.

The basic sciences and philosophies that have the human being as a central focus should also be applied to physical activity. The following briefs present a setting for the proposed projections in the next section.

Biological Sciences (Physiology). Physiology and anatomy have been part of the physical education profession for some seventy-five years in the United States and for longer in some European nations. Resultant studies in these areas have been primarily within the professional context of education as opposed to the disciplinary context of understanding physical activity in all its roles. Nevertheless, a considerable body of knowledge about physical activity as education has resulted.

More complete detail on biology as an applied discipline in physical activity is given in Chapter 4 but some generalizations are herein summarized. It is well established, from a biological point of view, that no two physical activities will produce the same end result. It is also well known that physiological changes in the organism are directly related to the intensity, duration, and frequency of physical activity. Being determined by the emphasis of the particular physical activity, changes within the organism are sufficiently different to be validly applied in ten professions that now use physical activity as the primary basis for achieving their goals. Hardly a system, organ, or function of the body is not influenced by physical activity. This includes the cardiovascular, muscular, skeletal, nervous, and endocrine systems. In addition, exercise has prophylactic effects. A more thorough review, in addition to Chapter 4, is found in a recent book published by the author and the International Committee of Physical Fitness Research.[1]

The biological sciences have also demonstrated the influences of physical activity on growth, development, and aging. In addition, knowledge of other phenomena, such as disease prevention and protection, prevention of injury, and rehabilitation from injury, has been provided as a result of biology in its physical education context. This work serves as a base for understanding the nature of physical activity and as a reference for projections into the future.

Sociology. The discipline of sociology involves the study of human behavior in a societal setting and, because man is a biological animal existing within such a setting, is closely related to biology. As a discipline, sociology does not dichotomize man into mind and body but recognizes both as an integral part of the functioning organism. Thus in its proper form this discipline deals with the whole person as a total personality in all its relationships.

Physical activity plays a significant role in society, serving within the total biosocial process. In the process of physical activity, individuals are

[1] Leonard A. Larson and Herbert Michelman, *International Guide to Fitness and Health* (New York: Crown, 1973), p. 10.

not only individuals but also members of the social groups that, to a large extent, determine the level of our national culture. Hence culture is the result of the behavior of individuals developed in groups. In physical activity the groups are the team, the game players, the physical activity classes, and numerous other groups in a plethora of professional contexts.

Physical activity can influence and contribute to social learnings, which in turn develop the social values that produce social interactions. It is the process of socialization and the ways in which people acquire their habits, attitudes, and social roles that determine their interrelationships with others in the social structure. There is hardly a sociological concept that does not apply to the social group in sports, athletics, and small-group physical activity. The socialization process is developed through the formation of rules and regulations, and through the structure of the team or group. Determining factors include the extent of competition and cooperation in physical activity; the degree of success or failure in play and in acquiring skills; the attitudes derived through vigorous competition and under stress; individual responsibility in the team context; and, above all, the human personality that exudes an enthusiasm about play that is vital to success.

Psychology. Psychology is the scientific study of the human mind, with all its powers, functions, and operations. It is also defined as the science of human behavior, which includes the study of perception, learning, and the emotional and personality structure.

Physical activity provides a setting for an applied psychological discipline. Many concepts applied in a sports and games context require psychological understanding. The emotions and the intellect as displayed in behavioral, cultural, and social practices, mental abilities and capacities, and mental deviations are only some of these phenomena. Human behavior resulting from the use of drugs, stimulants, and tobacco is a psychological matter because it is in conflict with accepted practices and facts. Tension and frustrations in play require psychological interpretations. Alertness, anxiety, bias, prejudice, confidence, staleness, and tolerance are some other basically psychological concepts that have significance for physical competition. Research on the slow learner, the champion, and the gifted is also needed.

There are many other phases of physical activity that demand the attention of the discipline of psychology. For example, aging in relationship to performance is thought to be more than a physical phenomenon, and the subjective aspects of fatigue apparently have a psychological, rather than a physical base. Similarly, excessive thinness or obesity resulting from psychological stress require further study, because they have profound implications for physical performance. Research into interests, motivation, attitudes, and social adjustment in physical activity is essentially psychological. In conclusion, the concepts of play, learning, and hard competition are factors that require study from more than a purely physical standpoint, important as this may be.

History. As a discipline, history has had deep roots in the domain of sports and physical activity, which have always been a part of civilization. Although the form of physical activity has differed, the physical aspects of man's life have long been recognized and emphasized for healthy living. The base was nearly entirely physical during the early pioneer days, when the United States was a newly developing country. In most cultures physical activity has been established and organized as a part of social living. History indicates that there was more physical activity in ancient civilizations than in the present era. However, regardless of historical period, it is clear that human activity is a biological requirement.

Knowledge of history is essential for understanding the present. It is necessary to understand the experiences of others in order to understand oneself. Some have said that there is little new in life, except in the environmental setting, with its varying human resources. The discipline of history is certainly a necessary part of sports and physical activity.

Nearly all sports and physical activities have their fundamental base in early life and civilization, with the early Greek and Roman periods being particularly noteworthy. In these and other pre-Christian periods, statements by great philosophers place the responsibility for the development of the physical body on society. During the past 2,000 years the history of civilization and philosophy shows that in most instances man's success in physical adaptation has determined the status of civilizations. In the past, physical activity and sports have been prominent in cultural, military, and political environments, contributing to the survival of governments and the strength of the military.

Physical Sciences. Physical sciences deal principally with inorganic matter, but chemistry and mechanics have components that apply directly to the human organism. Both play a fundamental part in understanding the human organism in physical activity. The study of human movement control can only be undertaken through the medium of physical activity. The general laws of mechanics are indispensable in the study of man-machine systems, because clear understanding of the movement mechanisms is not possible without such knowledge. The teaching of skills is based on mechanical laws and principles, of which the concept of feedback has become most prominent.

Philosophy. Philosophy is the search for understanding and explanation. It reflects social ideals and attempts to provide a rationale for the attitudes, practices, and ways of life of a people. Hence it is the discipline that provides explanation for behavioral action. The practices of the individual and society are based on their respective philosophies, which, in turn, provide a rationale for sports and physical activity. The latter lack purpose unless they are based on philosophical objectives.

Philosophy, being the relentless search for truth, provides man with guides for his thought, giving him basic direction. Philosophy includes several fields of study: logic, which deals with methods of thought; ethics, which deals with conduct; aesthetics, which is concerned with beauty; politics, which deals with social organization; and metaphysics, which is the study of the ultimate reality of all things. All the aforementioned phases of philosophy will find applications in sport and physical activity.

There have been many attempts to classify philosophies, the most common schools of thought suggested by philosophers being idealism, realism, and pragmatism. Idealism is a quest for the ideal. The mind and the spiritual self are considered central and independent of material relationships, because all that exists, exists in the mind. In the philosophy of realism, man is capable of perceiving external objects, which exist independently of the mind and spiritual being. Realism is a philosophic correlate of service; it directly opposes idealism. Pragmatism is a philosophy that advances the belief that if a thing works, it must be good. It is the school of thought that encourages anything that is practical, efficient, and satisfying, postulating an approach to truth through action. Present problems are important and problems of tomorrow will bring their own solutions.

There are many other philosophies—aesthetics (beauty), asceticism (spiritual excellence), dualism (independence of mind and body), empiricism (experience), essentialism (facts and skills), materialism (physical substance), perennialism (standards), naturalism (natural events), pluralism (multiple factors), and rationalism (reason).

Philosophies in a number of studies have been applied to physical activity as sports, athletics, and games, the results of which are summarized in Chapter 7 of this book.

Disciplines in Projection

The basis for projections of physical activity as applied or independent disciplines lies in evidence reflecting developmental trends over the last few years. Viewing physical activity in its disciplinary context, social order trends have been closely associated with the development of academic institutions, principally the colleges and universities. If resources are not available, or if institutional philosophy places less emphasis on physical activity as an important facet of the social order, the future will not be bright for further advancement. Fortunately, however, there are indications that considerable advances have been made in the disciplines of physical activity. There is no reason, at the present time, to believe that these developments will not continue. On the contrary, recognizing the modern need for physical activity and exercise, future developments would appear to be favorable in all the current disciplines. Evidence on how physical activity is likely to develop in the future will be briefly discussed (List 15).

List 15. Perspectives applied: Disciplines and professions

A. The disciplinary context.

1. Physical Activity (PA), because of its concern for the whole nature of man, has traditionally utilized the arts, the humanities, and the physical, social, and biological sciences in order to gain knowledge and understanding.
2. Man in PA is the focal point of interest, and knowledge of man in this capacity must cross disciplinary structures.
3. The disciplines are interested in basic, fundamental processes. Questions regarding the future role of PA will have to be structured with regard to the meaning of man's movement and his resultant behavior.
4. Emphasis in the disciplines related to PA must be on its nature as a biophysical and psychosocial phenomenon.
5. The key to the development of knowledge of PA lies in the consideration of human movement as a significant process.
6. Many PA's are taught without scientific evidence as to their effectiveness in meeting human demands.
7. The study of PA arises from the recognition of man in movement as the primary concern of the field. Hence the task of identifying the body of knowledge lies within the context of man in motion.
8. According to some views, the biophysical and social sciences have become too fragmented for use in the study of PA and human movement. Also, the historical disciplines have seldom considered moving man in a dynamic environment as a field of study.
9. With a unified scientific approach stressing interdisciplinary interaction, the traditional concept of a discipline may have to be abandoned as far as PA is concerned.
10. A tremendous need exists for a well-organized body of knowledge on the immediate and lasting effects of PA.
11. If the disciplinary domain of PA is to develop, the basic philosophic and scientific concepts of PA must be clarified.
12. One of the problems facing the domain of PA is its orientation; namely, whether PA should be studied for its own sake as a disciplinary concern or whether existing knowledge should be applied in a professional manner. A compromise appears warranted.
13. The body of knowledge of PA is considerable, yet diversified. Attempts must be made to build a structural framework of PA in order to focus the search for knowledge.
14. Because PA involves a broad spectrum of activity—e.g., exercise, games, sports, athletics, etc.—it has been difficult to develop a logical framework of PA within which to develop the "stuff" of disciplines; namely, concepts, hypotheses, theories, and laws.
15. A principal task of the future lies in explaining the multivarious be-

List 15. Perspectives applied: Disciplines and professions—Cont.

havior patterns of the individual and group as spectators and participants.[2]

B. The professional context.

1. The future impact of the professions in physical activity (PA) will be influenced by public policy affecting education, affluence, mobility, and the type of accessible resources.
2. The professional domain of PA must define its objectives and, more importantly, communicate them to the various publics.
3. There has been a shift of professional focus from the individual benefits of PA to conceptual concerns related to man in motion.[3]
4. Effective programs should be based upon facts about human PA.
5. Sport and dance are important facets of society and programs should provide for cultural participation by the individual.
6. Professional endeavors must reflect acceptance of the continuing need to examine knowledge and beliefs.
7. Evidence exists that present resources cannot support all forms of expressional PA. A major question for professionals in the area is the determination of priorities and the basis for such choice.
8. Knowledge gained from the study of man's participation in PA will be crucial in determining professional effectiveness.
9. The larger and more accessible the body of knowledge about human movement becomes, the better the professions related to PA can serve the needs of society.
10. The professional domain of PA must guard against any excessive preoccupation with the external symbols of sport and athletics that may detract from the more valuable experiences that can be achieved.
11. It is up to the professions to provide leadership in minimizing the environmental impacts of PA and their attendant equipment, facilities, and transportation requirements.
12. The professions in PA must have control in the establishment of policies and standards, because they are best qualified to assess present resources and future limitations facing participation in PA.
13. The professional domain of PA—preventive and sports medicine specialists, health educators, coaches, nutritionists, recreators, etc.—must work together to develop sound fitness programs and promote positive concepts about the relationship of exercise to health.
14. Professional associations of PA must stress leadership development and the need to organize and disseminate new knowledge of PA phenomena.
15. Professionals must make older people aware of the role of PA as a deterrent in the physiological process of aging. Similarly, PA's must be developed that are appropriate to changing life-styles that occur as a function of age.
16. Of growing significance is the leadership role in PA. This includes professional intrusion with regard to beneficial sports and PA forms for the individual and society.

[2] G. L. Rarick, "The Domain of Physical Education as a Discipline," *Quest*, **9,** 1967.

[3] J. Felshin, *Perspectives and Principles for Physical Education* (New York: Wiley, 1967).

List 15. Perspectives applied: Disciplines and professions—Cont.

17. In order to guarantee public commitment to PA programs, professionals in the area must ensure that the message about the importance of PA reaches voters and taxpayers when they are young and actively involved.

18. Professionals in the field must provide strong leadership and high-level expertise in the expansion of all kinds of PA's, of fitness programs in industrial and commercial as well as residential settings, of remedial and therapeutic services, and of continuing education and social welfare programs designed to benefit all segments of the population.[4]

Knowledge and Understanding. The need for scientific understanding of physical activity has caused the disciplines to promote study and research. Scientific inquiry into sports and physical activity is considered a rich and relatively untouched field of study for researchers. The role of the discipline is to study activity or movement directly, and then to formulate relationships into a generalizable body of knowledge.

A major concern of basic research is to develop a structural framework for a body of knowledge in order to encompass the whole realm of movement and activity. At the present time, with few exceptions, content on the knowledge and application of physical activity lacks organized structure.

It must be recognized also that, for the basic disciplines, it is necessary to establish that human movement is a significant process worth research and intensive study. What are its potential values in the larger realm of the problems in modern-day society and culture? Social significance is a major factor in determining if research is to be rapidly increased. Interest from the disciplines is also basic.

If the need for physical activity is recognized by the individual and society as a whole it would appear that studies of physical activity for the purpose of obtaining basic scientific knowledge will continue to grow. The disciplines will be established as having solid, applied functions and will be recognized, in time, as disciplines with a body of knowledge peculiar to physical activity.

Potentials of Physical Activity. At the present time the resources of knowledge and understanding of the philosophies and scientific potentials of physical activity are essentially found within the disciplines. The time appears far off when the disciplines can be truly established and research can be directed only within the context of physical activity per se. Until developments have reached the point of direct research, resources in understanding the potentials of physical activity must come from the basic disciplines, and from the motivations of basic scientists to perform research within the context of sports and physical activity.

[4] Ann Jewett, *Quest,* 1974.

It is unfortunate that physical activity is sometimes applied by public and professional leaders who are poorly informed of its potential value. From a pragmatic viewpoint, results demonstrate that physical activity will contribute to professional goals. Attempts, however, to differentiate the quantitative value of the various physical activities are considerably less successful (List 15).

Present and future research must focus on the biophysical and psychosocial nature of man in sports. Information is needed on participants in physical activity and on the various activities and combinations of activities that exert changes in man. The approach must be *process*- and not product-oriented.

Developments in the future will place increasing emphasis on knowledge and understanding of the worth of physical activity to humanity. The professions will become increasingly oriented toward and grounded in the sciences and philosophies. It will be less possible to develop programs lacking adequate scientific foundations. These trends will lead also to the development of additional professions that employ physical activity and sports as the developmental medium.

Disciplines of Physical Activity. The developments of the scientific foundations of sports and physical activity have come largely from the disciplines during the past seventy-five years. Physical activity, because of its concern for the holistic nature of man, has traditionally utilized the arts, the humanities, and the physical, social, and biological sciences in order to gain knowledge. Man has been the focal point of interest to a large degree in most of these disciplines, and in recent years this interest has extended to man in physical activity. The trend is indeed evident, and interest will, no doubt, continue.

Further classification is needed of scientific concepts, elements, qualities, and functions. The domain of physical activity in the life of the people must be more clearly defined and structured to provide direction for disciplinary research. Qualified professionals in the area of physical activity are best equipped to establish a structural framework. This process is under way, and the future will, no doubt, establish a close working association between the professions of physical activity and the basic scientific and philosophic disciplines.

A major concern, of course, for the domain of physical activity is the direction of its orientation. Whether research should be contained within the sports context directly, or whether a larger perspective is required within the sports context directly, or whether a larger perspective is required within the basic scientific fields has always posed a problem for those interested in determining the value and worth of physical activity. It would seem that the full resources of sciences and philosophies should be used, even if knowledge cannot be immediately applied. It is essential for any field of endeavor that emphasis, at least initially, should be placed on basic research. Holding research fully within professional walls will ultimately limit its scope. It would appear reasonable to assume that in the future, interest and emphasis will continue as they are now programmed.

Sociocultural Values and Relationships. Sports and physical activity have deep roots within the culture of many peoples and exert a strong influence on the culture itself. The task of the future is to understand the behavioral roles assumed by people toward sports as spectators and participants, as related to individual personality and behavioral patterns and traits. Research contributions from all the disciplines and philosophies appear to be required for the analysis and determinations of such behavioral patterns.

Human Development and Physical Activity. The fundamental purpose of physical activity and sports is broad human development, ranging from a purely physical function and encompassing the well-being of the individual. Because of the large scope of physical activity, a single basic or applied discipline is inadequate as a resource for the knowledge needed to direct all its professional applications. The traditional concept of a subdiscipline as simply an adjunct to the principal purposes of the discipline will need to be discarded. Subdisciplines must become well established within the structural framework of physical activity but with the full content associated with the basic disciplines. The fragmented approach is no longer adequate. In the future, six well-established disciplines will be developed within the context of sports and physical activity. Leadership preparation and research will come from the universities through the integration of resources from the basic sciences and philosophies, medicine, athletics, and physical education. In this connection the term *physical education* will cease to be a meaningful designation except as one of the ten professions (List 15).

Probably the most significant projection for physical activity and sports is that of its advancement to disciplinary status. If present trends continue, the rate of development will be rapid. One example will be sufficient. In the United States, sports medicine was born only twenty years ago. It was developed by a group that recognized sports as requiring resources from medicine, science, and education. It is now a well-established profession and there are also a number of scientists working in sports medicine as a discipline.

The potentials of physical activity are so vast that if society continues to be interested in its worth to the individual for his mental, social, and emotional well-being, the future is indeed bright. In this present age of reduction in work and consequently in physical effort, sports and physical activity can be expected to assume an increasingly large role.

Physical Activity as Professions: Projections

Physical activity currently is organized into ten professions, which are now operational to various degrees. The professions of physical education and sports and athletics are probably the largest and exert an influence on nearly every person in the United States and most other countries. Although they are strong professions, further development is required. Eight other professions are also reported on in the present book. For example, recreation as a profession includes a large following and many professional workers. It is now fragmented into a number of professional groups with differing emphases and specializations, and physical activity is only a part of the profession of recreation. With future developments it could become a specialized facet of total recreation programs. To present a current status setting for projections of physical activity as professions, briefs will be presented from each of the ten chapters of Part III. Reference should be made to each chapter for additional content.

Current Status Briefs on the Professions

In Part III we define a profession as "a formally organized group, with its own internal controls, designed to render a public service that represents a need or a requirement for individuals and society constituting the culture." It is recognized that the life and worth of a profession are determined by the people. If professional services are essential and of acceptable quality, the profession will be assured of success.

Athletics and Sports. Athletics are organized into informal structures or groups as sports, but are highly organized and structured as athletics. Although no single profession exists for sports and athletics, there are numerous organized groups that are developed around aspects of both. There are coaches' associations in nearly all sports, professional associations on regulations for sports, athletic trainers, administrators of college and university athletics, and numerous others. Each of these many groups operates in a professional manner, with accompanying offices, membership, fees, and so on, to resolve issues and to exert control on their respective organizations.

Culture and Leisure. Physical activity is a large and growing part of culture and leisure. Programs in physical recreation for special groups (for example, the aged) represent a part of organized leisure for services to the people that it would be impossible to provide on an individual basis. There are numerous organizations for leisure programs that are structured and organized as professions.

Dance. Dance is rooted basically in physical movement. It is a highly specialized activity with many groups organized around particular interests and with varying responsibilities for the different dance forms. There are dance groups within the cultural (e.g., ballet), artistic and creative (e.g., aesthetic), personal (e.g., social), and sociocultural (e.g., ethnic) domains that are structured to direct and apply dance for precise goals. The number of professional groups and disciplines in the wide variety of dance forms at local, state, national, and international levels is large indeed.

Education. Education is probably the largest and most formally organized profession that utilizes physical activity for at least the partial achievement of educational goals. The AAHPER is the most prominent professional organization in physical education. It has its greatest membership (some 60,000) among the schools and colleges. There are other professional groups organized for sports for both men and women, of which the American College of Physical Education Association is only one. Men and women in sports are also organized into groups directing work within the context of sports programs.

Health. Health is constituted in numerous professional groups, there being no single profession. There are so many facets for health that a single profession would become much too diffuse to render quality services. These groups are organized around physical activity and represent a sports contribution to health under several roles: educational, growth and developmental, psychological, sociocultural, and physical. The health potential of physical activity is large, and there is growing recognition, based on research, of its contributions to mental, emotional, and physical health.

Institutions. In the United States the growth of professional organizations within institutions has probably been the most rapid for physical activity and sports. These are classified into eight institutions that program sports and physical activity, with employees being categorized into professional groups with various degrees of formal structure. It is significant to note that the growth in each of these groups is rapid. A classification system that includes religious, health and welfare, military, industrial and commercial, penal and correctional, sport clubs and social organizations, governmental, and educational organizations appears to cover most of the institutions.

Preventive Medicine. Preventive medicine involves the "whole-man" concept and incorporates all intellectual, emotional, physical, genetic, and chemical components for the early detection and correction of deteriorative trends. The components of physical activity as professions of preventive medicine are comprised of injury prevention, health maintenance, mental and emotional factors, rehabilitative and therapeutic factors, and disease prevention and control.

Recreation. Recreation involves considerably more than sports and physical activity, which, nevertheless, represent a large part of the recreational interests of the people. The professional domain that includes sport and physical activity is comprised of programs, government involvement, leadership, and philosophic aspects and professions within physical recreation. The role of physical recreation in leisure is increasing because of more free time and the recognized need for physical activity. As a result, professional workers have had to organize around their interests and specializations as professional groups.

Rehabilitation. Rehabilitation is constituted by leaders of sports and physical activity with professional goals for the restoration of the handicapped individual to the fullest physical, mental, social, and economic usefulness he is capable of reaching. The conceptual domain of sport and physical activity in rehabilitation includes physical, psychological, social, and medical factors.

Sports Medicine. The sports medicine profession, with several groups of specialization, is organized on the foundations of the basic sciences and medicine as essential for the understanding of physical stresses in sports and medicine. The various branches, which encompass medical, scientific, and educational objectives, are concerned with correction and protection of the human organism. They are also responsible for the direction of sports so that favorable outcomes will result.

Professions in Projection

The present status of the professions of physical activity was reviewed in the preceding section. It seems clear that all are in the developmental stage. At the present time, they all fall short of the criteria for a profession. This does not mean that they are not operational and are not rendering services to the population. It *does* mean that they have not reached a desirable stage of professional development such that the members can regulate the requirements for standards that represent the highest level of public service. For example, the medical schools (which are not always of high quality) cannot license graduates to practice medicine, but are regulated by the profession through the state regulating agency. If the medical graduate cannot meet the state requirements, through examination, he cannot practice medicine. There are many who fail, particularly those graduates from countries where medical education does not have the overall standards that are found in most universities in the United States. This regulation is not found in any of the ten professions of physical activity, except for medical practitioners in the profession of sports medicine. Of course, there are professional standards within each profession, but they represent guidelines rather than enforced regulations.

From the preceding review, we now present projections on what can be expected in professional development for physical activity. Summary statements, gleaned from the literature and considered to be representative of current trends, represent the basis for the projections (List 15).

Philosophy. The future of the professions of physical activity will be influenced by developments that affect such areas as education, affluence, and mobility, and certainly by the resources essential for a profession. From a philosophical viewpoint, incorporation of physical activity into the lives of the people is now highly favored. It is recognized that the need for exercise and its importance in weight control play an essential role in health. Professional services will therefore be needed from all of the ten professions now organized. No doubt, other professions will develop on the basis of recognized needs and as the degree of specialization increases.

It is essential, however, if developments in the professions are to occur, that the professions themselves influence the public. They cannot wait for the public to request services. On the contrary, they must continuously make the public aware of their need for the services that can be provided by the physical activity professions.

The internal work of the current professions must be extensive and intensive if favorable developments are to occur. Although services must be communicated to the public, of equal importance is the presentation of a scientific and medical rationale for their utilization. This must be provided through research and clinical practice to ensure acceptance. This applies to all services, but particularly those that personally affect the individual. Sports and physical activity must have a scientific base that supports their value to the individual. The evidence now provides only partial support, and full understanding of the role of physical activity is still at a distance. Current research, however, is continuously closing the gap. There are few carefully planned and controlled studies that do not support physical activity favorably.

Social Institutions. Physical activity is rapidly growing in its various professional roles in social institutions. Current roles, with few exceptions, are nevertheless only at the beginning stages. A very recent example is found in professional sports, which are organized by commercial institutions. Here the promotion of sports not only as vocations, but also for entertainment purposes is only about forty or fifty years old. The most rapid developments have occurred within the past two decades.

The prospects for future applications of physical activity within social institutions are indeed bright. The formal programs in schools and colleges will continue to advance their leisure emphasis on sports, but the major developments will be within the other social institutions within society. Some examples and projections follow.

1. *Athletics and sports.* The advancement of women in sports is a prime example. Furthermore, there have been rapid developments among social institutions in the programming of sports as part of the social program for employees.
2. *Culture and leisure institutions.* There has been an increased emphasis on leisure and the preparation of people for a life of physical activity to sustain the body and to give pleasure within an informal activity.
3. *Dance.* Professional applications of the dance will increase, emphasizing both participation and spectator roles.
4. *Education.* Physical activity will become more completely integrated into school programs as preparation for leisure life. There will be special emphasis on knowledge of the human organism and the skills essential to sustain health and advance health levels. Roles in preventive medicine will increase significantly.
5. *Health.* Research into the health potentials of physical activity is now at its highest level. The positive results of physical activity for both the normal and the handicapped will produce significantly increasing interest in further studies and applications in institutional programs.
6. *Institutions.* Those now programming sports and physical activity range from informal groups to professional sports institutions. Community activity within institutions will increasingly apply physical activity for institutional goals.
7. *Preventive medicine.* The application of physical health and fitness for preventive measures has significantly increased in the past ten years. With modern experimental techniques all research results and programs will be advanced for preventive purposes.
8. *Recreation.* A rapid increase is now noted in the utilization and planning of sports and physical activity in recreation for the sedentary and the aged, who previously have been unable to participate satisfactorily.
9. *Sports medicine.* Physical activity is fundamental to sports medicine, which is a relatively new profession that has grown rapidly during the past twenty years in the United States, and will continue to grow because of the increased involvement of people in sports.

Thus in social institutions utilizing the current professions that now employ physical activity to achieve goals, trends point to the advancement of services. Increased use of sports is a major factor in this development, as are advances in knowledge of their worth.

Individual and Society. In addition to the philosophy and social institutions that provide the foundations for projections on physical activity, the individual and society must be considered as a fundamental reference. Sports, dance, and other social forms of physical activity are important facets of society and the culture. The sociocultural status of sports has improved in the many societies of the United States as well as throughout the world. It is rapidly becoming a cultural medium for the improvement of understanding between peoples.

Emphasis is now placed on knowledge about the effects of physical activity on the individual, society, and culture. This represents a changing focus of professional emphasis from outcomes to understanding. Implicit is the belief that the larger and more accessible the body of knowledge on physical activity becomes, the better services will be in meeting demonstrated needs. Objectives are directed toward an improvement in these services to the individual and society.

Professional interest is now directed toward the promotion of physical activity in leisure and health programs. The individual and society will require increasing opportunities for sports in the future, and the rate of growth will most likely be rapid in the next two or three decades.

Programs. The relatively recent development of physical activity programs as disciplines and professions is indicated in this book. The progress has been so rapid that, at the moment, one cannot truly conceptualize what has happened. Most professionals have come through school and college programs viewing physical activity only within the context of physical education. Many have been confused when physical activity was used as athletics, attempting to interpret and classify athletics as physical education. They now are beginning to realize that athletics is a unique profession, related to but quite independent of physical education. As indicated, at present this growth is reflected in the development of six disciplines and ten professions within this short period of time.

Today programs of physical activity are rooted in the sciences and are based upon facts about their potential for human development. Regardless of the purpose, little progress can be made unless the objectives behind the use of physical activity can be supported. Even allocating open space in a community for free play must now be rationalized on the basis of its value to the taxpayer. Does it contribute to the well-being of the people in the community? Is it worth the cost? These are the questions that have to be answered. If the response is positive, the chances of support will be favorable, since most communities are interested in upgrading community life.

Advancements of programs in physical activity are based on the participation of the people. Recreation departments keep precise records of the uses made of their facilities, and it is these that will provide financial support for their programs. The test of whether such programs have value is determined by the desire of the people to participate and the positive experiences they derive from them.

In the coming years, and especially among older people, the professions of physical activity must make people aware of the importance of physical activity for healthy living. Only within the past five or ten years have efforts been seriously made to bring scientific knowledge to older people on the importance of physical activity and physical work. Work alone, even when physical in nature, applies largely to the muscular system. This is certainly not enough for those in the fifty and older age bracket. The effect of physical activity on the physiology of aging is now evident; it appears to be essential for sustaining the organism as well as delaying the aging process.

Leadership. The most drastic changes within the disciplines and professions of physical activity will be in leadership. The day is almost over where someone who participated in athletics can take over leadership in programs of physical activity as disciplines or professions. Only in professional sports does this practice continue, and this also will not last. The sophisticated knowledge required for leadership in sports now demands systematic study.

Advancements in the issue of leadership qualifications must come from the professional associations. These must set standards for leadership preparation and implement procedures for licensing the practitioner in each phase of specialization. This now appears to be the only way that leadership can be elevated to a level capable of providing proper guidance. Professional self-regulation to upgrade personnel is essential because of the high degree of specialization needed by people engaged in leadership activities.

Leadership requires specialized preparation in skills and understanding about the role of physical activity within society and the culture. Professional understanding of behavior within societal and cultural contexts is essential. It is also important that leadership preparation go beyond a single discipline or profession. Leaders must understand the full potentials of physical activity even if they specialize in only one phase. Overlap within the disciplines and professions is very large, and no discipline or profession is so specific as to be limited to any single application of physical activity.

Of course, specialization has just begun in the disciplines and professions of physical activity, and the peak of development is not in the foreseeable future. The time is coming when specialization for practices within a discipline or profession will become standard. The need for specialized preparation is now recognized by most professional leaders, but the implementation process will take time.

Administration. The administration of all facets of physical activity as disciplines and professions is becoming a complex leadership function that involves not only knowledge about physical activity, but also understanding of the human being per se. A specialist is now required in the various areas. A director of athletics, for example, cannot easily qualify as a director of physical education. This is true also for administration in programs of rehabilitation and preventive medicine, to name but a few. In the future, higher qualifications will be necessary for administrative personnel.

There are numerous problems to be resolved in the administration of the various forms of physical activity. There is evidence that community resources will have difficulty in providing support for all the disciplines and professions of physical activity. All activities in the community will become a matter of priority. No community, apart from the large metropolitan areas, will have resources to render services to all the population. It appears unlikely that universities and colleges can provide all the administrative requirements for all the specialized phases of leadership preparation. Each university will have to select its own emphasis to cover all the specialization needed.

One of the dangers in working with physical activity is the possibility of becoming preoccupied with the external symbols of athletics and sports, with losing sight of the developmental values for the individual and society. Sports and athletics, in administration, can easily become an end in themselves. The director of athletics must go beyond external requirements. A major goal for the administration of all phases of physical activity should be to establish policies and standards that will guarantee full value from participation. The basis should be the individual, society, and the culture, and the goal the upgrading of life through desirable participation practices. This is indeed the true purpose of administration. If sports is for the public, the administrator is then a public servant. Thus he or she must convey to the public the values that they can derive from physical activity programs. This is the prime responsibility for the administration of all the disciplines and professions of physical activity.

The day is now about over when the athlete can become a coach or administrator with little more preparation than the sport itself provides. Administration of physical activity in the future will become a highly specialized function, with university programs planned for the preparation of leaders.

An Overview

This book reviews the current status of physical activity as disciplines and professions. Of more significance, however, is its extension of the status of physical activity, with all its potentials and developments, to applications for the future. The study of the current status of physical activity is indeed needed, for many citizens do not see physical activity as having a role beyond the activity itself. This is true even for many college graduates who study physical activity in its most prominent application, physical education. The roles of physical activity extend, however, considerably beyond those of physical education. The present chapter (and the entire book) is essentially a review of physical activity with its perspectives and projections in their applied form. Projections for the administration of physical activity are also presented and deal primarily with the requirements for the achievement of long-range goals.

Developments during the past few years leave little doubt about the direction applications are taking. When we view the present rate of development, there is also little doubt as to future development. The evidence indicating the basic need for physical activity as well as the culturally amenable setting for sports is sufficient to project favorable developments into the future. A most interesting development is the popular attitude that activity alone is not sufficient; it must have further value. Basic science has the responsibility of making scientific studies of physical activity. Whole new groups of applied scientists are now being prepared within the professions of physical activity as disciplines. This development will lead to programs similar to those of other academic disciplines.

References

American College of Sports Medicine, *Encyclopedia of Sport Sciences and Medicine.* New York: Macmillan Publishing Co., Inc., 1971.

Bothwell, P. E. *A New Look at Preventive Medicine.* London: Pitman, 1965.

Boyle, R. H. *Sport—Mirror of American Life.* Boston: Little, Brown and Company, 1963.

Broer, M. R. *Efficiency of Human Movement.* Philadelphia: W. P. Saunders Company, 1973.

Brown, C. "The Structure of Knowledge of Physical Education," *Quest,* **9,** 1967, 73–79.

Browne, C. G., and T. S. Cohn. *The Study of Leadership.* Danville, Ill.: Interstate Printers and Publishers, 1958.

Carlson, R. E., T. R. Deppe, and J. R. MacLean. *Recreation in American Life.* Belmont, Calif.: Wadsworth Publishing Co., Inc., 1972.

Cassidy, R. "Societal Determinants of Human Movement: The Next Thirty Years," *Quest,* **16,** 1971, 48–54.

Clark, K. G. (Ed.) *Preventive Medicine in Medical Schools,* Report of Colorado Springs Conference, November, 1952. Baltimore: Waverly Press, 1952.

Corbin, H. D. *Recreation Leadership.* Englewood Cliffs, N.J.: Prentice-Hall, Inc., 1970.

Cowell, C. C., and W. L. France. *Philosophy and Principles of Physical Education.* Englewood Cliffs, N.J.: Prentice-Hall, Inc., 1963.

Cozens, F. W., and F. C. Stumpf. *Sports in American Life.* Chicago: University of Chicago Press, 1953.

Davis, E. C. (Ed.) *Philosophies Fashion Physical Education.* Dubuque, Iowa: William C. Brown Company, 1963.

Davis, E. C., and D. M. Miller. *The Philosophic Process in Physical Education.* Philadelphia: Lea & Febiger, 1967.

Feibleman, J. K. *The Institutions of Society.* London: Allen & Unwin, 1956.

Felshin, J. *Perspectives and Principles for Physical Education.* New York: John Wiley & Sons, Inc., 1967.

Fleishman, Edwin A. *The Structure and Measurement of Physical Fitness.* Englewood Cliffs, N.J.: Prentice-Hall, Inc., 1967.

Halpin, A. W. (Ed.) *Administrative Theory in Education.* New York: Macmillan Publishing Co., Inc., 1967.

Halpin, A. W. *Theory and Research in Administration.* New York: Macmillan Publishing Co., Inc., 1966.

Hertzler, J. O. *Social Institutions.* Lincoln: University of Nebraska Press, 1946.

Hook, Sidney. "The Crisis of Our Democratic Institutions," *The Humanist,* July–August, 1969.

Jewett, Ann. *Quest,* 1974.

Jokl, E. *The Scope of Exercise in Rehabilitation.* Springfield, Ill.: Charles C Thomas, Publisher, 1964.

Jokl, E. *What Is Sports Medicine?* Springfield, Ill.: Charles C Thomas, Publishers, 1964.

Kaplan, Max. *Leisure in America: A Social Inquiry.* New York: John Wiley & Sons, Inc., 1960.

King, B. G., and M. J. Showers. *Human Anatomy and Physiology.* Philadelphia: W. B. Saunders Company, 1969.

Knowles, M., and H. Knowles. *How to Develop Better Leaders.* New York: Association Press, 1955.

Krusen, F. H. *Concepts in Rehabilitation of the Handicapped.* Philadelphia: W. B. Saunders Company, 1964.

Larson, L. A., M. R. Fields, and M. A. Gabrielsen. *Problems in Health, Physical and Recreation Education.* Englewood Cliffs, N.J.: Prentice-Hall, Inc., 1953.

Larson, L. A. *Curriculum Foundations and Standards for Physical Education.* Englewood Cliffs, N.J.: Prentice-Hall, Inc., 1970.

Larson, L. A., and H. Michelman. *International Guide to Fitness and Health.* New York: Crown Publishers, 1973.

Lave, W. R., R. G. Corwin, and W. G. Monahan. *Foundations of Educational Administration.* New York: Macmillan Publishing Co., Inc., 1967.

Lederberg, J. "Health in the World of Tomorrow," Pan American Health Organization, Sanitary Bureau, WHO.

Loy, J. W. "The Study of Sport and Social Mobility," Monograph paper, University of Wisconsin, 1968.

Loy, J. W., and G. S. Kenyon. *Sport, Culture and Society.* New York: Macmillan Publishing Co., Inc., 1969.

McGlynn, G. H. (Ed.) *Issues in Physical Education and Sports.* Palo Alto, Calif.: National Press Books, 1974.

McNamara, R. S. "The Searching Mind," *Today's Education,* Washington, D.C., 1969.

Marxer, W. L., and G. R. Cowgill (Eds.) *The Art of Predictive Medicine.* Springfield, Ill.: Charles C Thomas, Publisher, 1967.

Molt, P. E. *The Organization of Society.* Englewood Cliffs, N.J.: Prentice-Hall, Inc., 1965.

"Moral and Spiritual Values in the Public Schools," Educational Policies Commission, Washington, D.C., NEA, 1951.

Munroe, A. D. *Pure and Applied Gymnastics.* London: Edward Arnold & Co., 1959.

Nash, J. B. *Philosophy of Recreation and Leisure.* St. Louis: The C. V. Mosby Co., 1953.

Neumeyer, M. H., and E. S. Neumeyer. *Leisure and Recreation.* New York: A. S. Barnes & Co., Inc., 1949.

Nixon, J. E. "The Criteria of a Discipline," *Quest*, **9**, 1967, 42–49.

Proceedings of Rehabilitation Conference, Chicago, September, 1966, C. D. Shields, Chairman.

Rarick, G. L. "The Domain of Physical Education as a Discipline," *Quest*, **9**, 1967, 49–53.

Ross, M. G., and C. E. Henry. *New Understandings of Leadership*. New York: Association Press, 1957.

Ryan, A. J. "History of the Development of Sport Sciences and Medicine," *Encyclopedia of Sport Sciences and Medicine*. New York: Macmillan Publishing Co., Inc., 1971.

Schurr, E. *Movement Experiences for Children*. Englewood Cliffs, N.J.: Prentice-Hall, Inc., 1975.

Scott, G. M. *Analysis of Human Motion*. New York: Appleton-Century-Crofts, 1963.

Shivers, J. S. *Leadership in Recreational Service*. New York: Macmillan Publishing Co., Inc., 1963.

Simon, H. A. *Administrative Behavior*. New York: The Free Press, 1966.

Steinhaus, A. "The Disciplines Underlying a Profession," *Quest*, **9**, 1967, 68–73.

Taylor, H. "The Crisis of Our Democratic Institutions," *The Humanist*, July–August, 1969.

Ulrich, C. *The Social Matrix of Physical Education*. Englewood Cliffs, N.J.: Prentice-Hall, Inc., 1968.

Webster, R. W. *Philosophy of Physical Education*. Dubuque, Iowa: William C. Brown Company, Publishers, 1965.

Zamir, L. J. (Ed.) *Expanding Dimensions in Rehabilitation*. Springfield, Ill.: Charles C Thomas, Publishers, 1969.

Zeigler, E. F. *Philosophical Foundations for Physical, Health and Recreation Education*. Englewood Cliffs, N.J.: Prentice-Hall, Inc., 1964.

Index

of specialization, 351–352
of sports, 315
See also Sociocultural aspects
Customs, 78

D

Dance, 162–176
American social, 171
ethnic, 171
modern, 171
professional status of, 163–166
professions in, 364
Defects
functional, 198
physical, 198
structural, 198
See also Handicapped individual
Delinquent behavior, 77–78
Democracy, 4, 8–9, 27–28, 33, 45, 146, 265
Determinism, 107
Developmental potentials of physical activities, 16, 18 (*See also* Human development)
Direction abilities of human organism, 62
Disability. *See* Handicapped individual; Injuries
Discipline
education as, 186
in human development, 39
in physical activity, 17, 19–20, 50–51
projections on, 352–362
Disease, 198, 207
prevention of, 235, 243, 246–247
in sports medicine, 310–311
rehabilitation and, 275, 276, 295
See also Health
Diurnal variations, 22
Drugs, as medical aids, 290
problems in using, 333
in rehabilitation, 290
in sports medicine, 307

use of, in sports, 24, 25, 209, 317
Dualism, 106
"Dynamic interactions," in environment, 335–338

E

Economic factors
in human development, 37
in physical activity, 32–33
social responsibility in, among nations, 9, 11
Education
and human development, 37
as institution, 223–224, 228
leisure and, 157–158
physical activity and, 29, 33–34, 157–158, 223–224, 228
as profession, 181–196, 364
(*See also* Physical education)
as profession, 181–183
in recreational programs, 256
in rehabilitation of handicapped individual, 291–292, 296–297
social responsibility in, among nations, 9–10, 12–13
Educational rehabilitation, 148
Efficiency, physical work, 129
Emotional factors, in physical activity, 23–25, 54, 64, 318, 333 (*See also* Psychological aspects)
Empiricism, 108
natural, 109
Encyclopedia of Sport Sciences and Medicine, 299–301, 303, 313, 314
Endurance, 312, 323
general, 58, 62
muscular, 58
Energy expenditure, 18, 21
Energy principles, 53